# INSPIRE

## HAIR FASHION FOR SALON CLIENTS

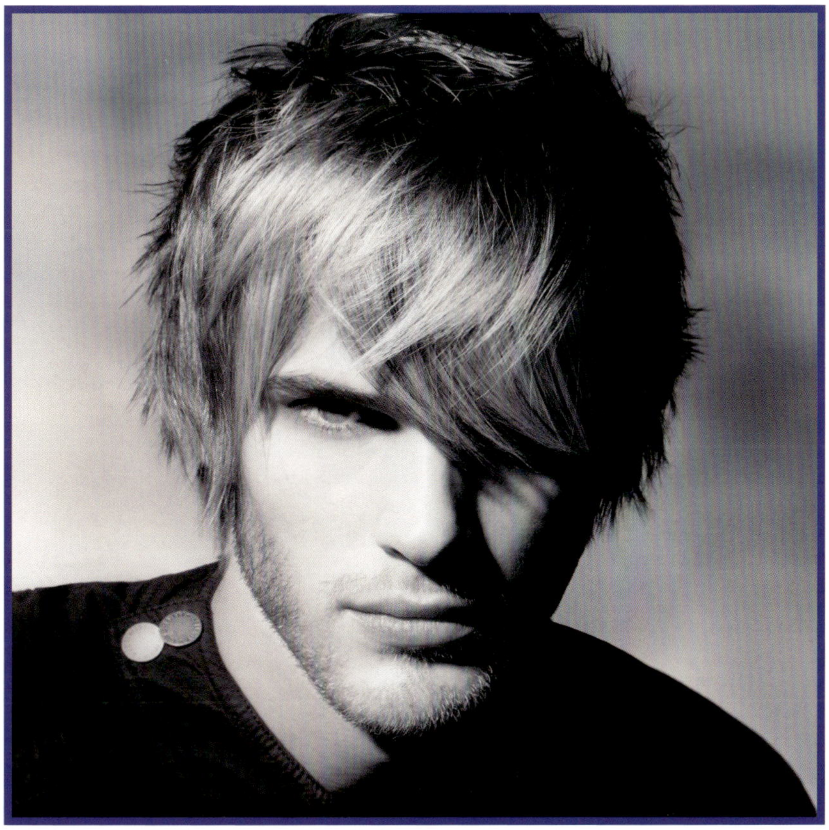

**Goldwell** — Hair: Goldwell Styling Team

# INSPIRE
HAIR FASHION FOR SALON CLIENTS

Featuring
## Men, Women & Children

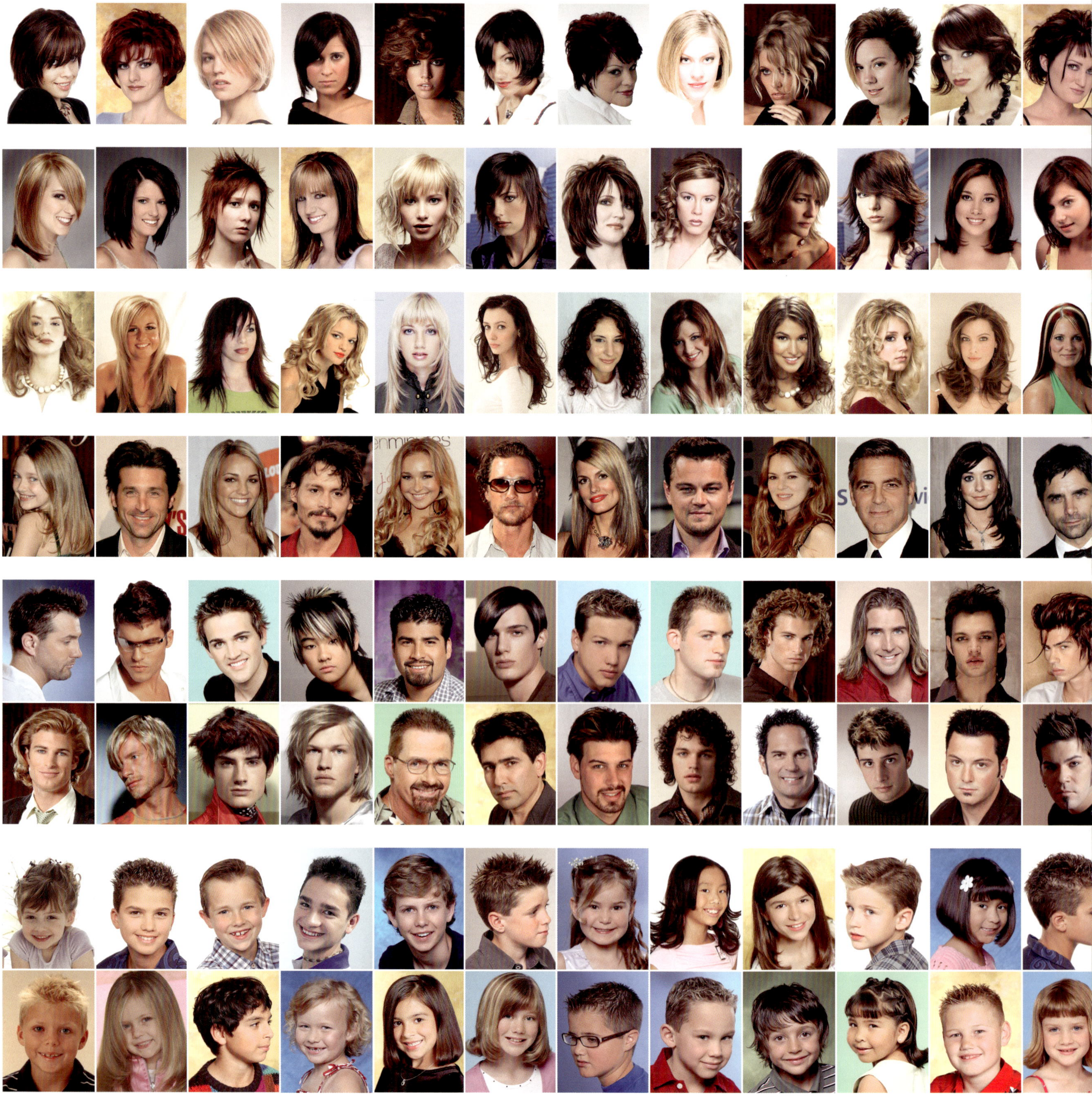

# TABLE OF CONTENTS VOL. 60

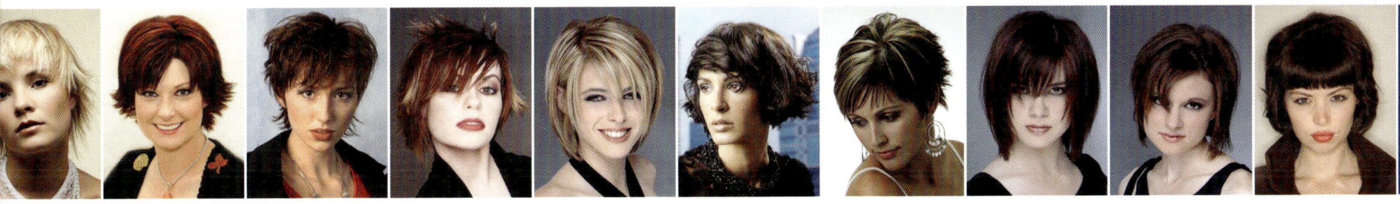



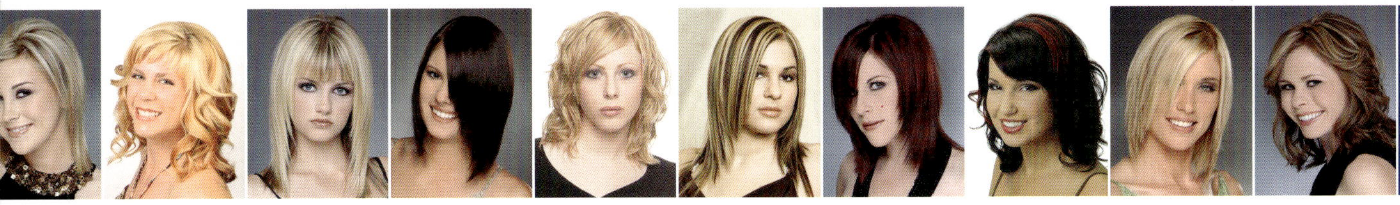



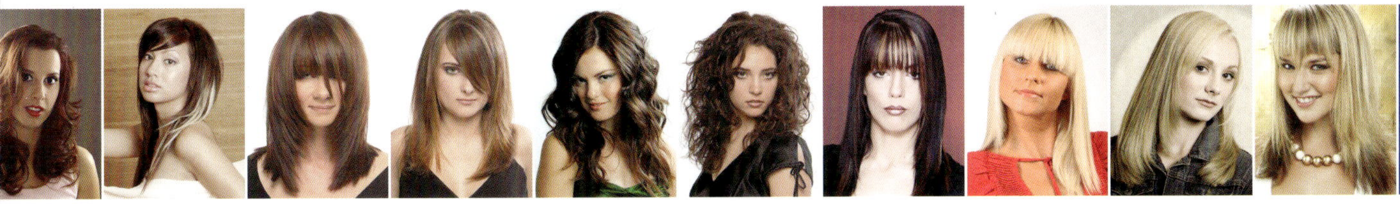



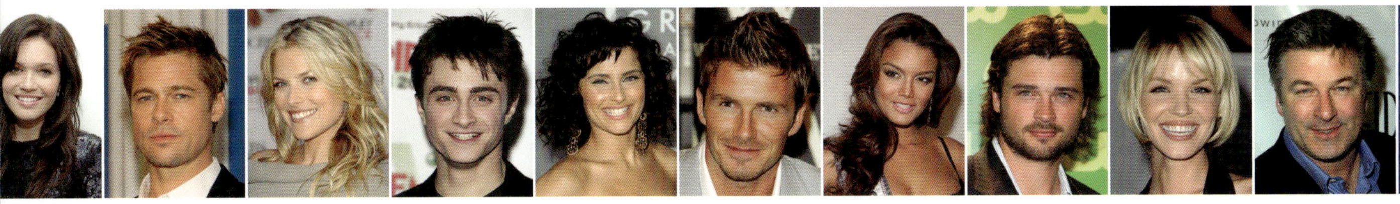



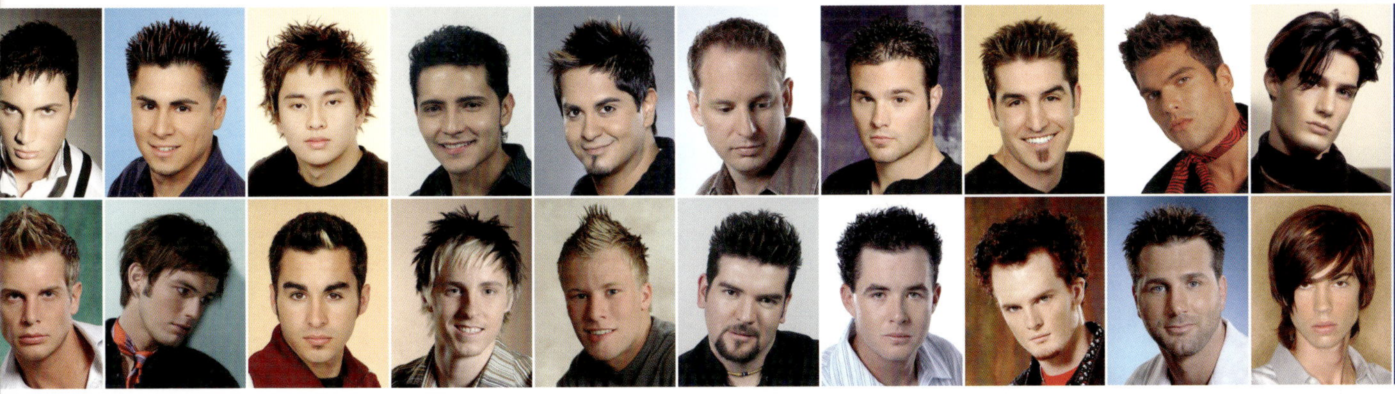



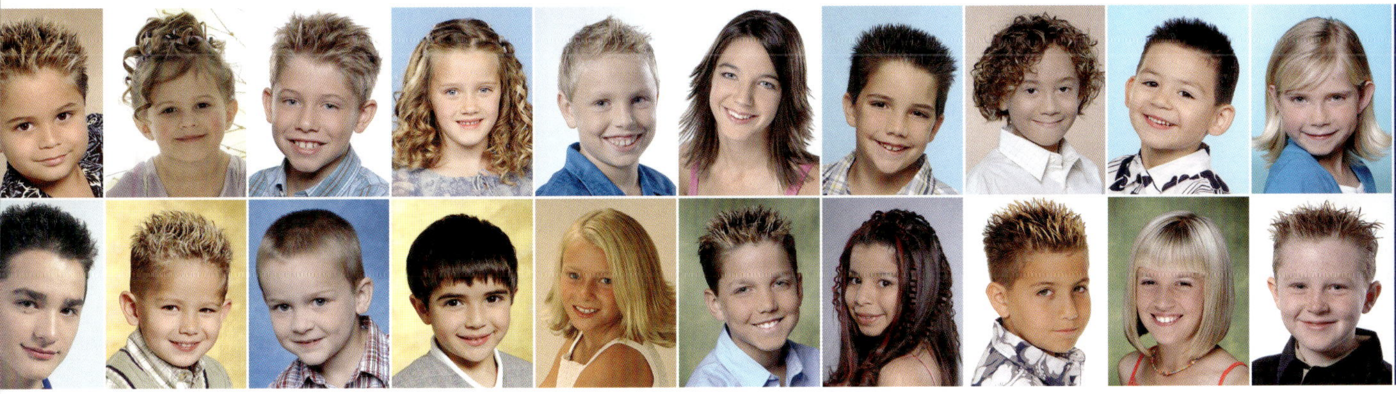

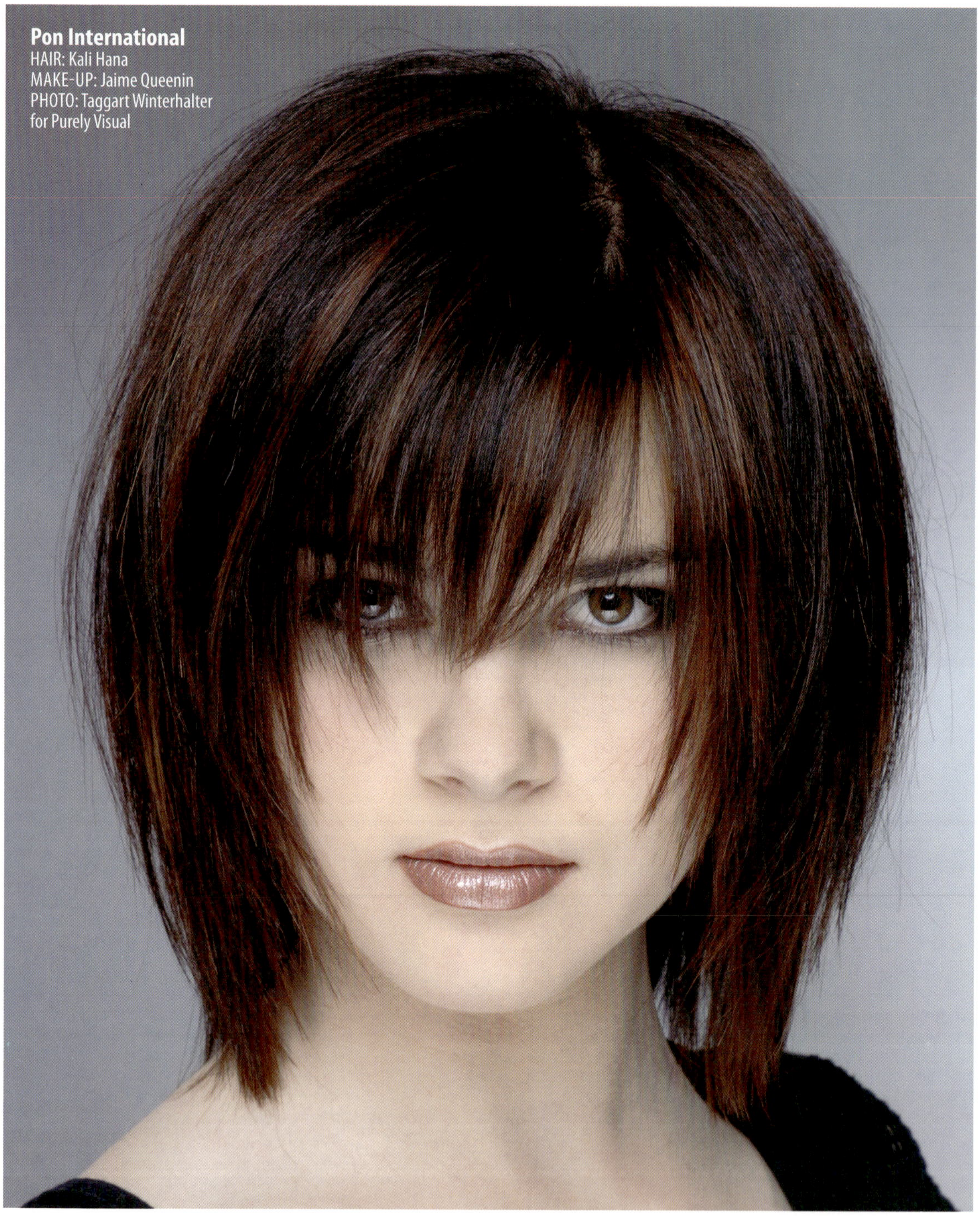

**Pon International**
HAIR: Kali Hana
MAKE-UP: Jaime Queenin
PHOTO: Taggart Winterhalter for Purely Visual

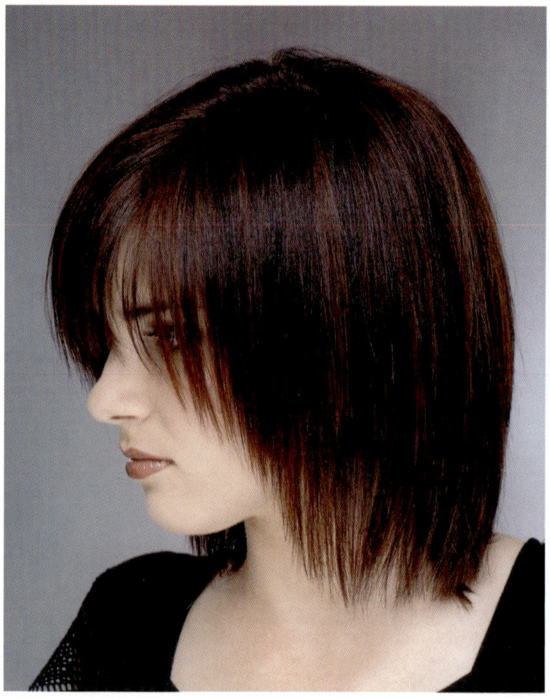

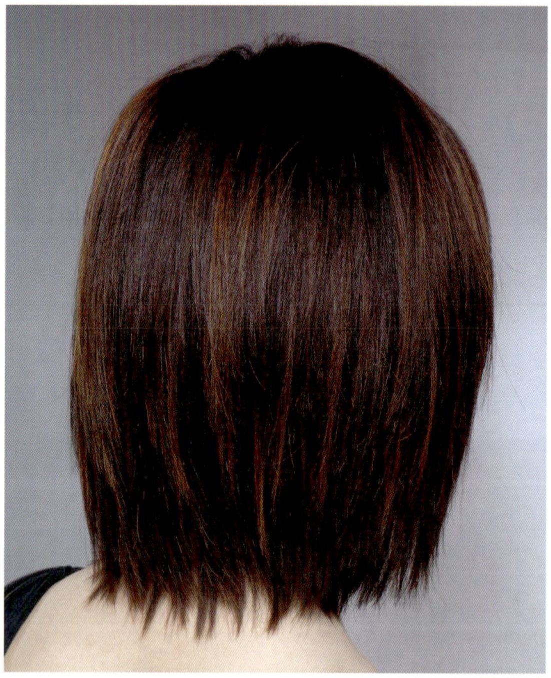

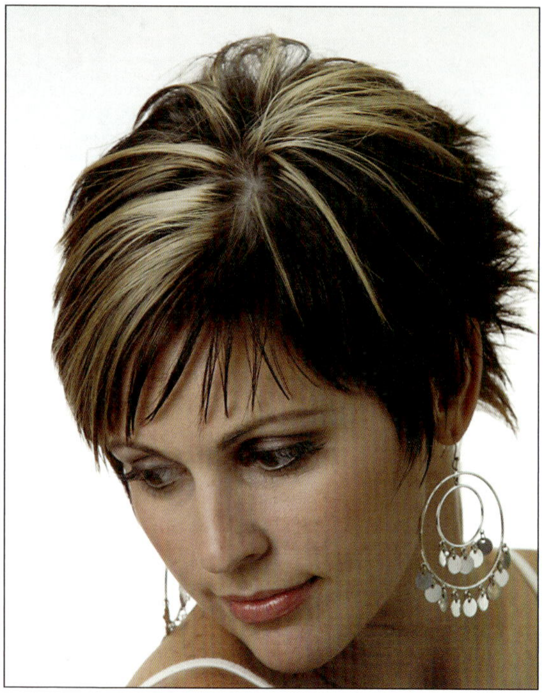

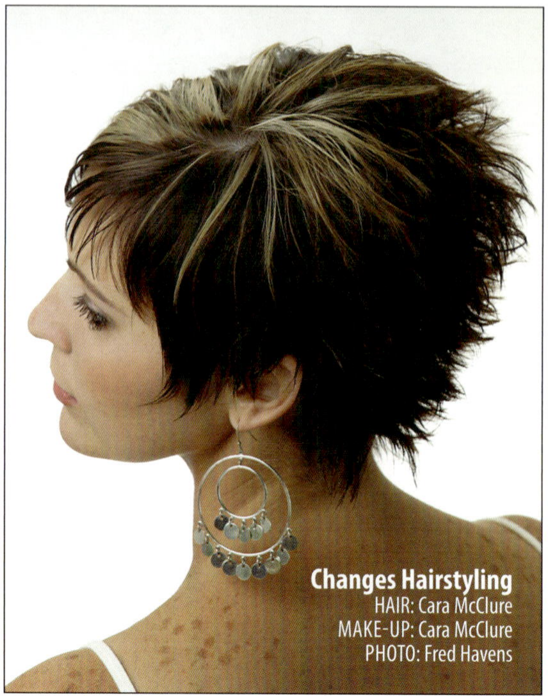

**Changes Hairstyling**
HAIR: Cara McClure
MAKE-UP: Cara McClure
PHOTO: Fred Havens

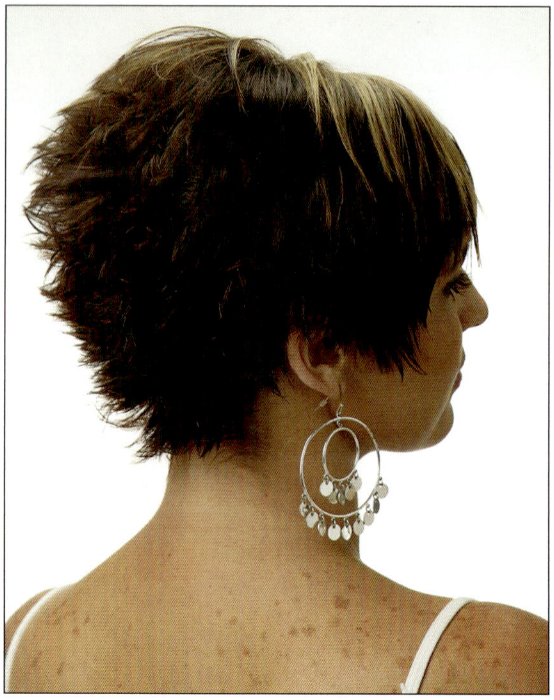

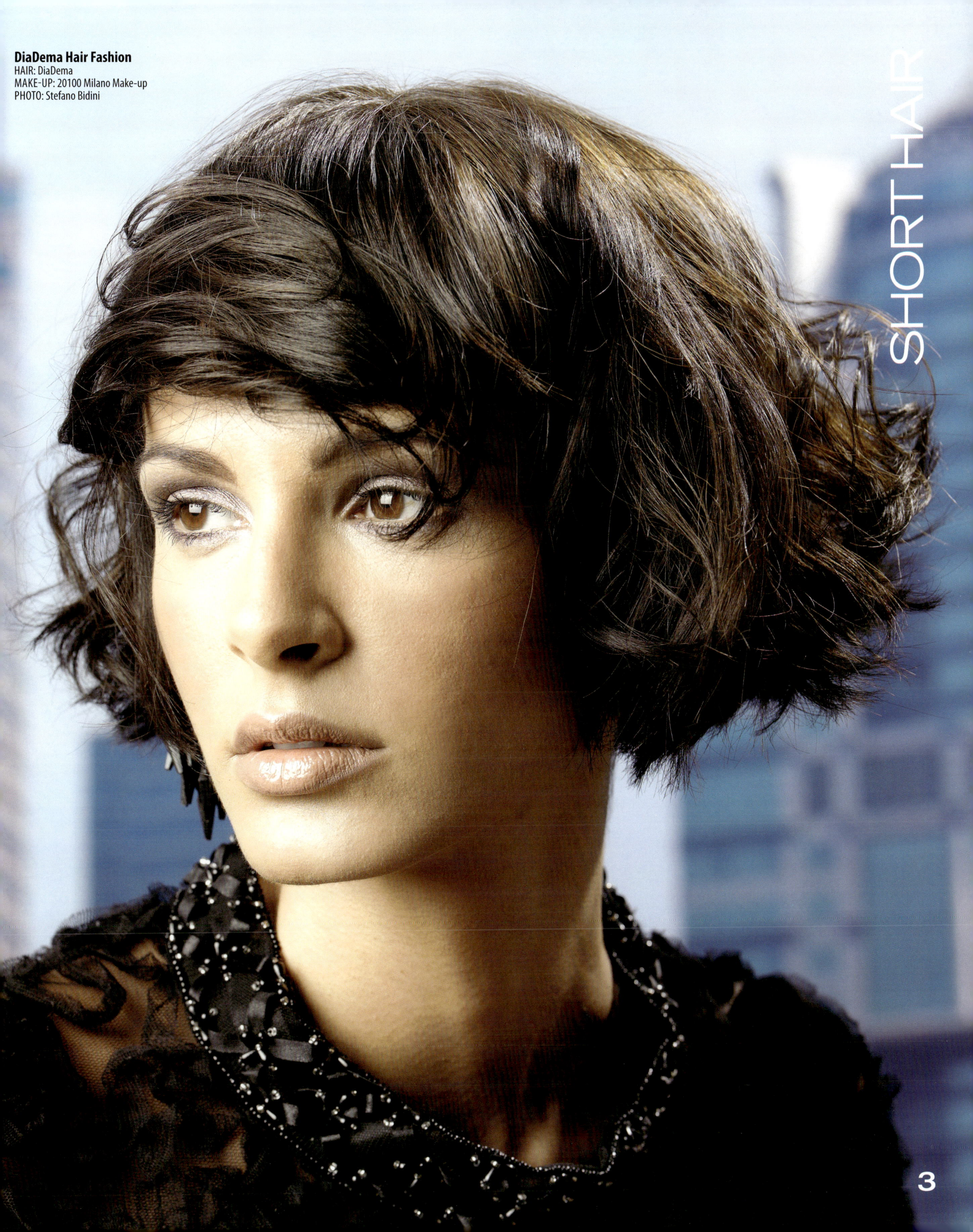

**DiaDema Hair Fashion**
HAIR: DiaDema
MAKE-UP: 20100 Milano Make-up
PHOTO: Stefano Bidini

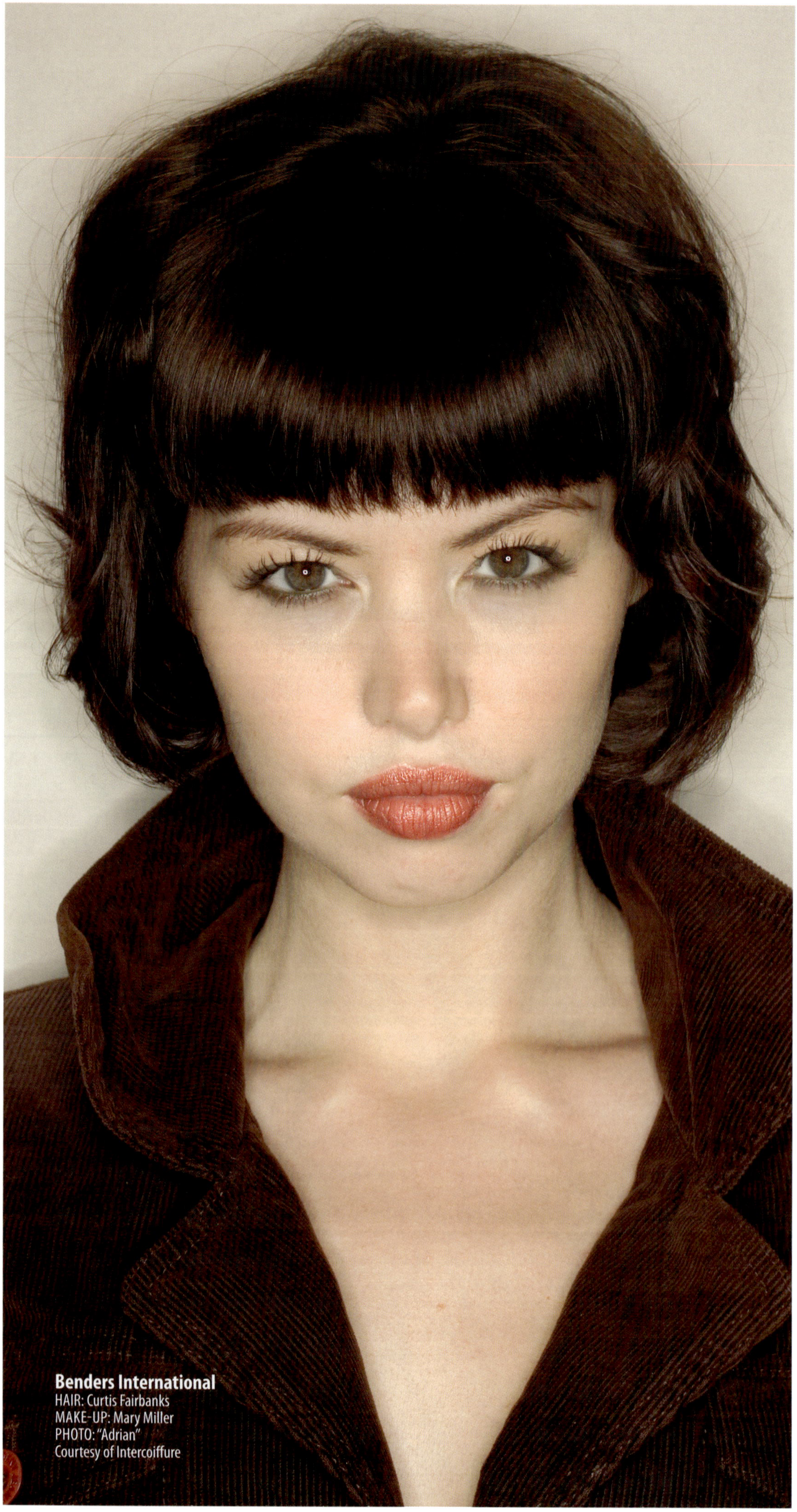

**Benders International**
HAIR: Curtis Fairbanks
MAKE-UP: Mary Miller
PHOTO: "Adrian"
Courtesy of Intercoiffure

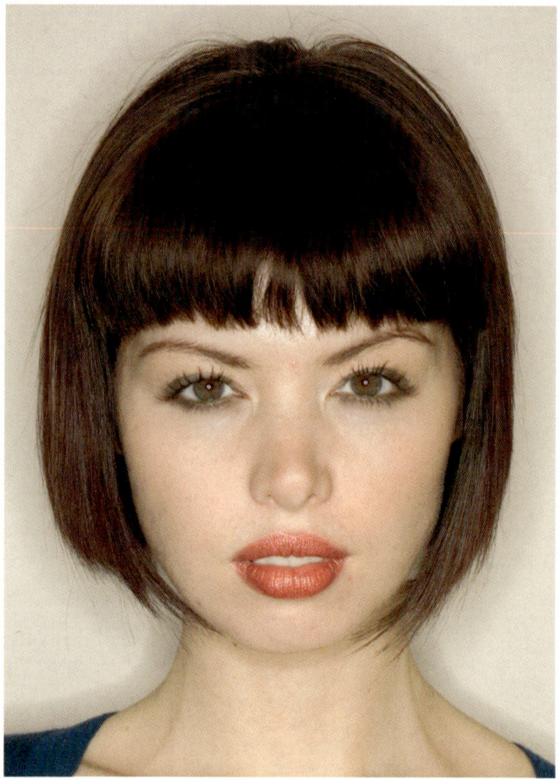

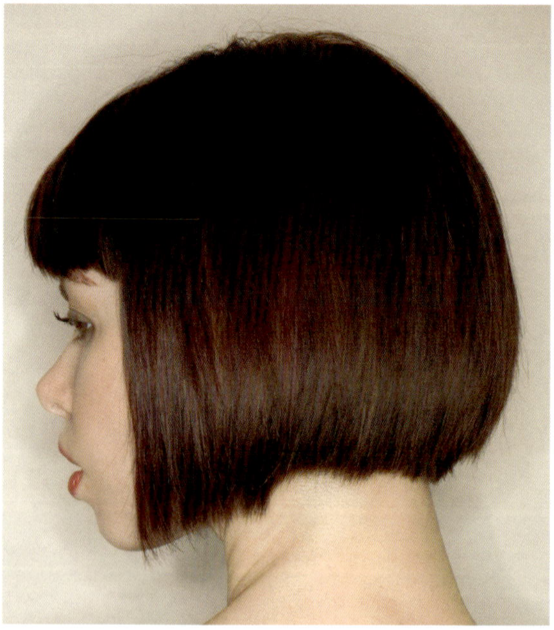

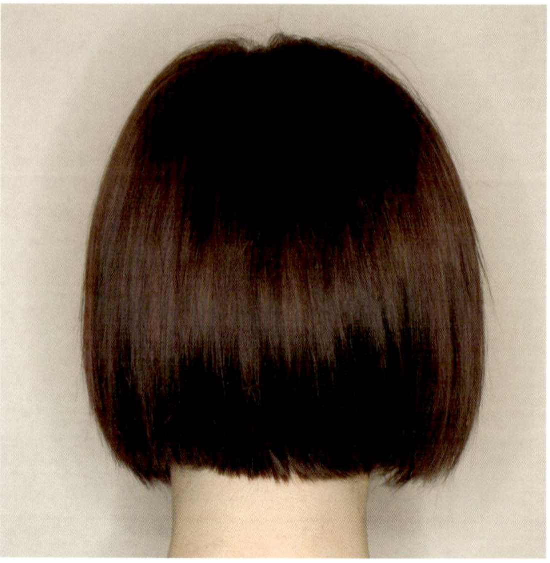

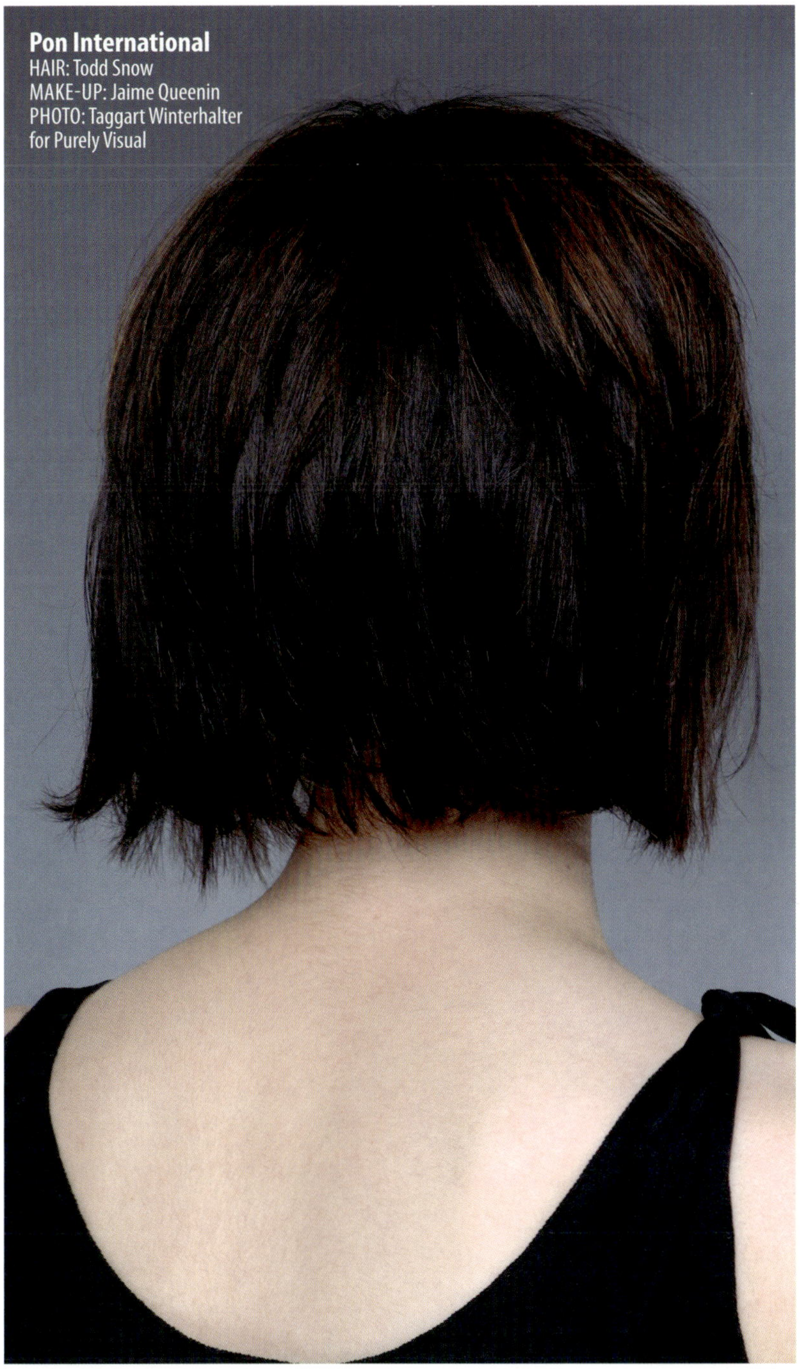

**Pon International**
HAIR: Todd Snow
MAKE-UP: Jaime Queenin
PHOTO: Taggart Winterhalter
for Purely Visual

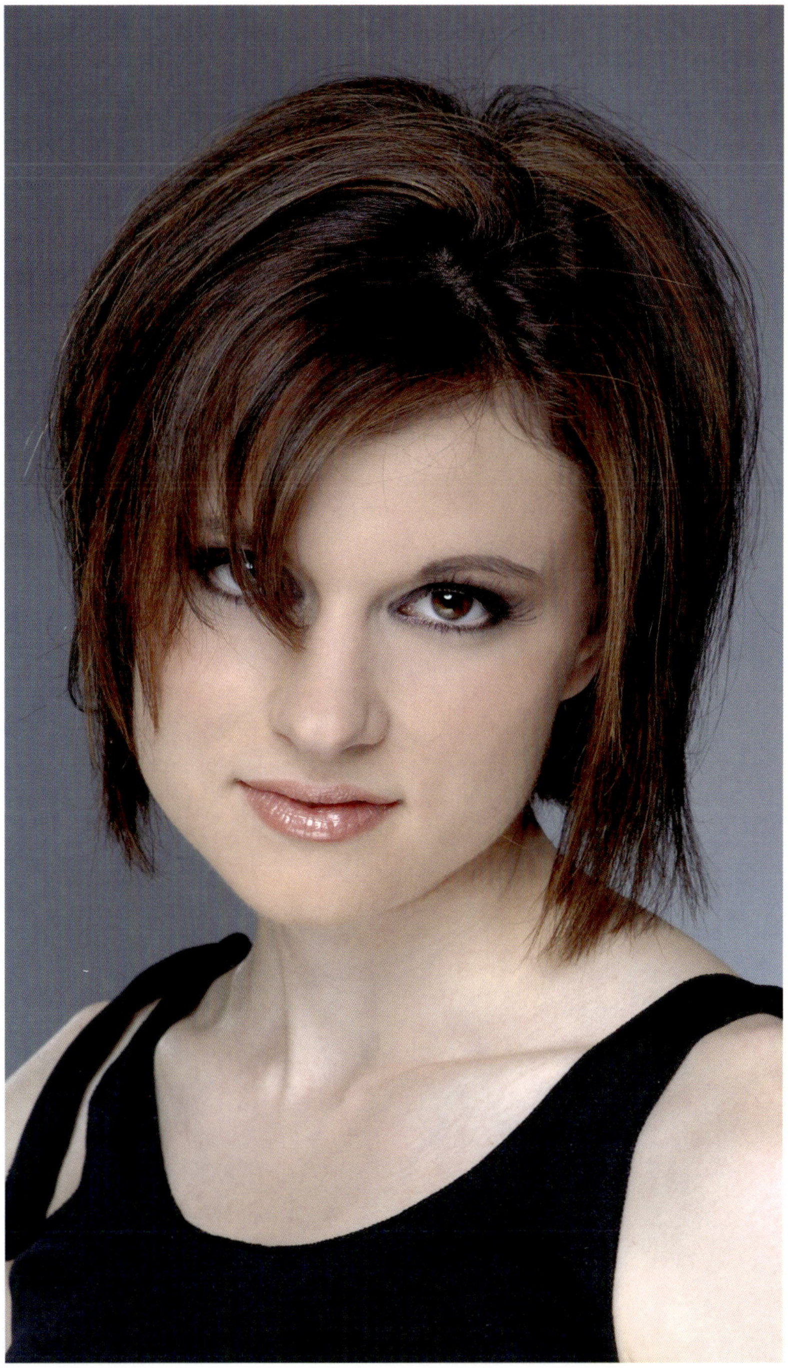

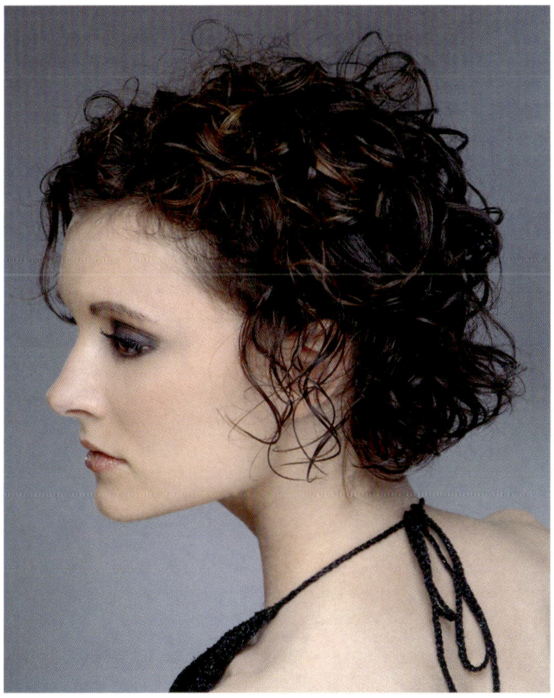

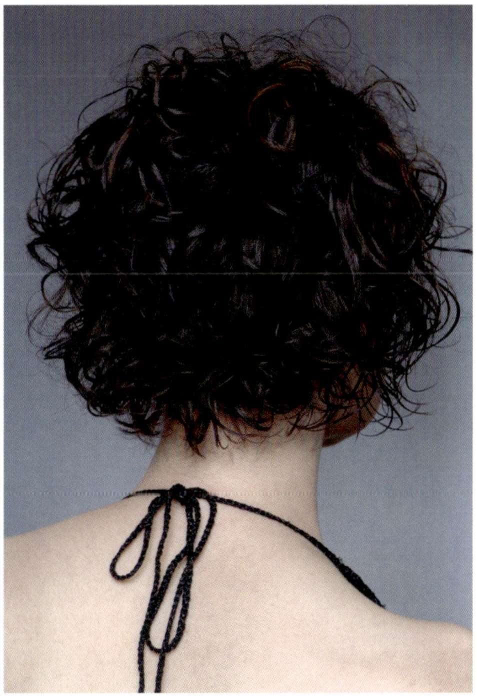

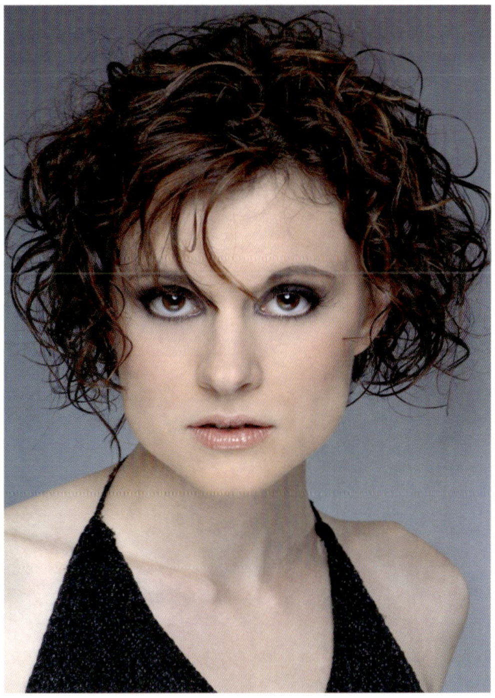

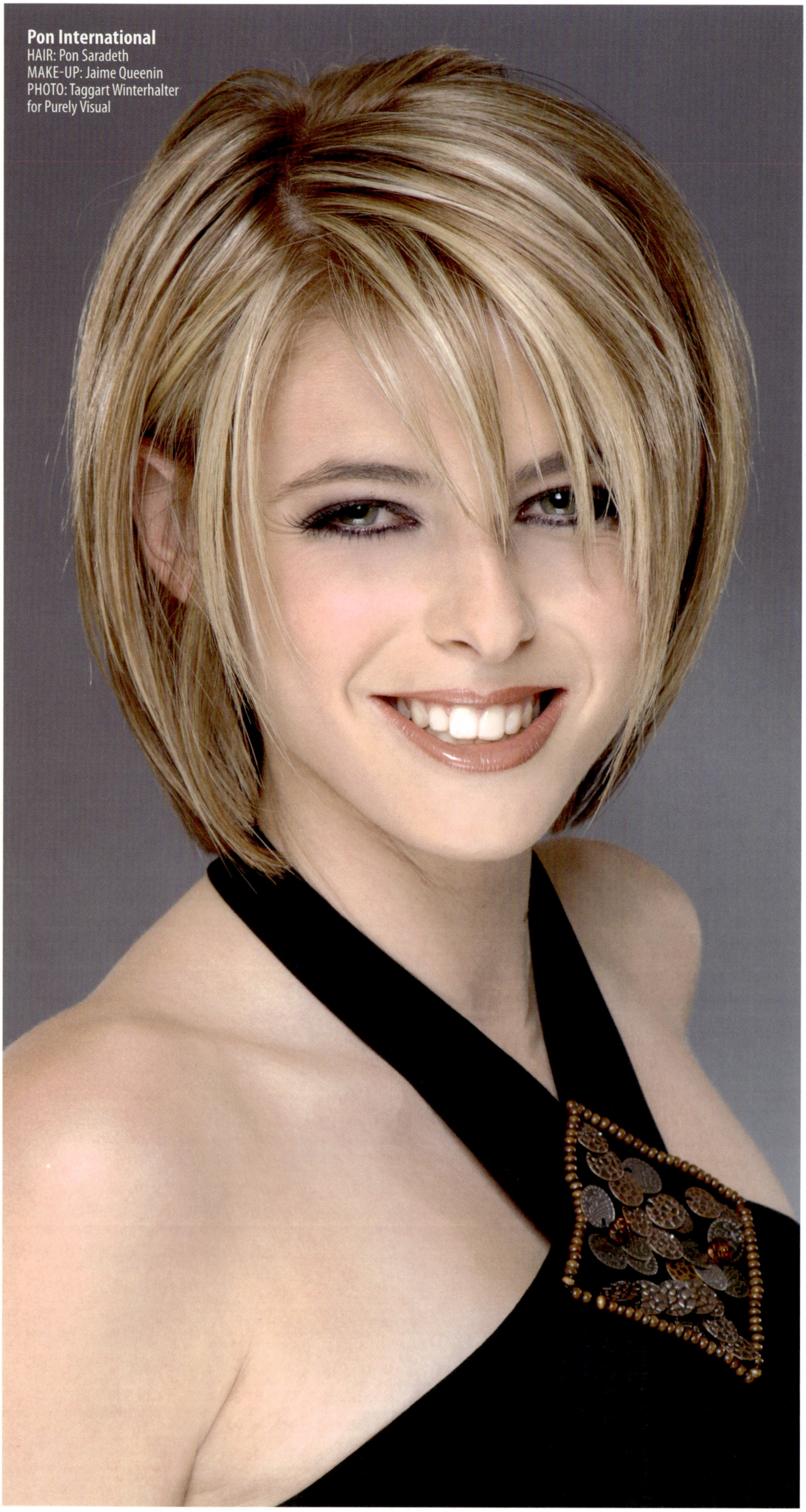

**Pon International**
HAIR: Pon Saradeth
MAKE-UP: Jaime Queenin
PHOTO: Taggart Winterhalter
for Purely Visual

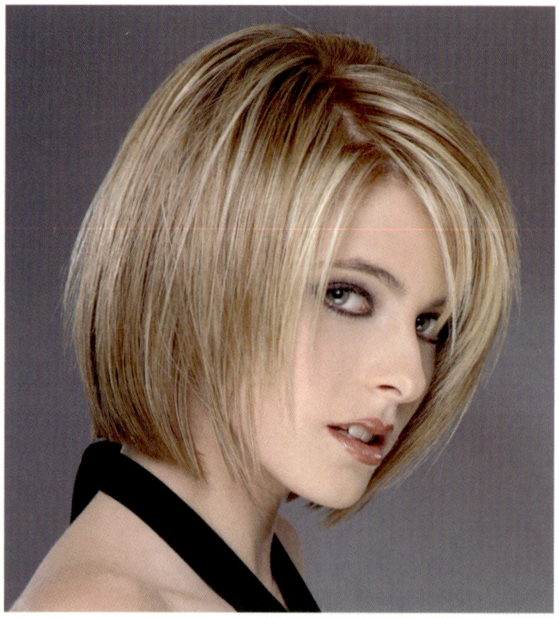

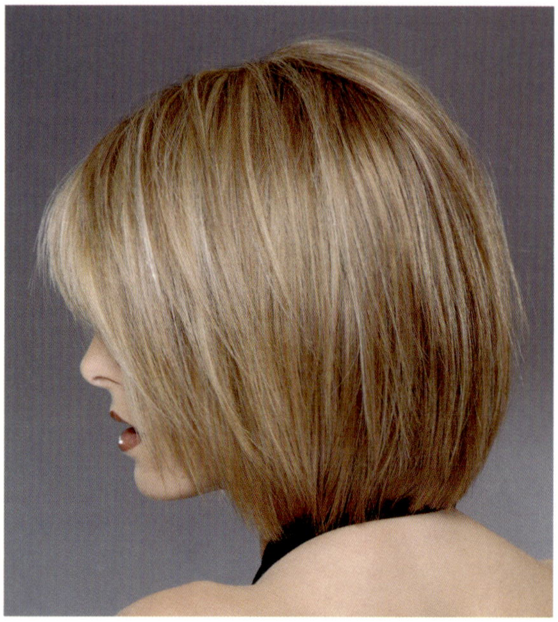

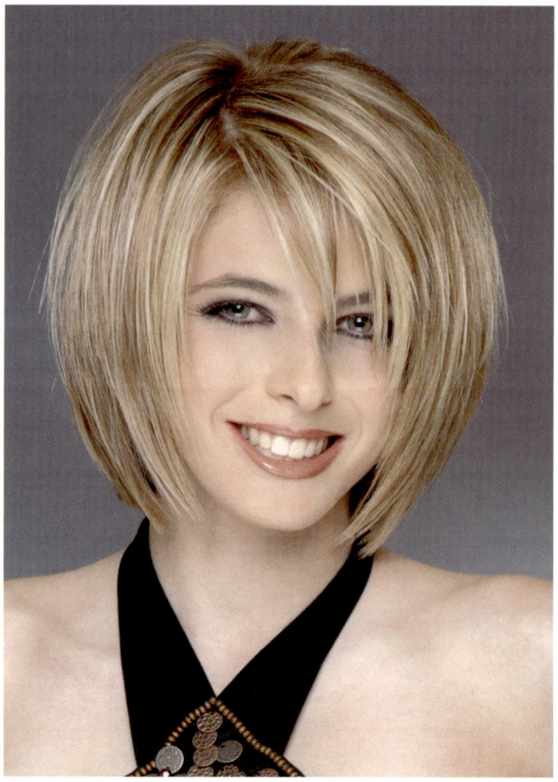

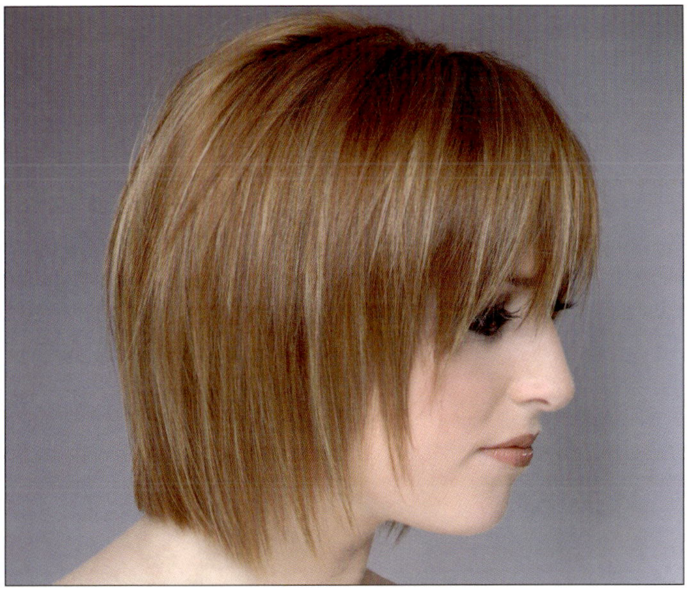

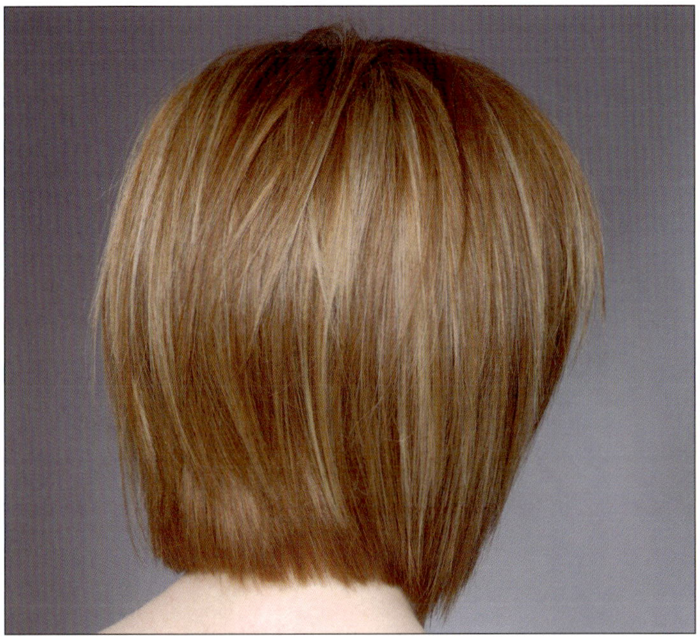

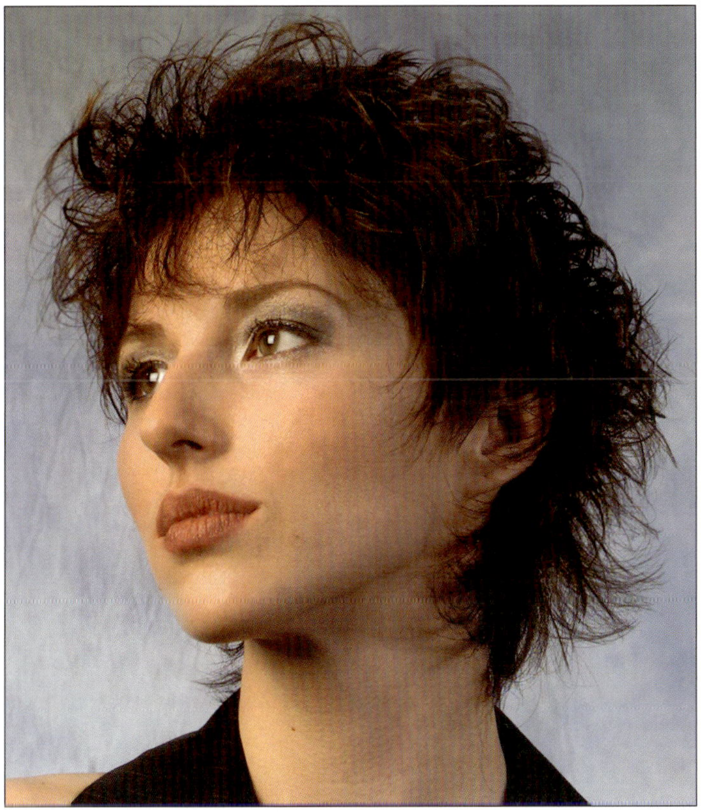

**Pon International**
HAIR: Pon Saradeth
MAKE-UP: Jaime Queenin
PHOTO: Taggart Winterhalter
for Purely Visual

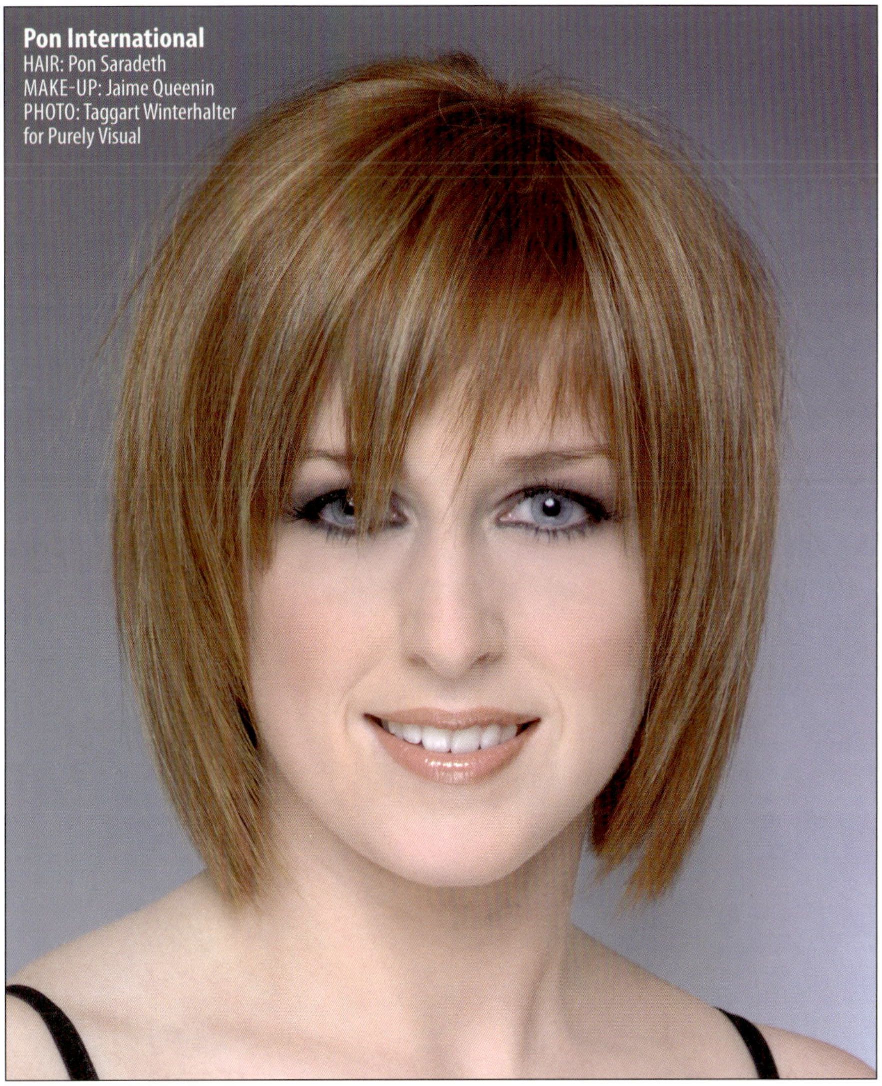

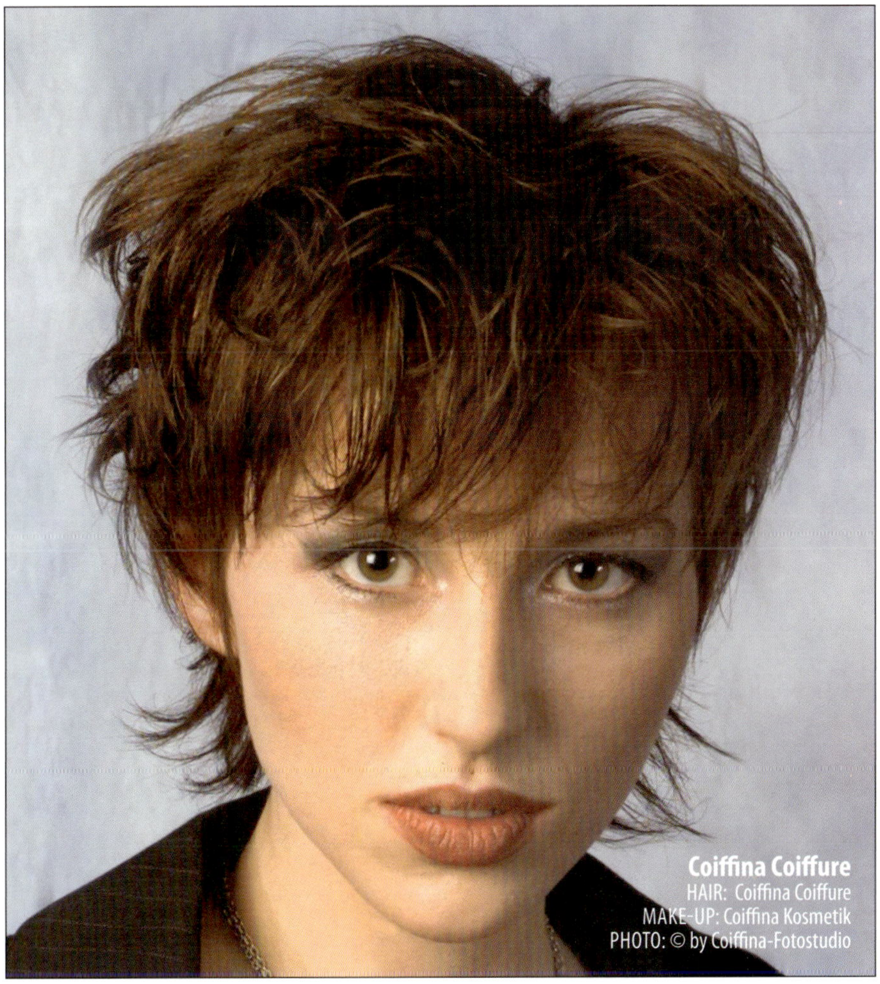

**Coiffina Coiffure**
HAIR: Coiffina Coiffure
MAKE-UP: Coiffina Kosmetik
PHOTO: © by Coiffina-Fotostudio

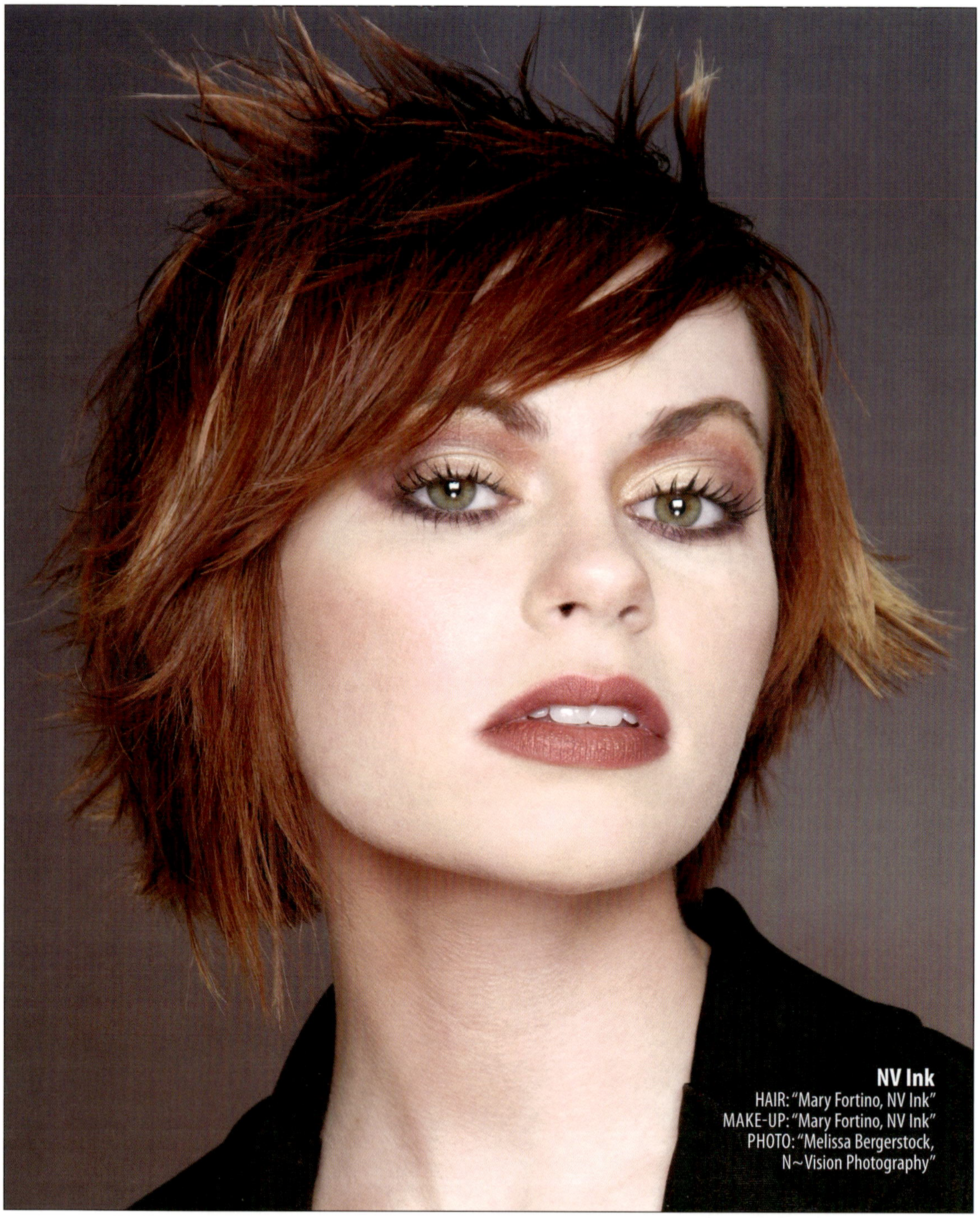

**NV Ink**
HAIR: "Mary Fortino, NV Ink"
MAKE-UP: "Mary Fortino, NV Ink"
PHOTO: "Melissa Bergerstock, N~Vision Photography"

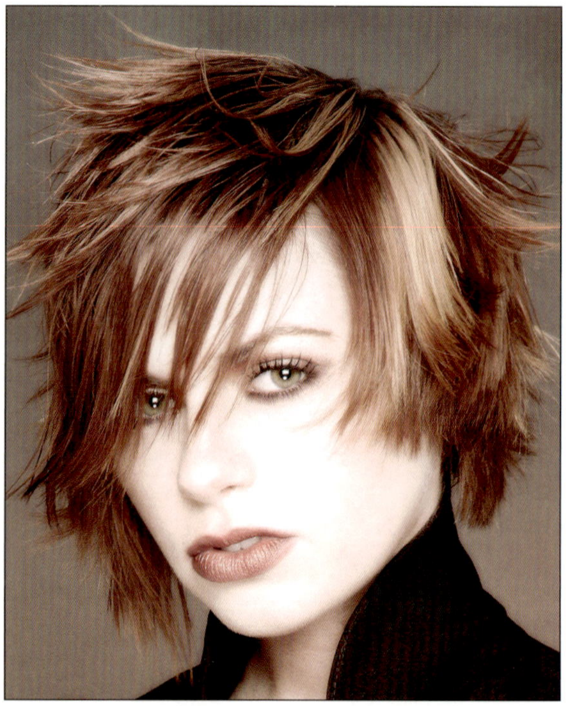

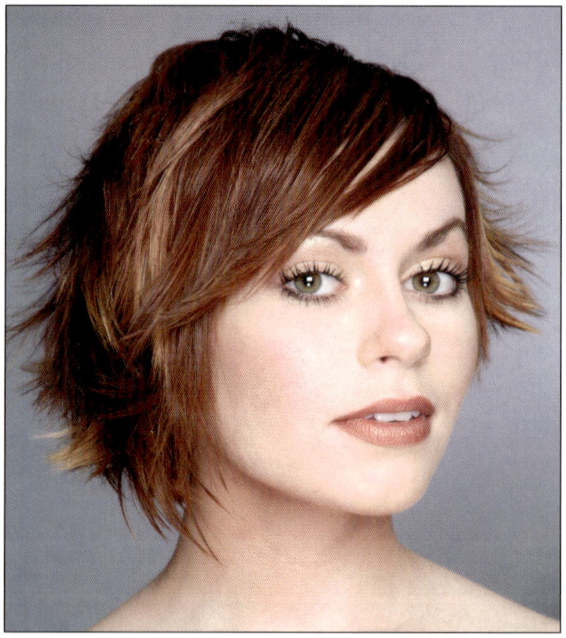

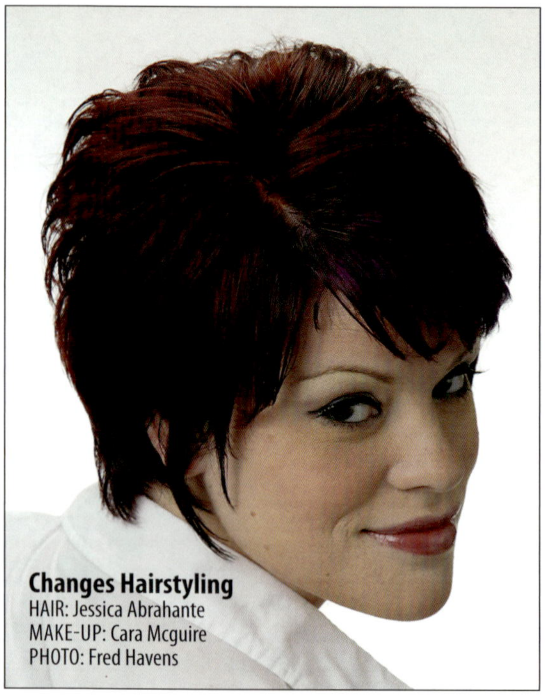

**Changes Hairstyling**
HAIR: Jessica Abrahante
MAKE-UP: Cara Mcguire
PHOTO: Fred Havens

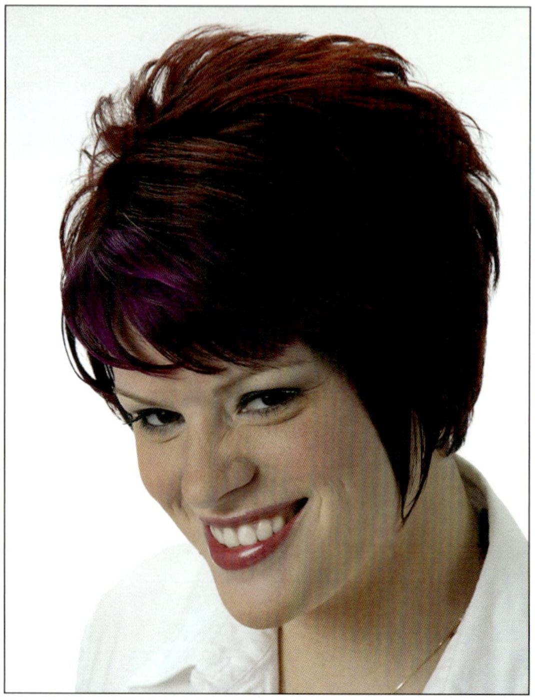

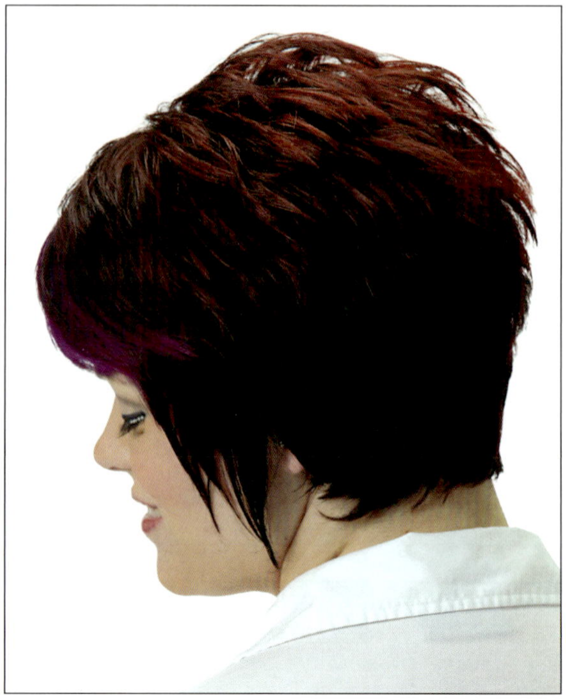

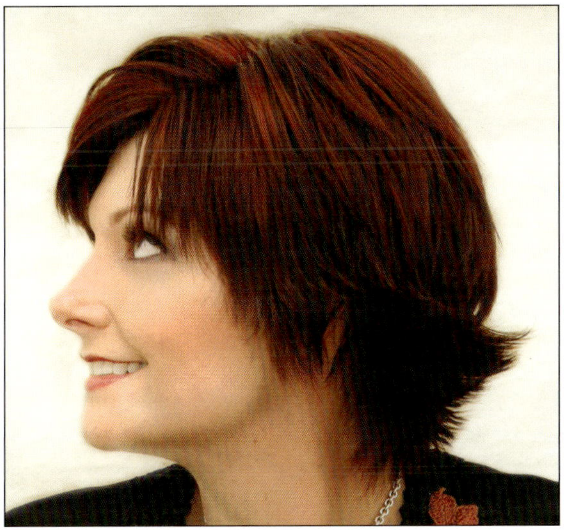

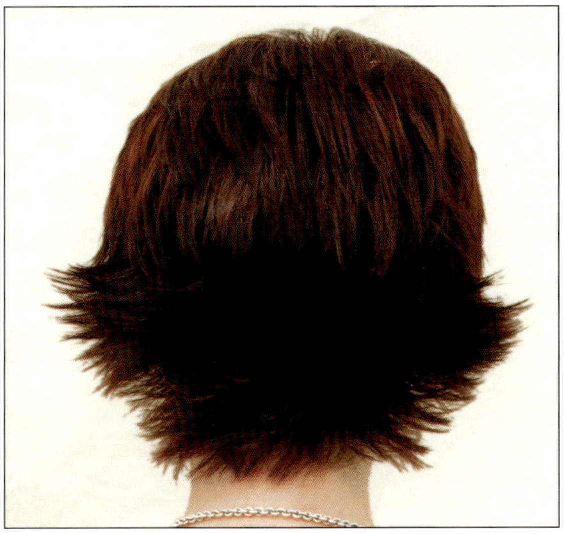

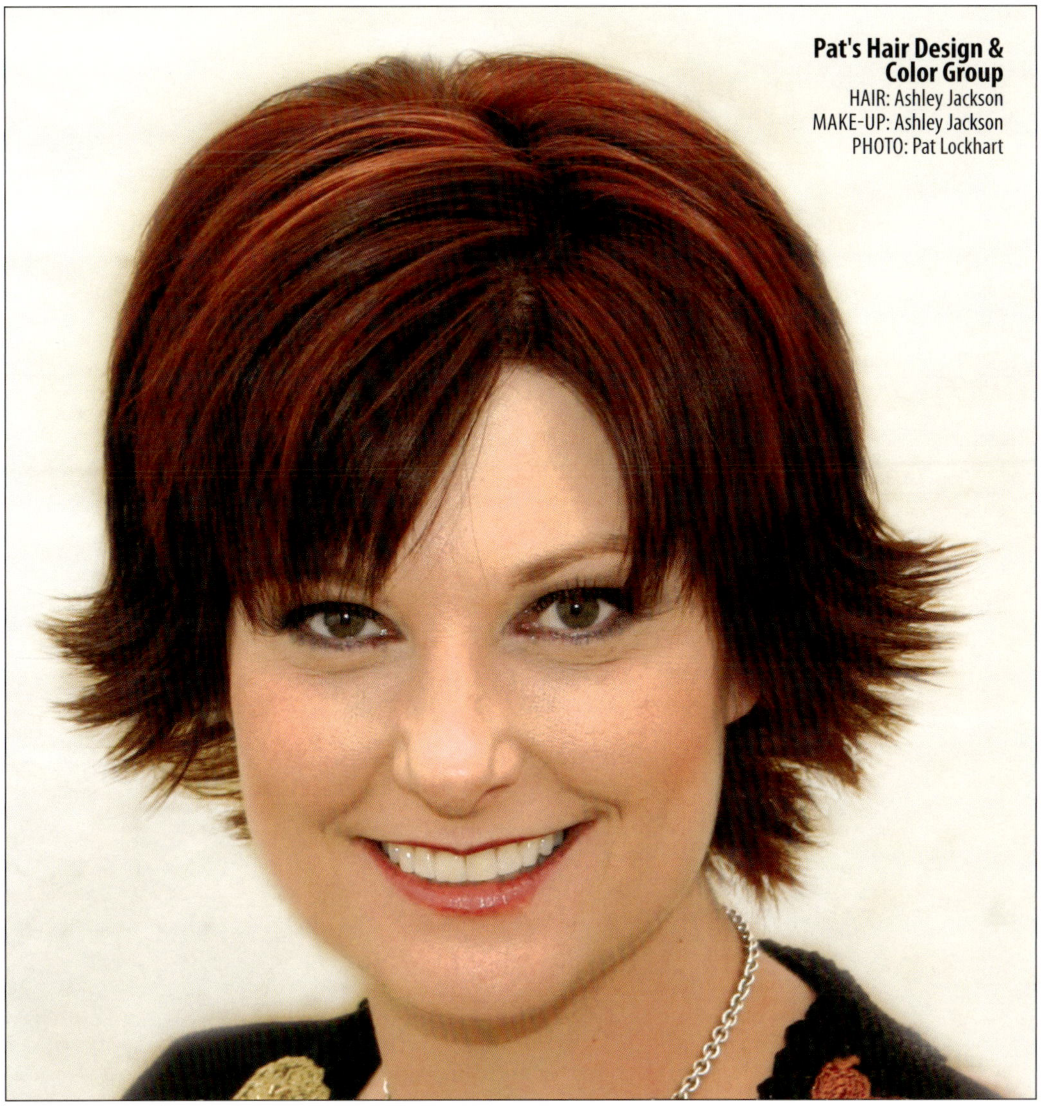

**Pat's Hair Design & Color Group**
HAIR: Ashley Jackson
MAKE-UP: Ashley Jackson
PHOTO: Pat Lockhart

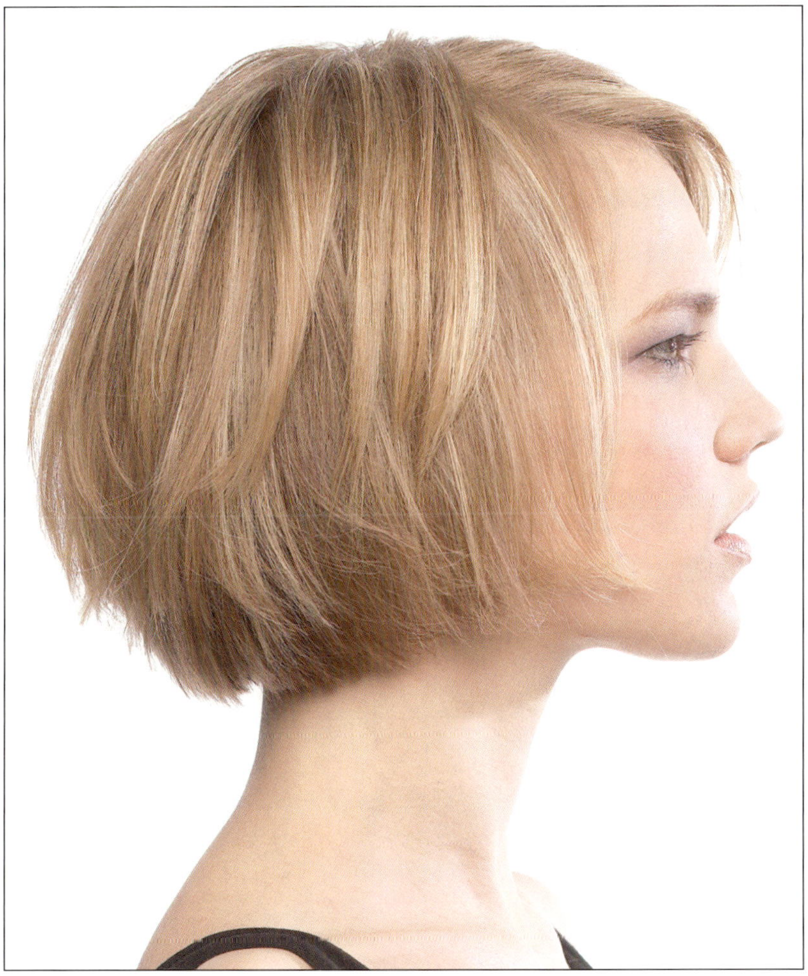

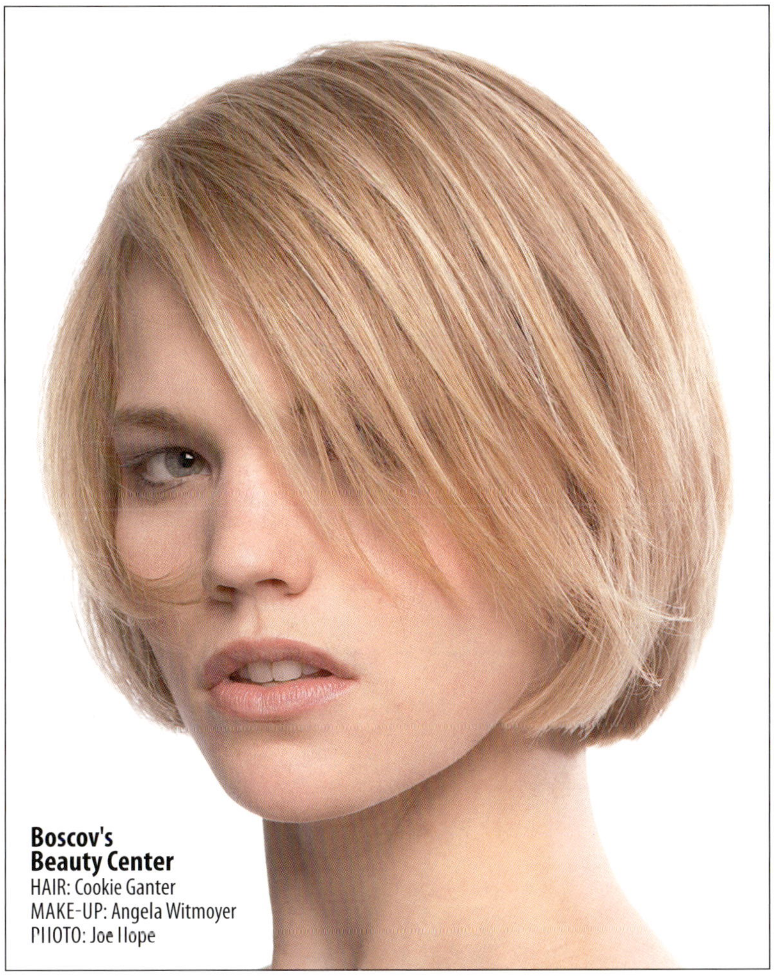

**Boscov's Beauty Center**
HAIR: Cookie Ganter
MAKE-UP: Angela Witmoyer
PHOTO: Joe Hope

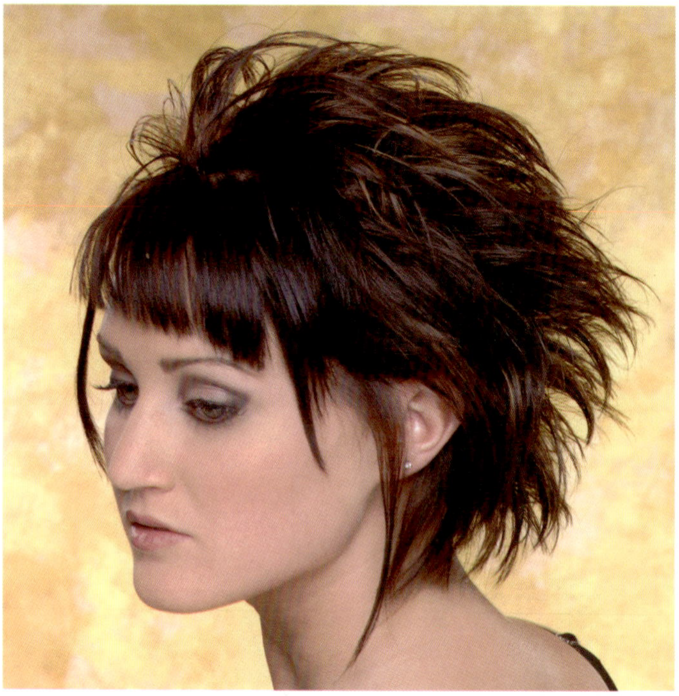

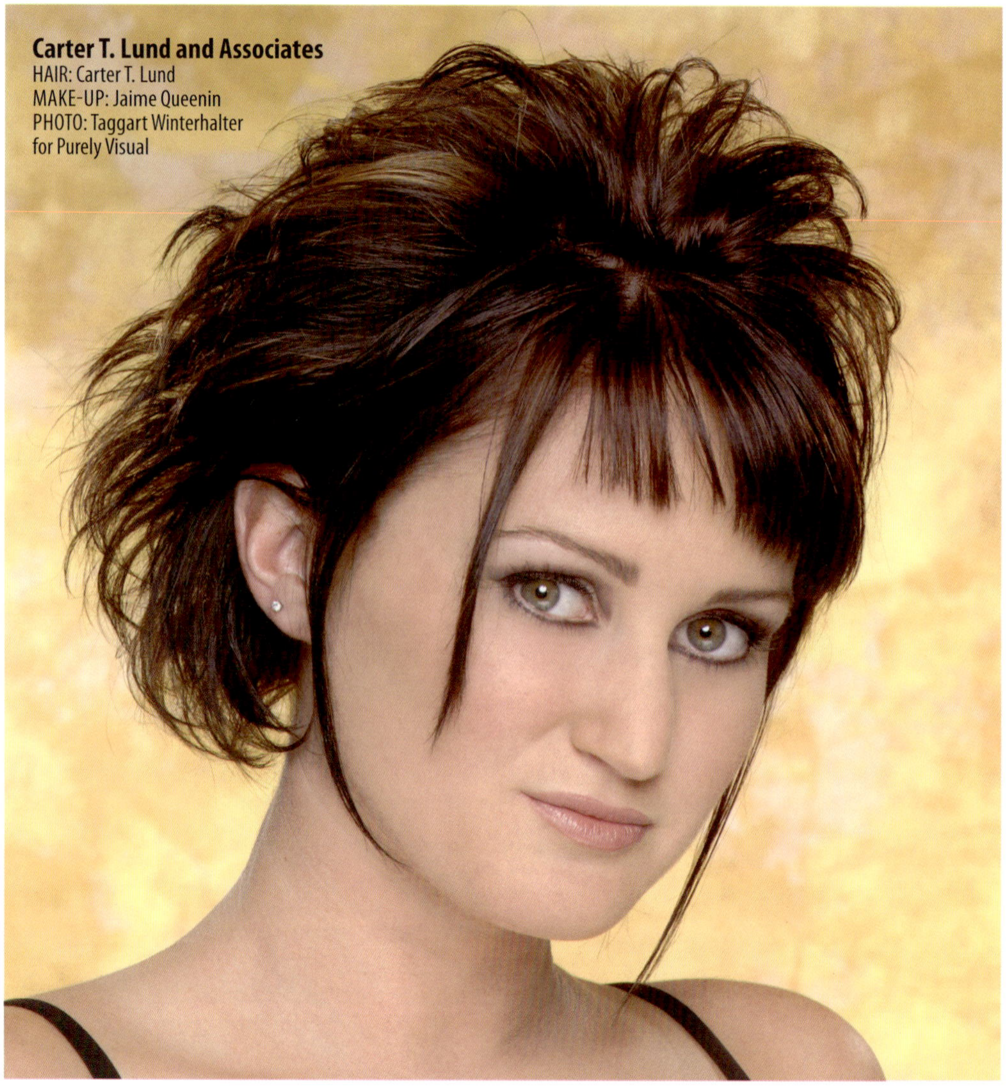

**Carter T. Lund and Associates**
HAIR: Carter T. Lund
MAKE-UP: Jaime Queenin
PHOTO: Taggart Winterhalter
for Purely Visual

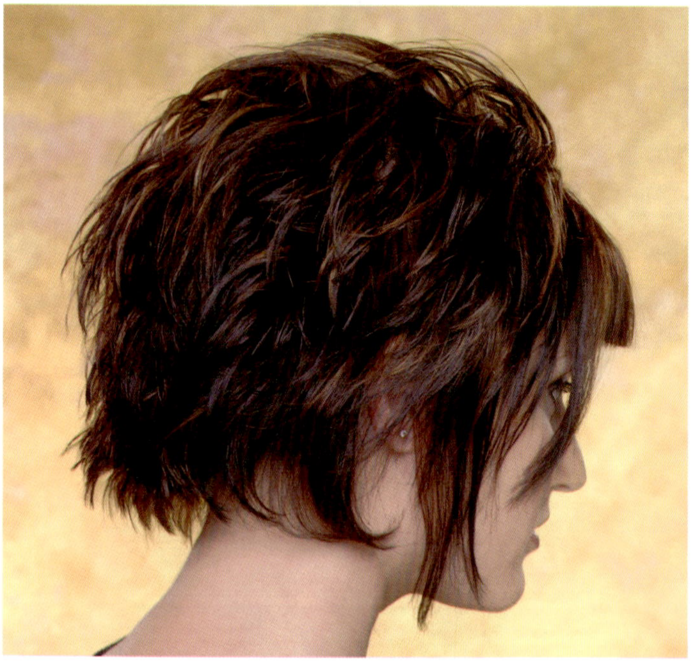

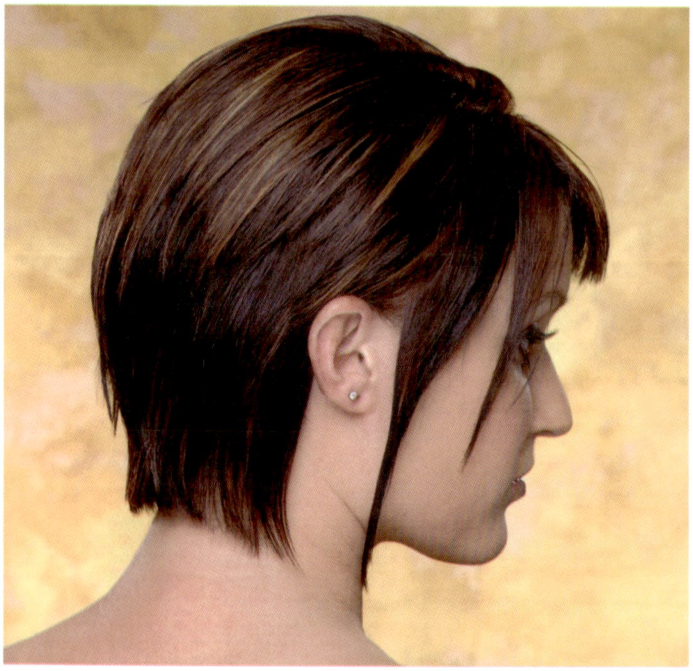

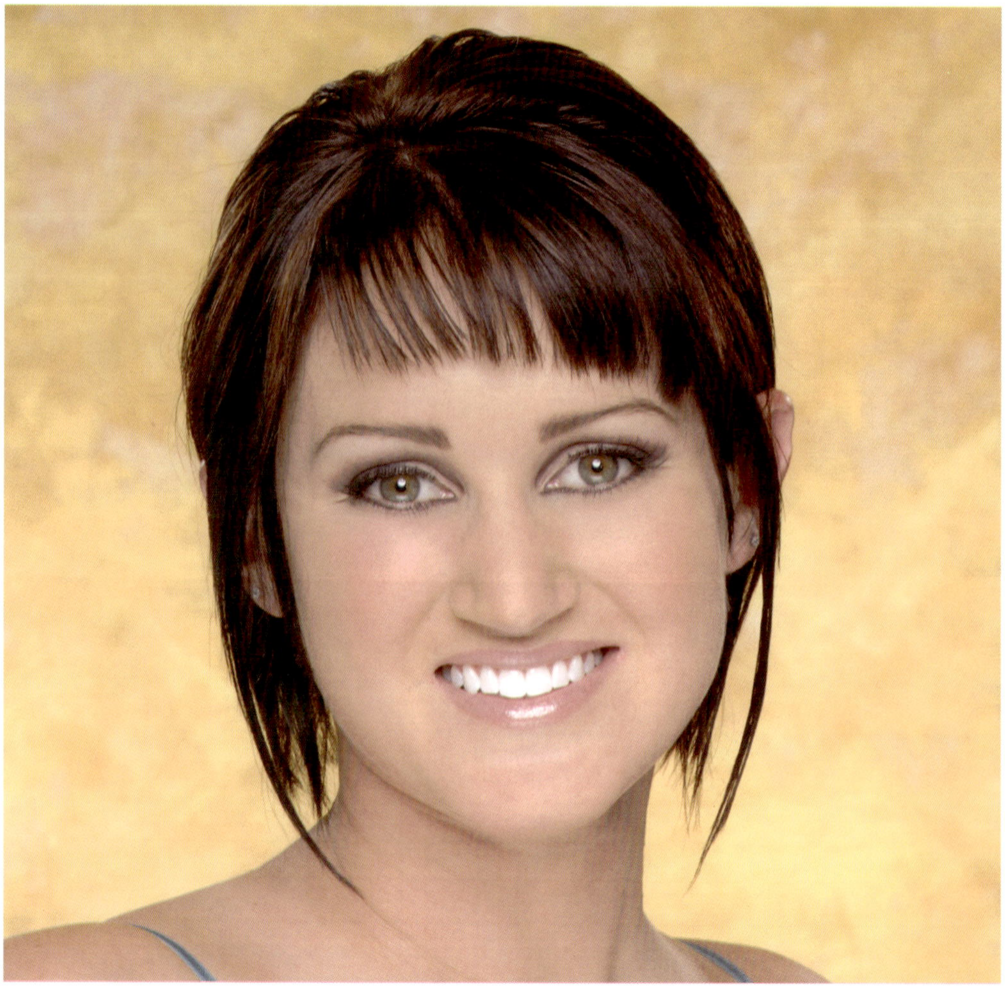

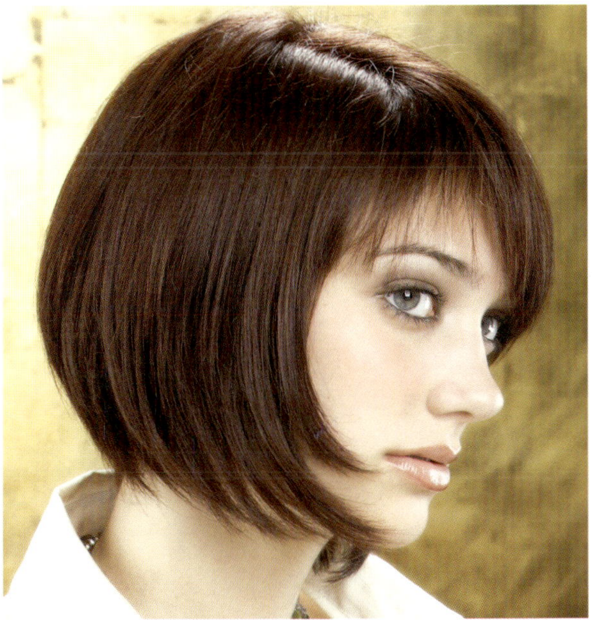

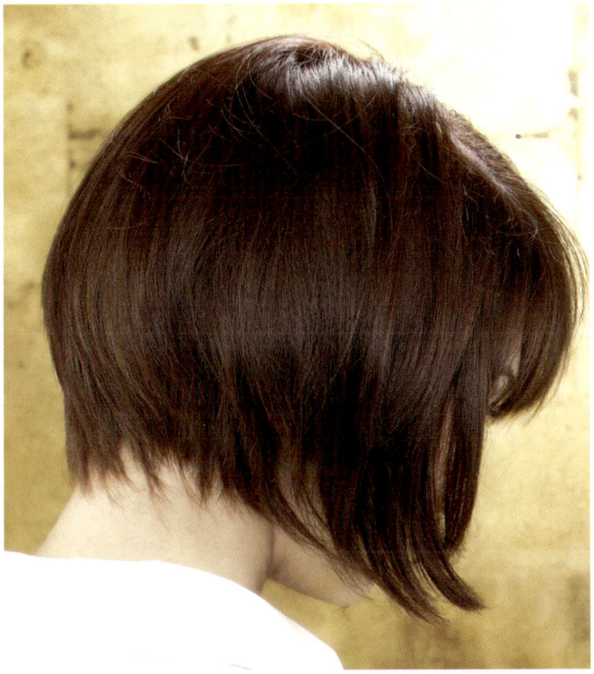

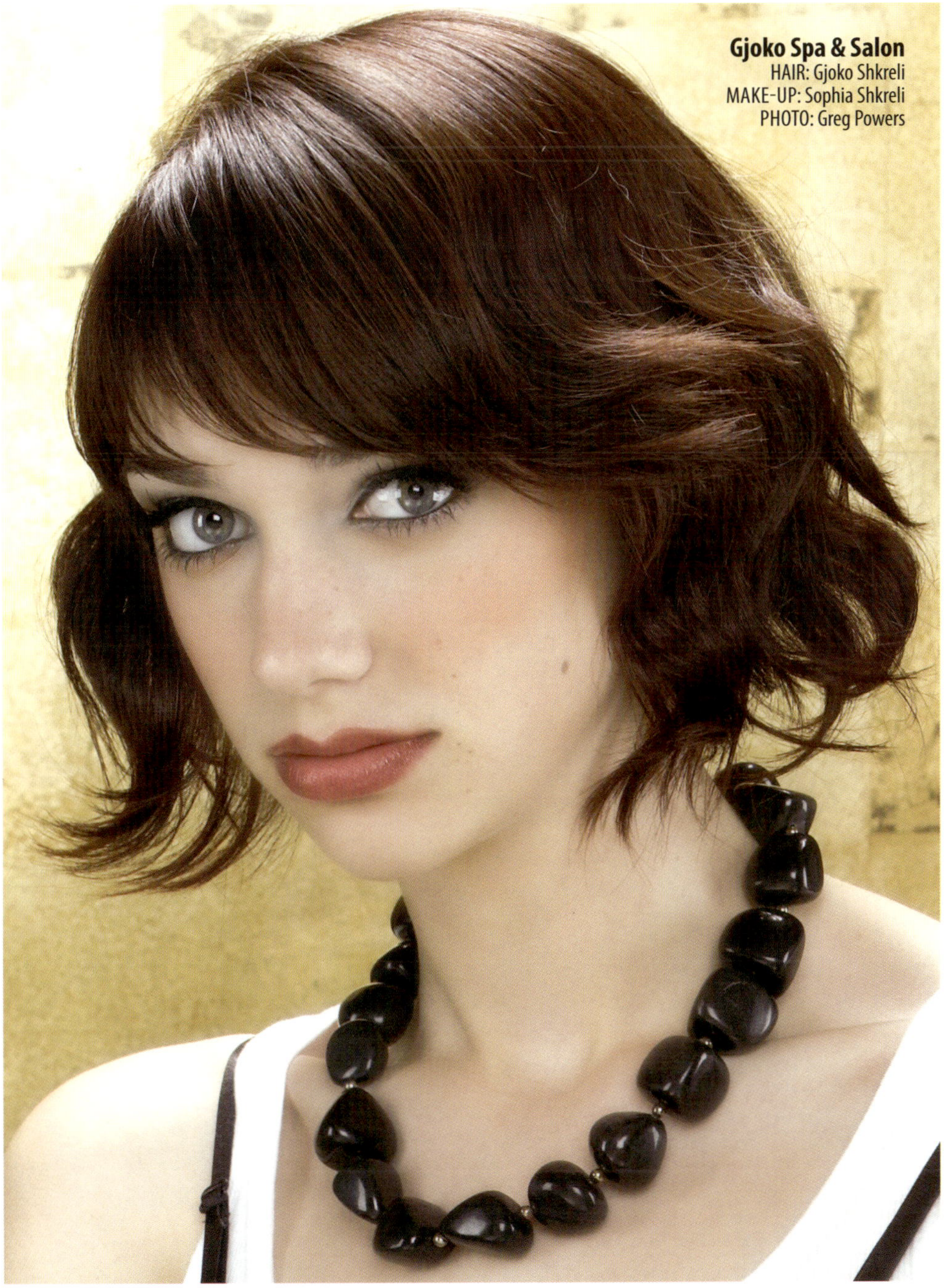

**Gjoko Spa & Salon**
HAIR: Gjoko Shkreli
MAKE-UP: Sophia Shkreli
PHOTO: Greg Powers

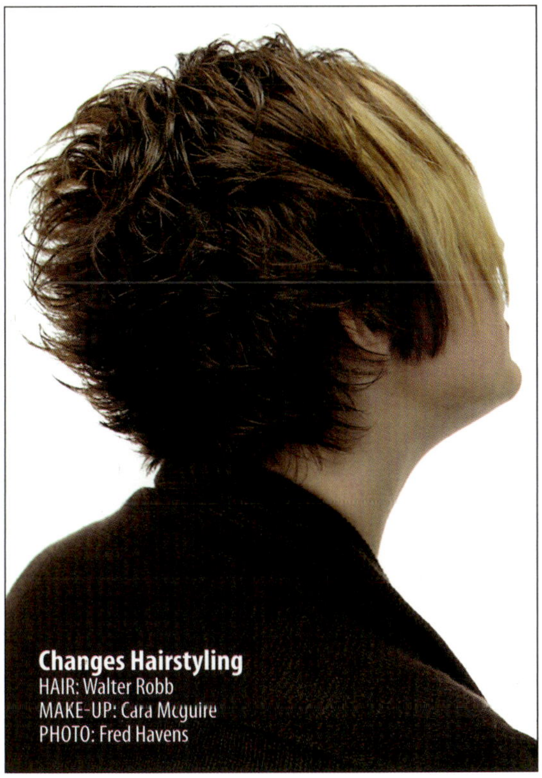

**Changes Hairstyling**
HAIR: Walter Robb
MAKE-UP: Cara Mcguire
PHOTO: Fred Havens

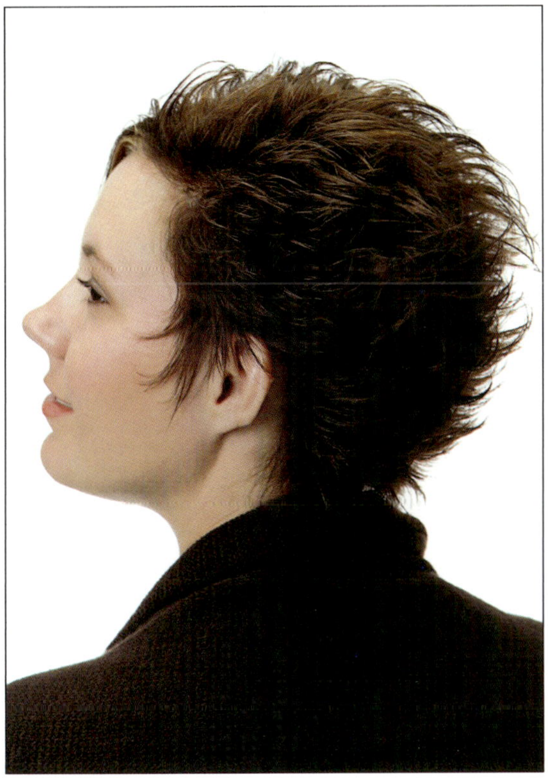

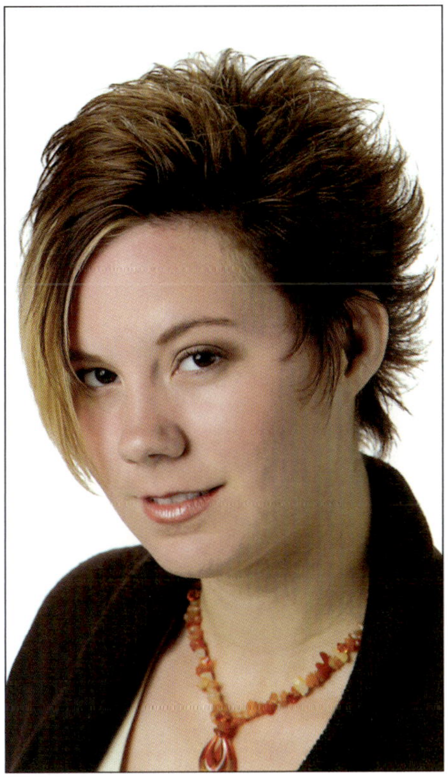

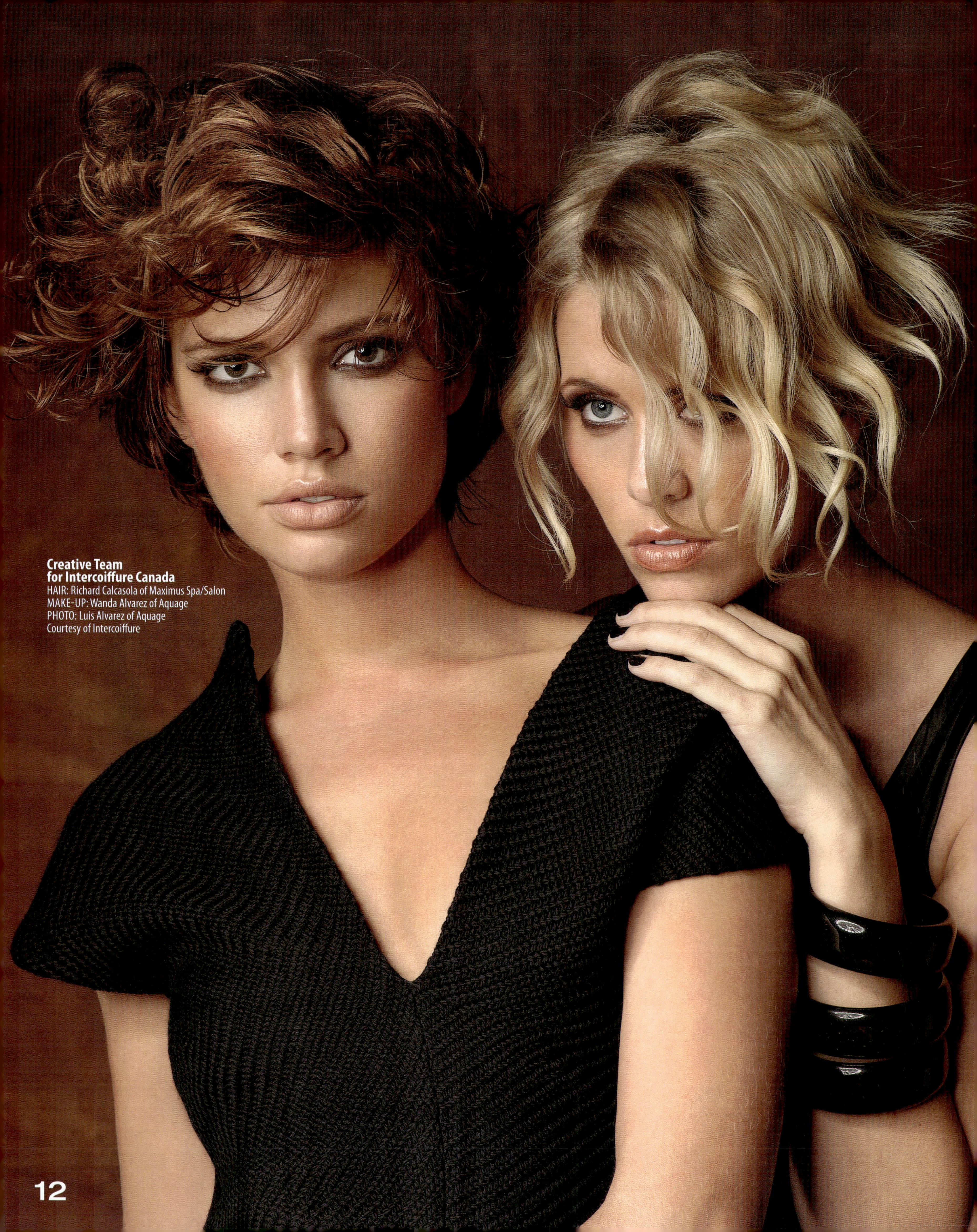

**Creative Team for Intercoiffure Canada**
HAIR: Richard Calcasola of Maximus Spa/Salon
MAKE-UP: Wanda Alvarez of Aquage
PHOTO: Luis Alvarez of Aquage
Courtesy of Intercoiffure

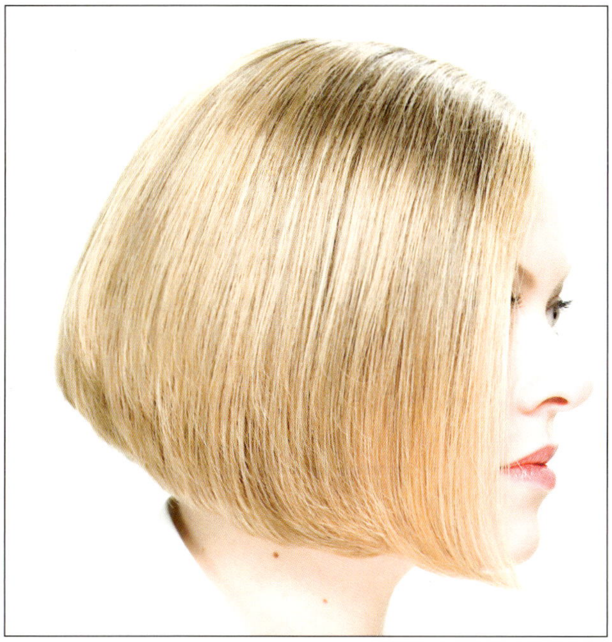

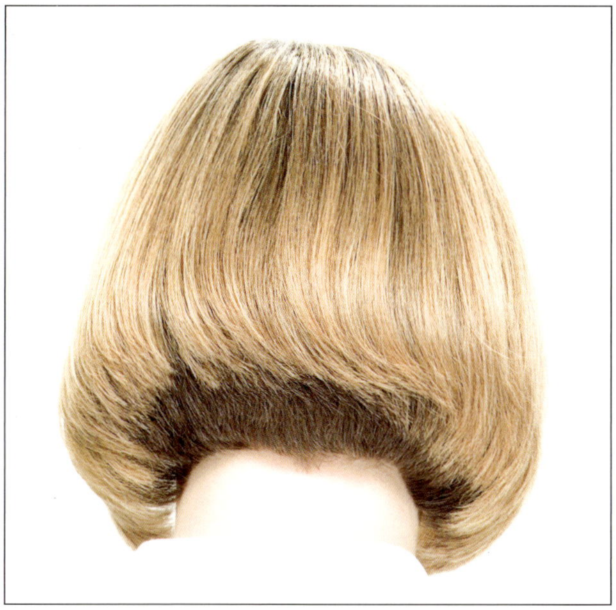

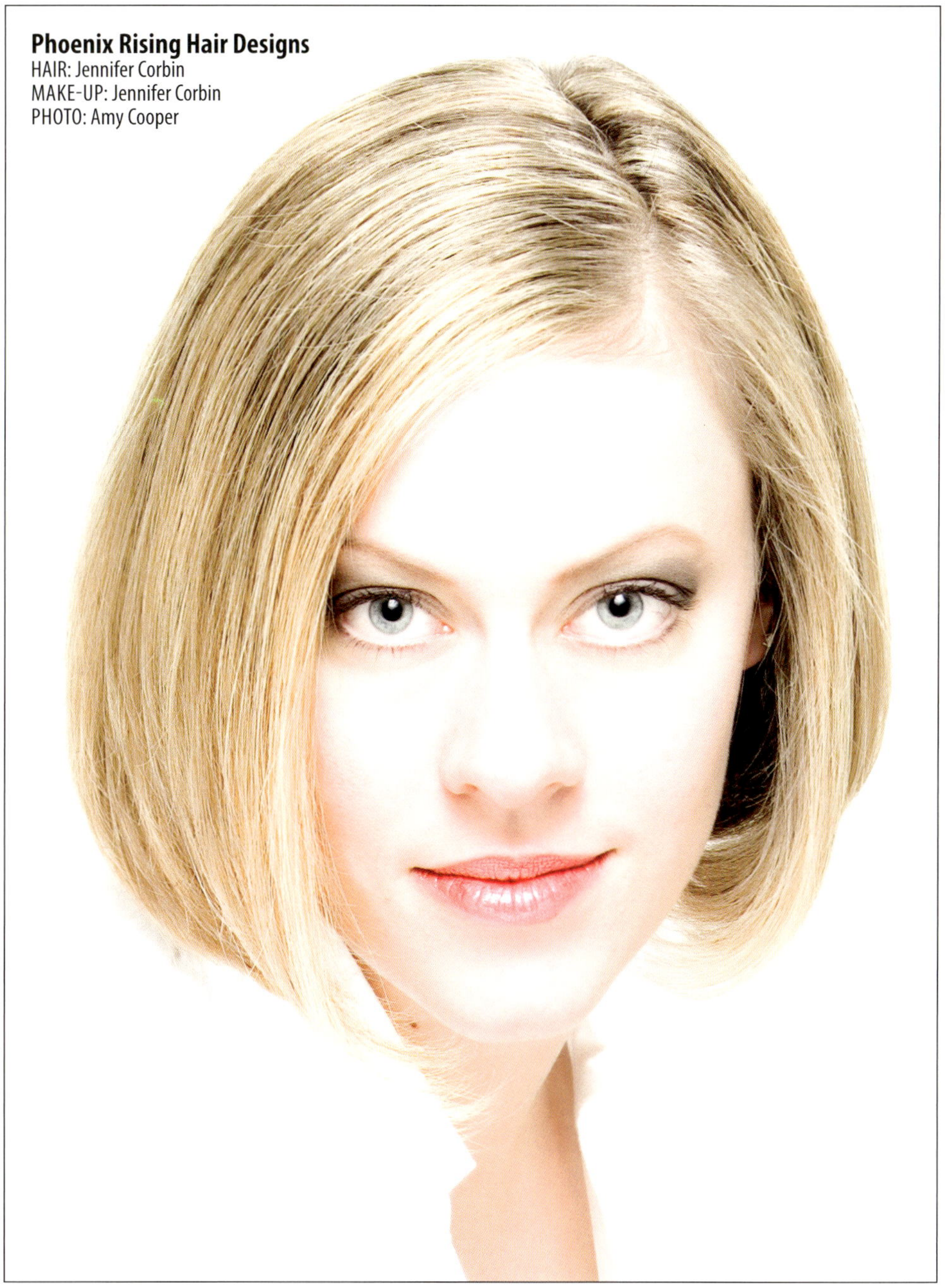

**Phoenix Rising Hair Designs**
HAIR: Jennifer Corbin
MAKE-UP: Jennifer Corbin
PHOTO: Amy Cooper

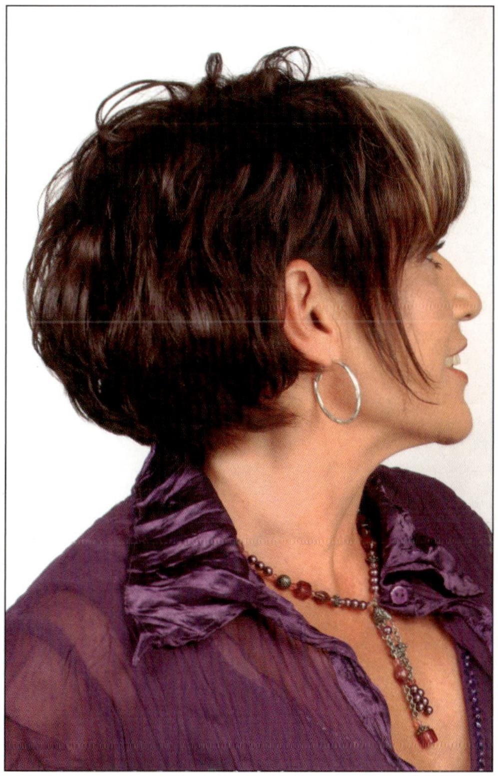

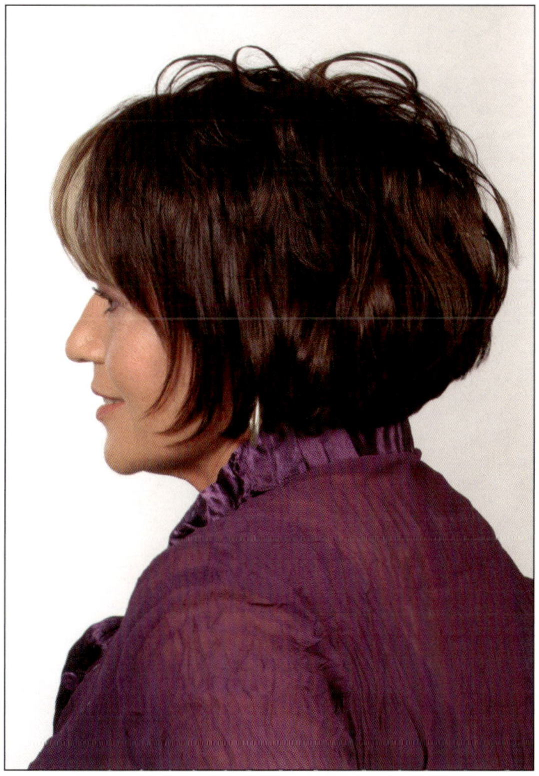

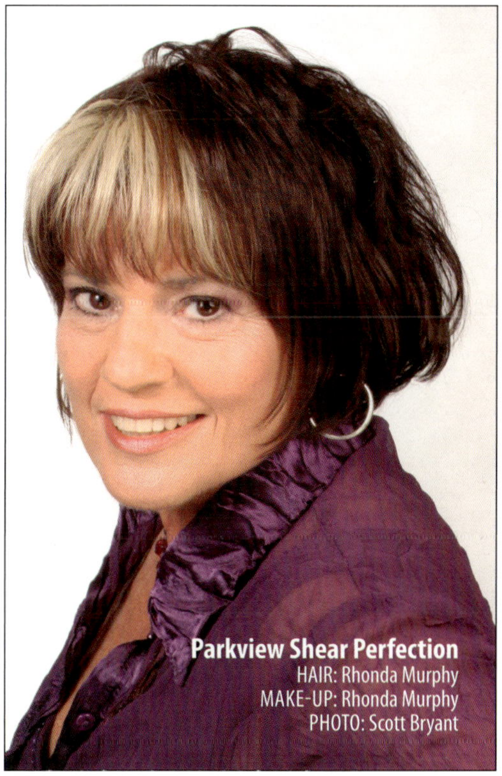

**Parkview Shear Perfection**
HAIR: Rhonda Murphy
MAKE-UP: Rhonda Murphy
PHOTO: Scott Bryant

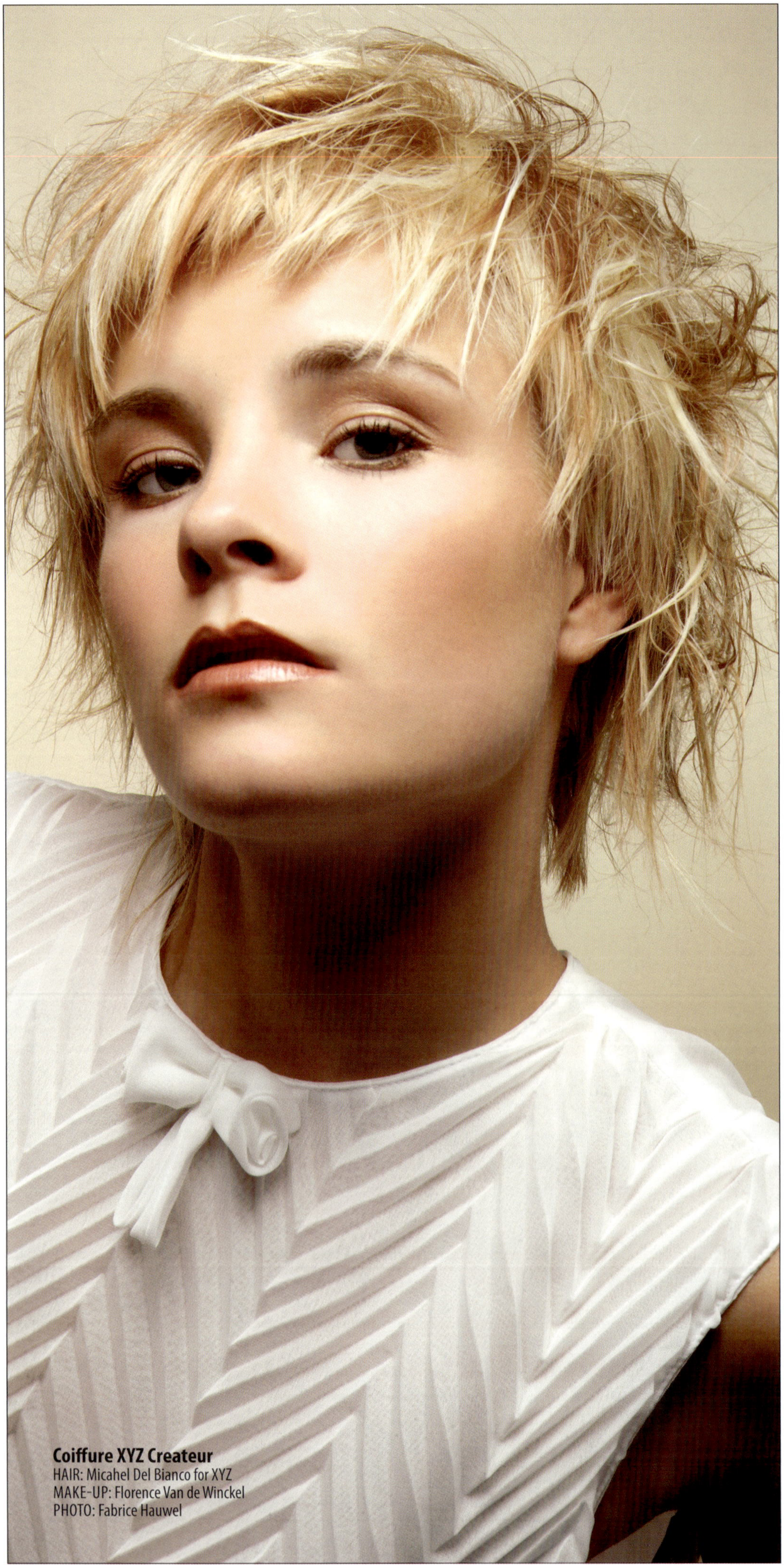

**Coiffure XYZ Createur**
HAIR: Micahel Del Bianco for XYZ
MAKE-UP: Florence Van de Winckel
PHOTO: Fabrice Hauwel

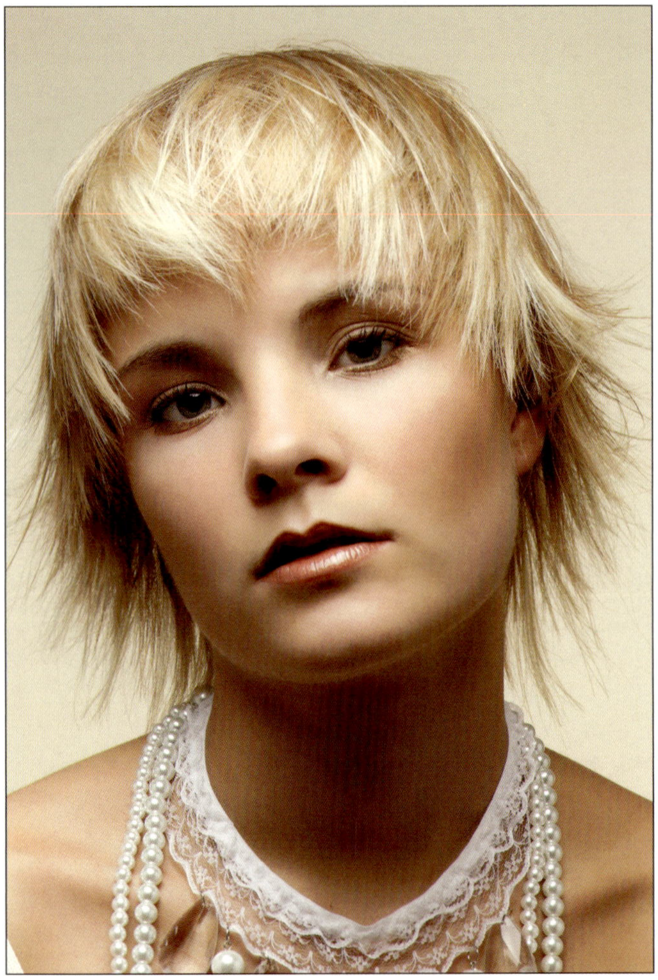

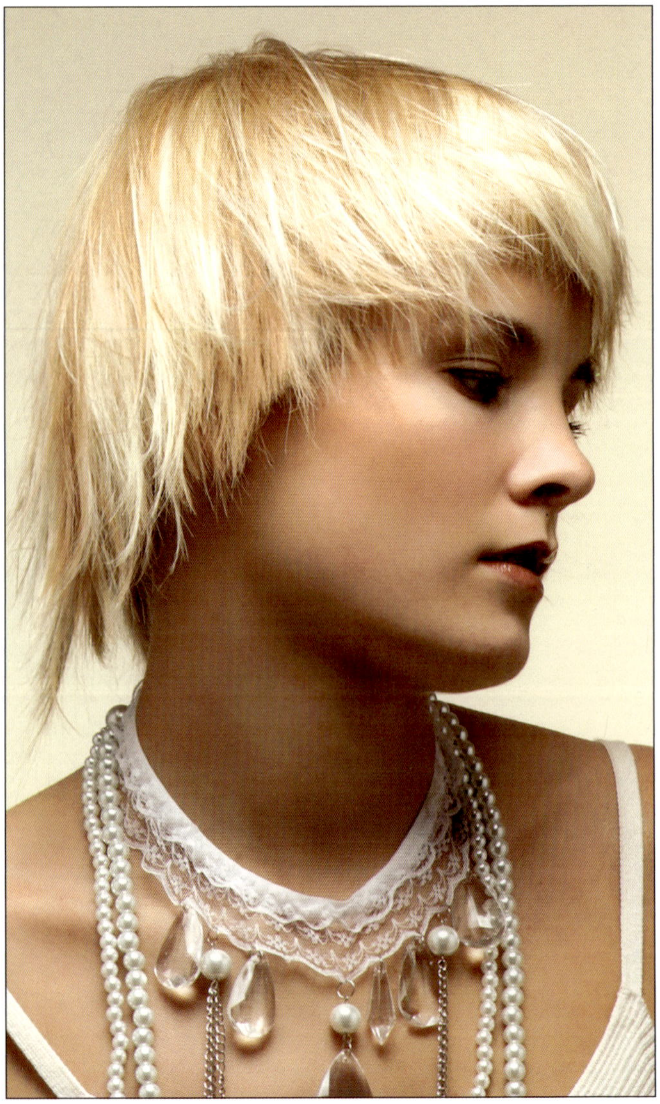

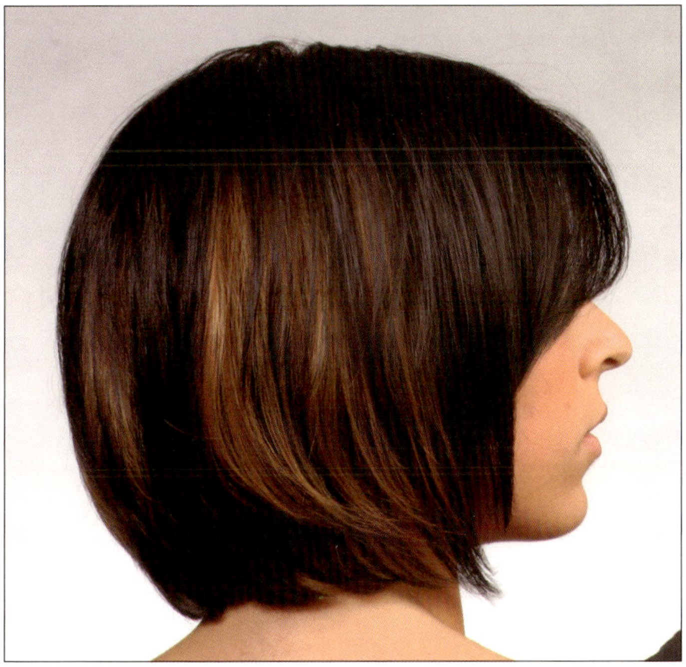

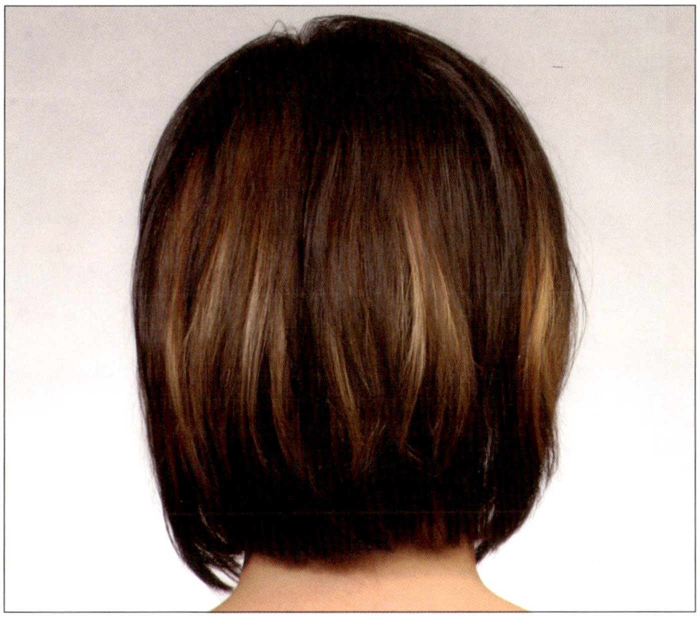

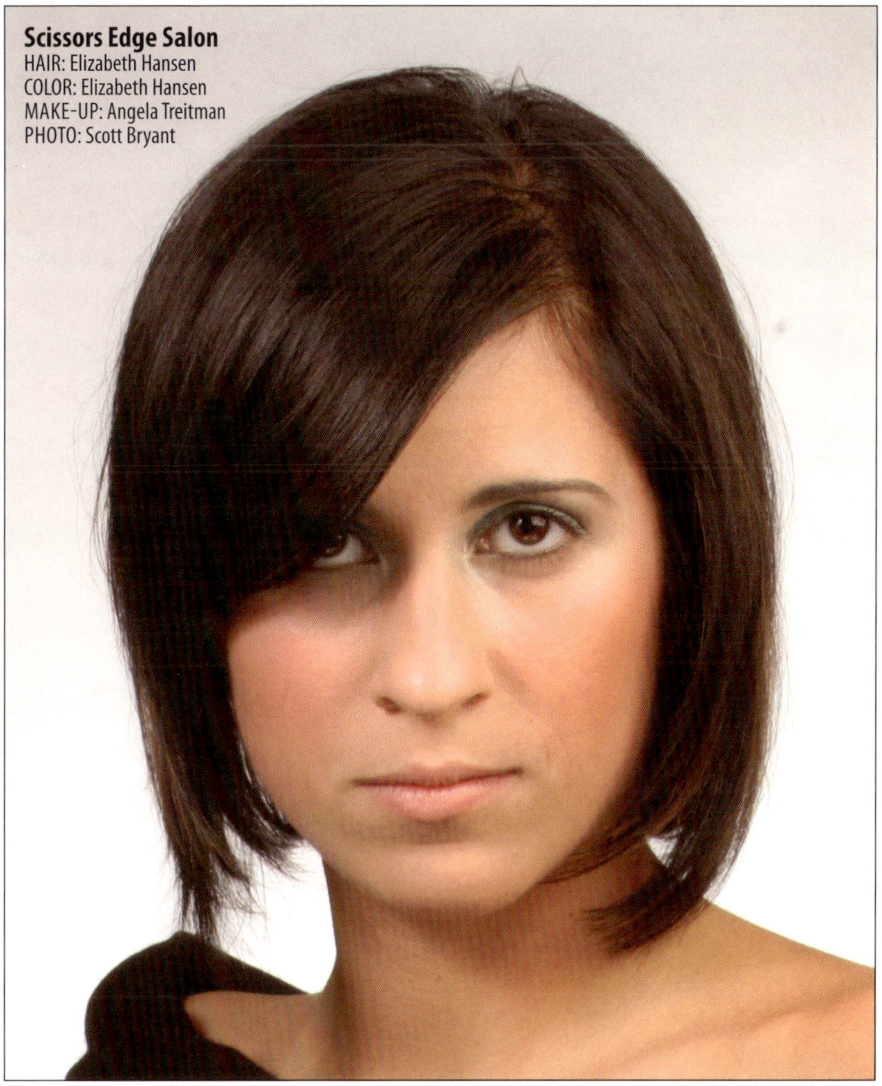

**Scissors Edge Salon**
HAIR: Elizabeth Hansen
COLOR: Elizabeth Hansen
MAKE-UP: Angela Treitman
PHOTO: Scott Bryant

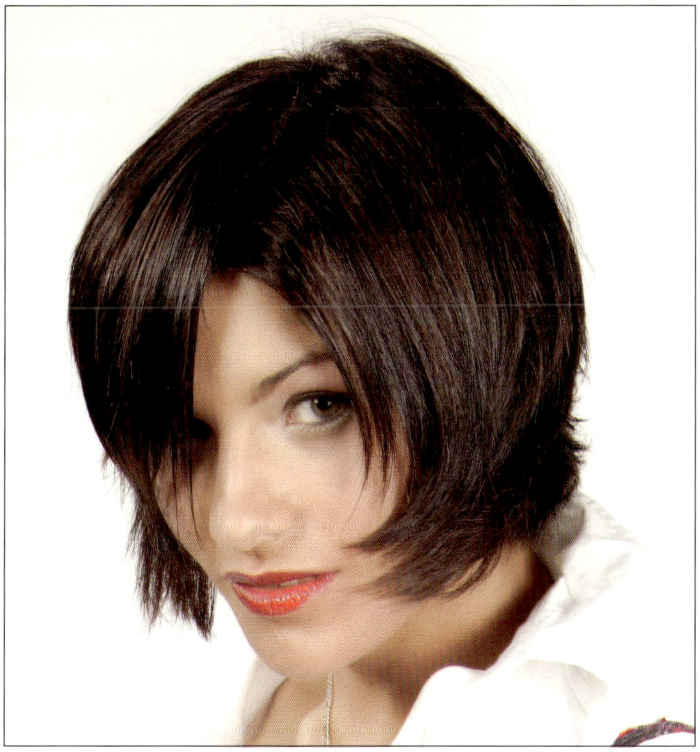

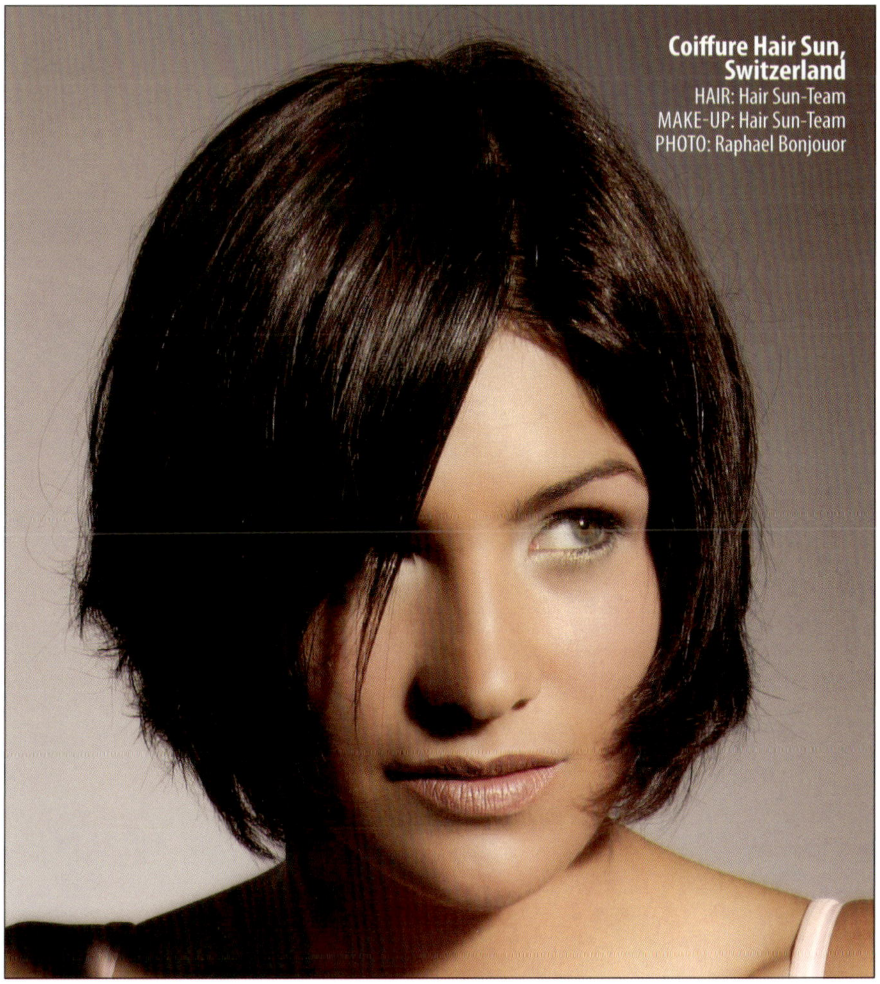

**Coiffure Hair Sun, Switzerland**
HAIR: Hair Sun-Team
MAKE-UP: Hair Sun-Team
PHOTO: Raphael Bonjouor

**Joseppi & Mimmo Hair Design**
HAIR: Dao Van
MAKE-UP: May Nguyen
PHOTO: Anthony Giang

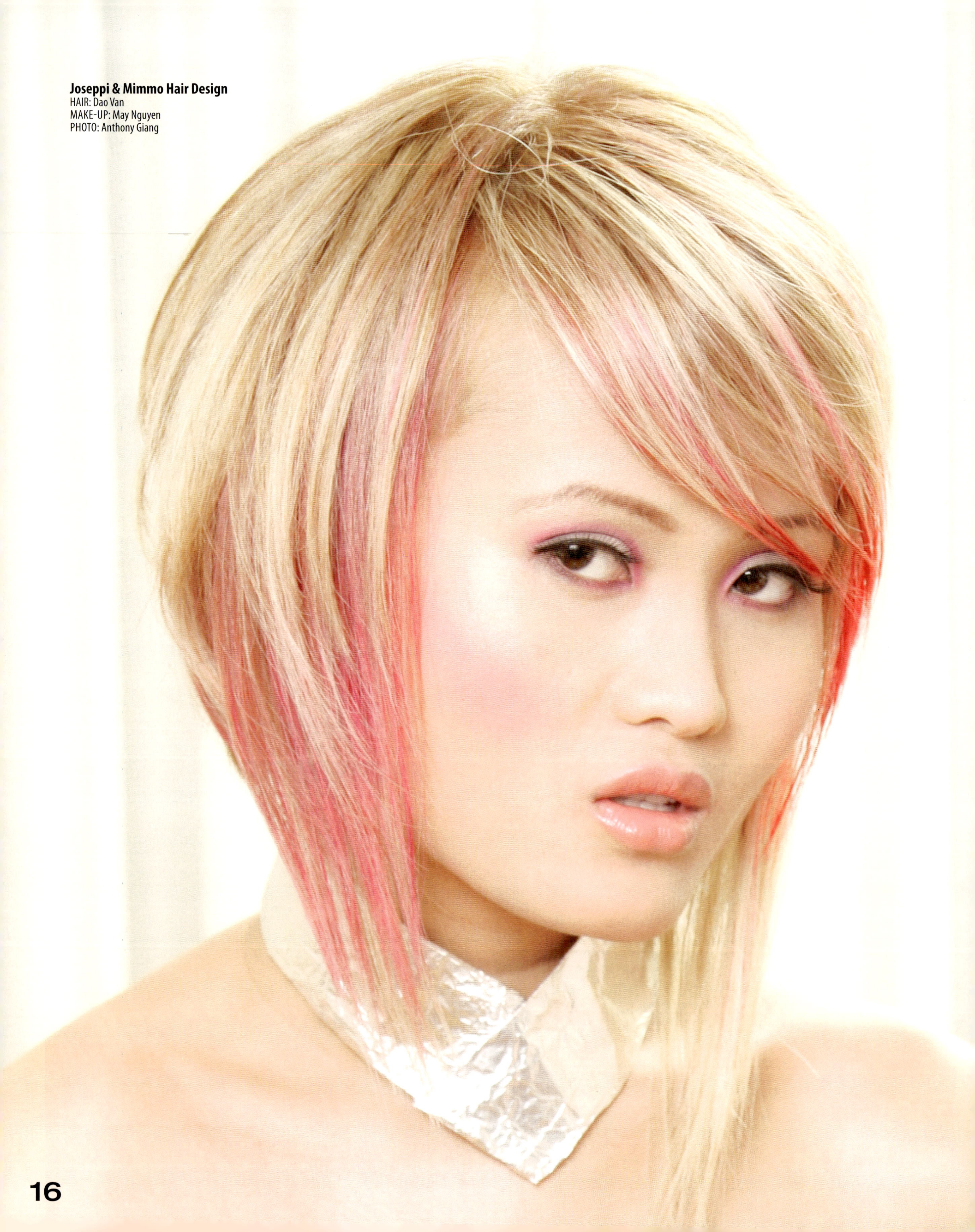

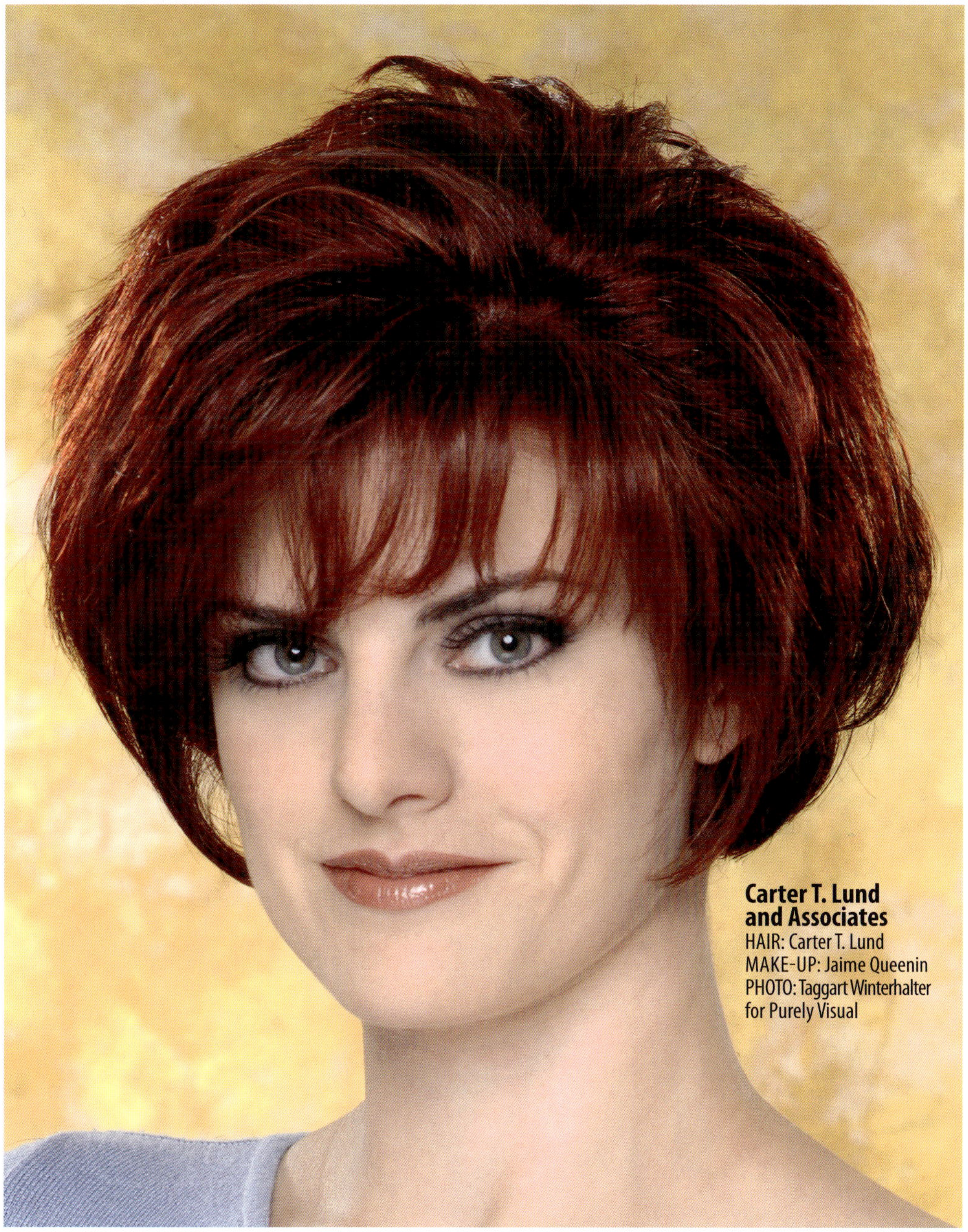

**Carter T. Lund and Associates**
HAIR: Carter T. Lund
MAKE-UP: Jaime Queenin
PHOTO: Taggart Winterhalter for Purely Visual

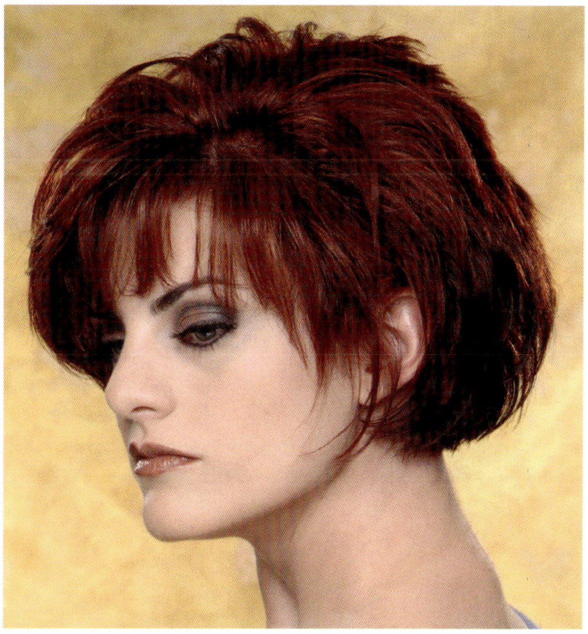

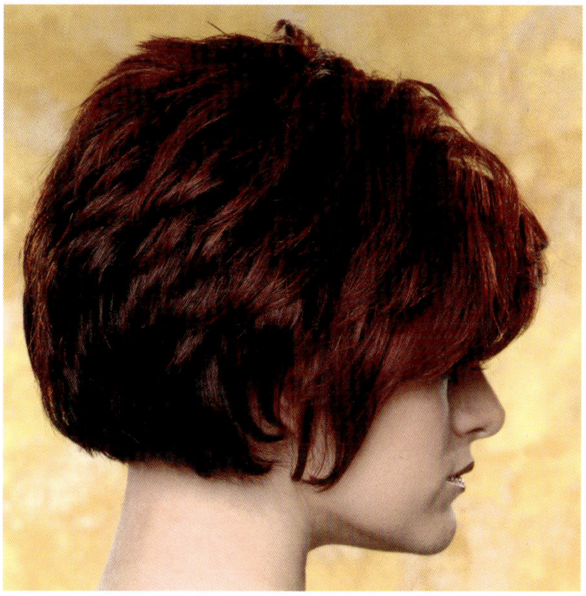

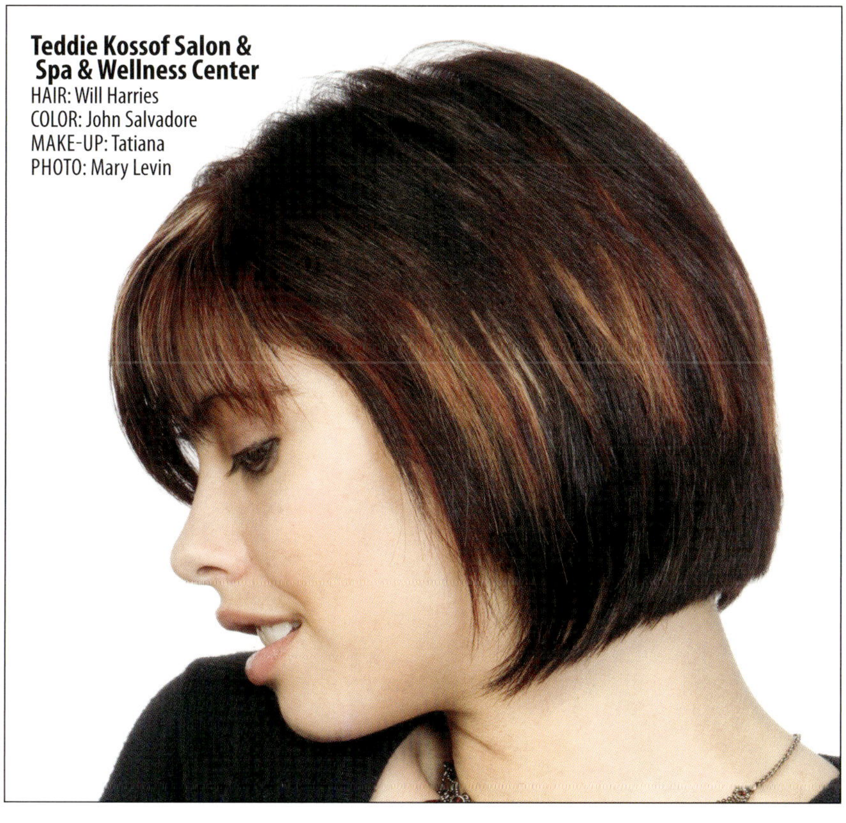

**Teddie Kossof Salon & Spa & Wellness Center**
HAIR: Will Harries
COLOR: John Salvadore
MAKE-UP: Tatiana
PHOTO: Mary Levin

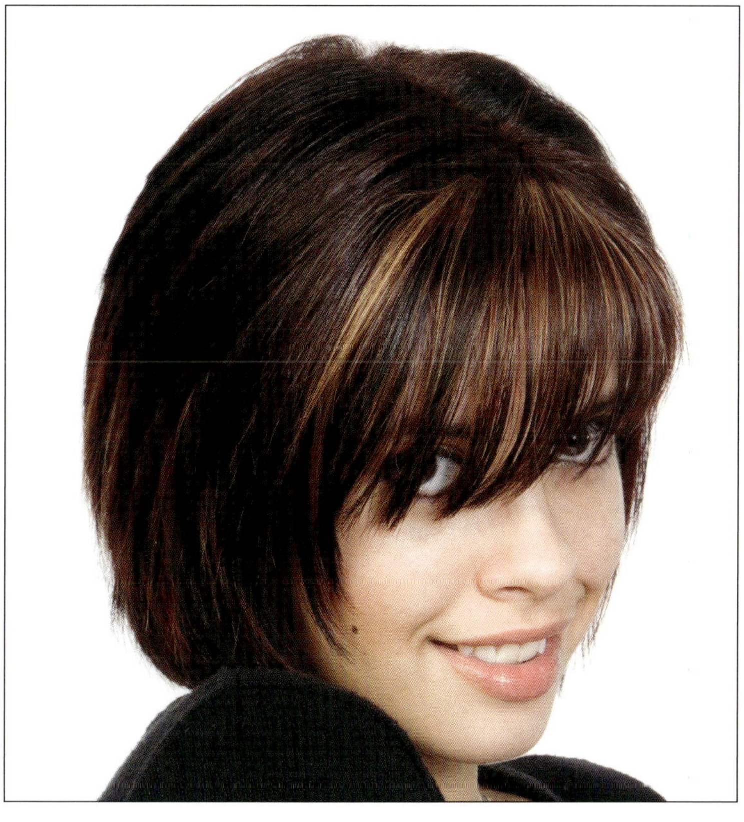

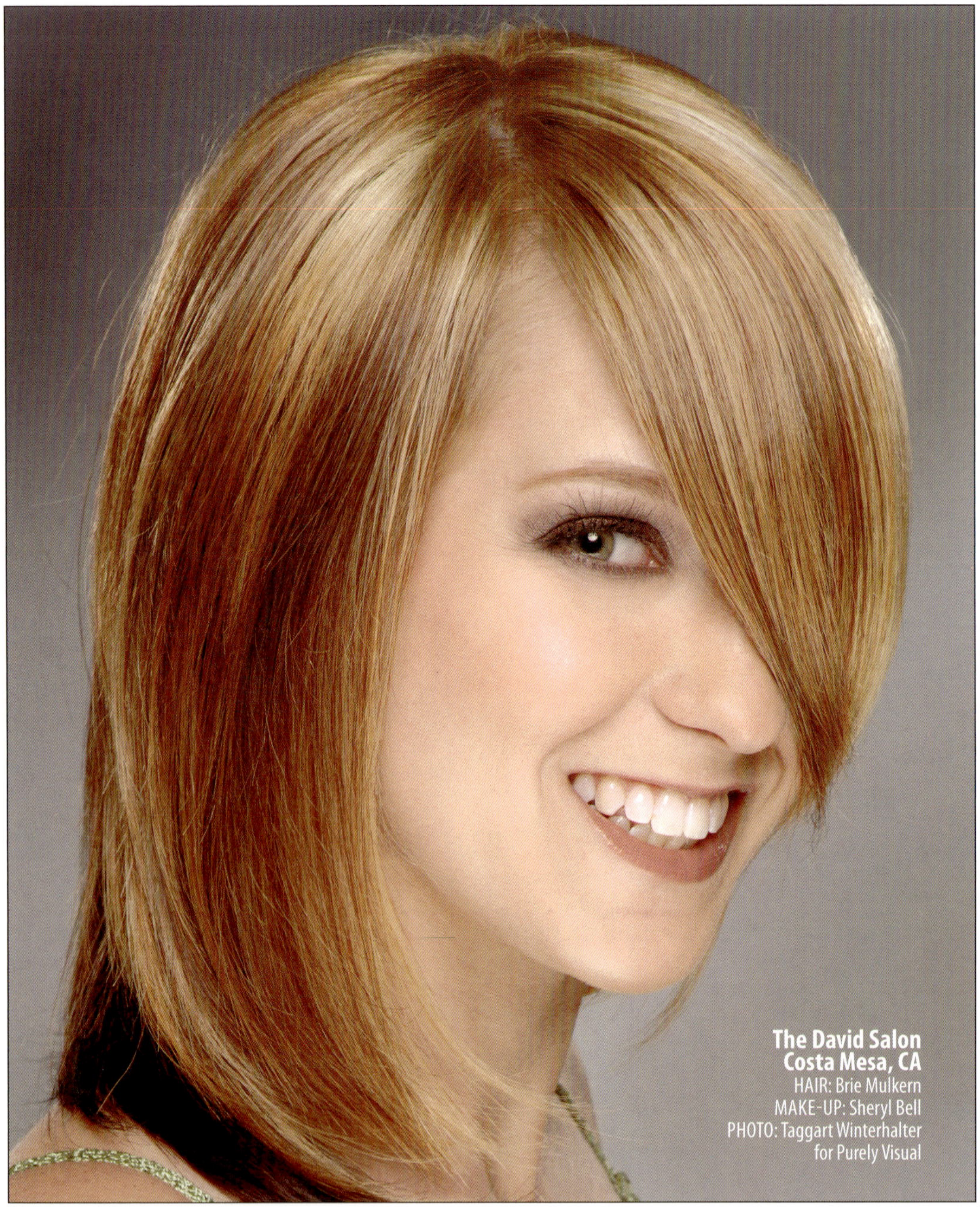

**The David Salon**
**Costa Mesa, CA**
HAIR: Brie Mulkern
MAKE-UP: Sheryl Bell
PHOTO: Taggart Winterhalter
for Purely Visual

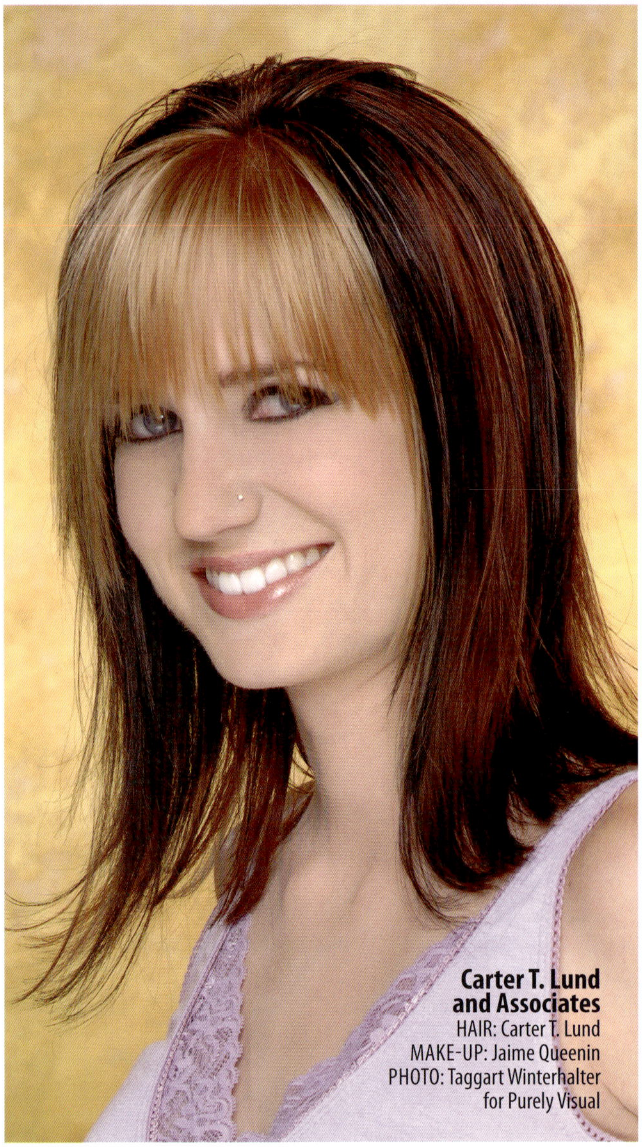

**Carter T. Lund**
**and Associates**
HAIR: Carter T. Lund
MAKE-UP: Jaime Queenin
PHOTO: Taggart Winterhalter
for Purely Visual

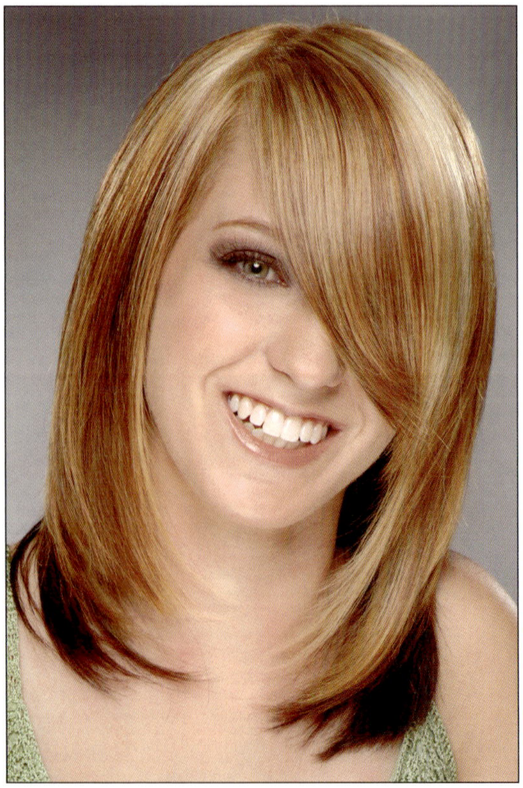

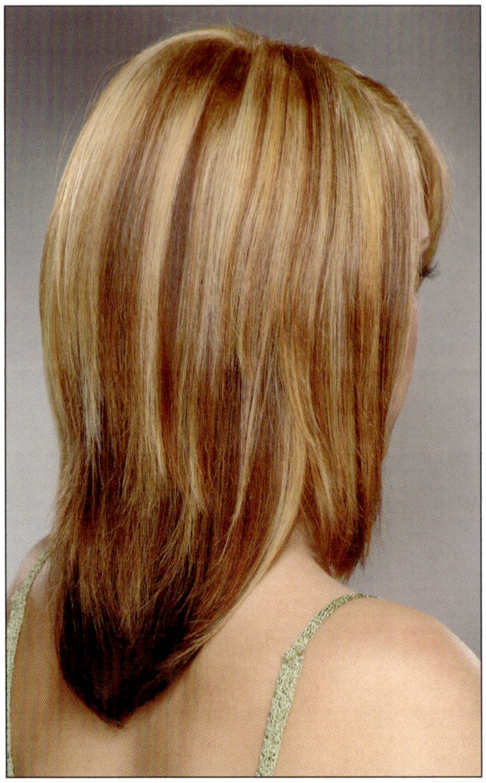

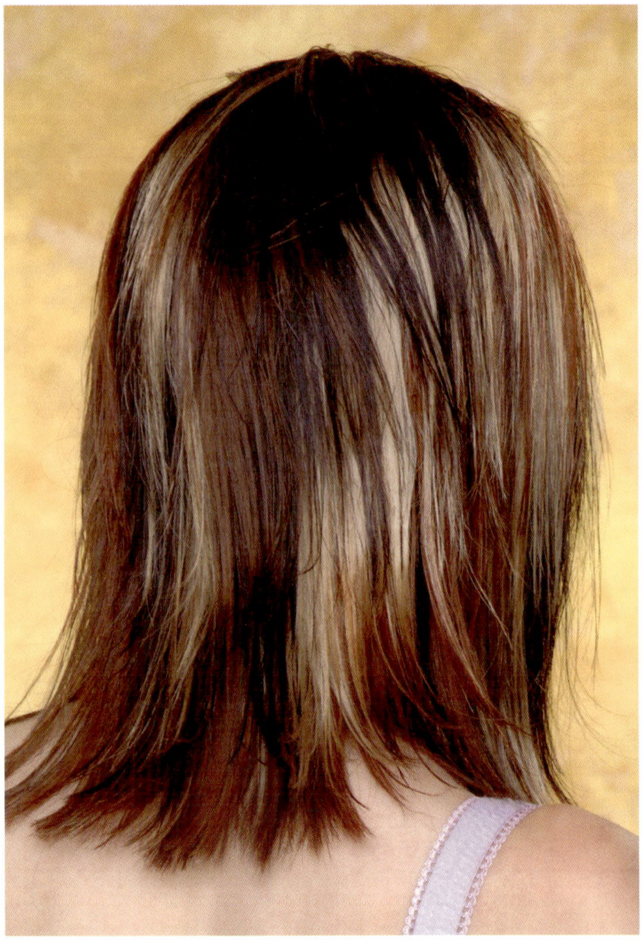

**DiaDema Hair Fashion**
HAIR: DiaDema
MAKE-UP: 20100 Milano Make-up
PHOTO: Stefano Bidini

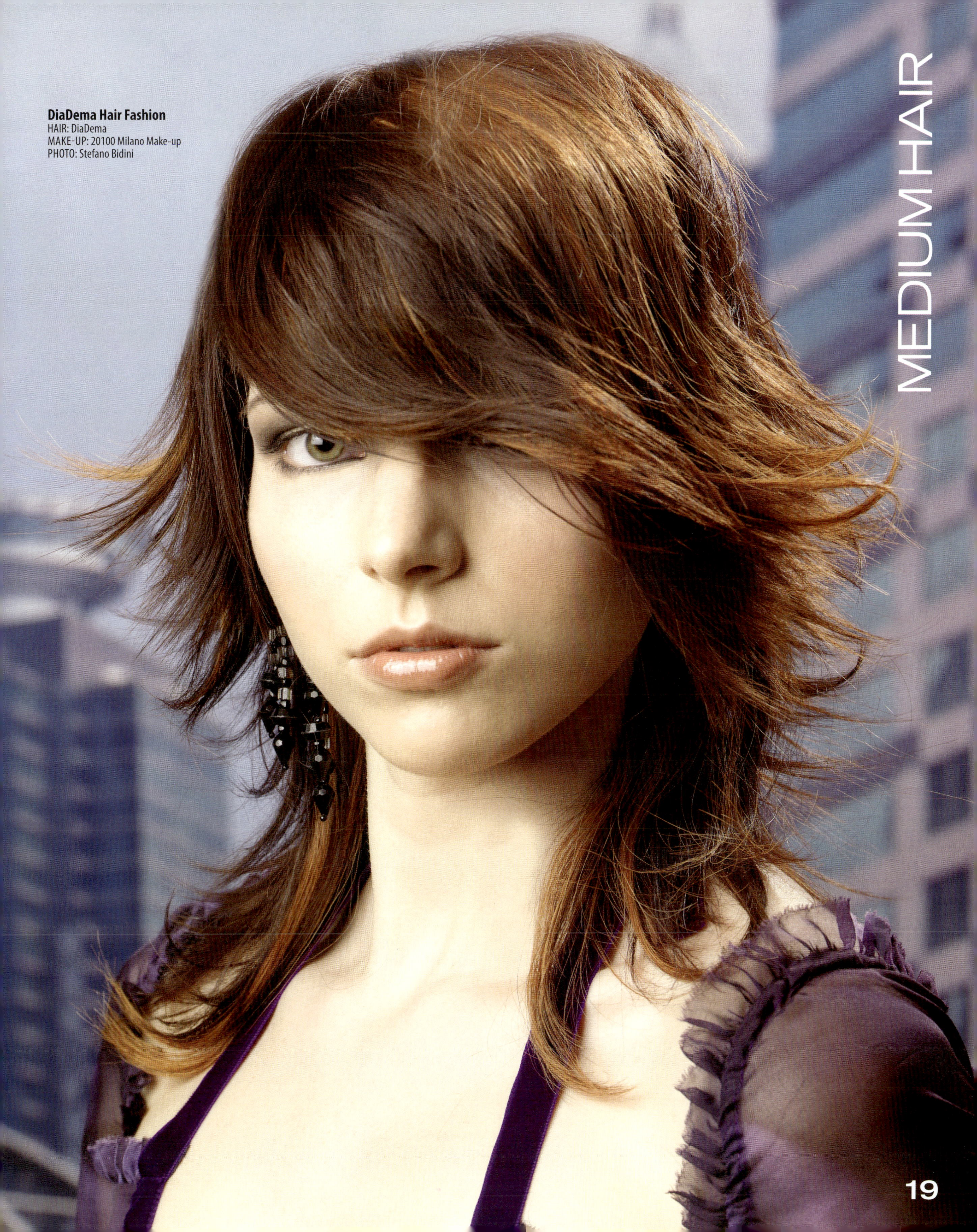

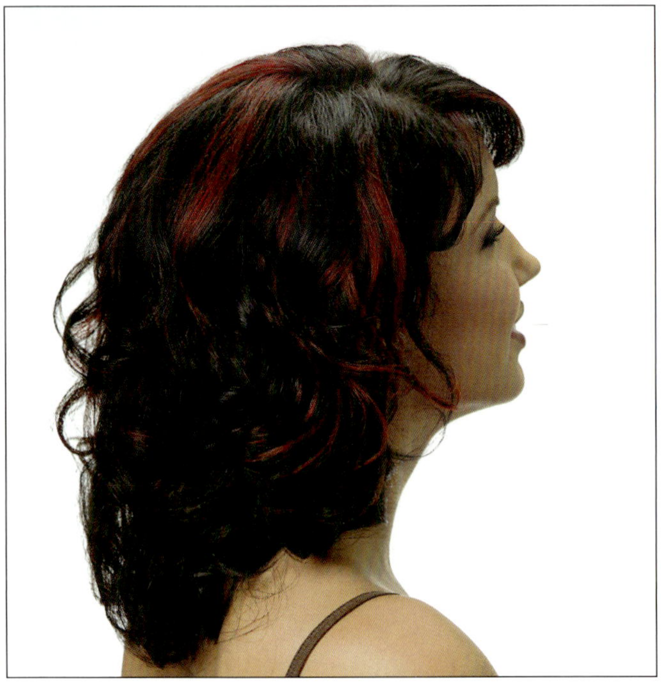

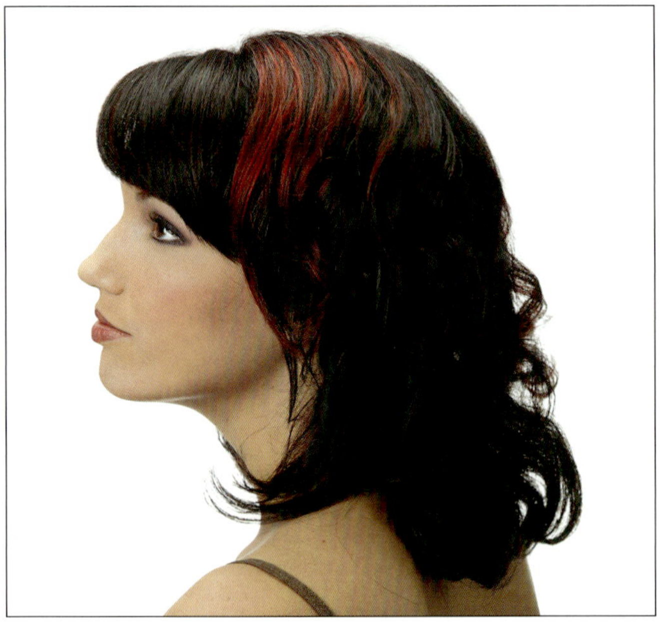

**Changes Hairstyling**
HAIR: Gil Trautman
MAKE-UP: Gil Trautman
PHOTO: Fred Havens

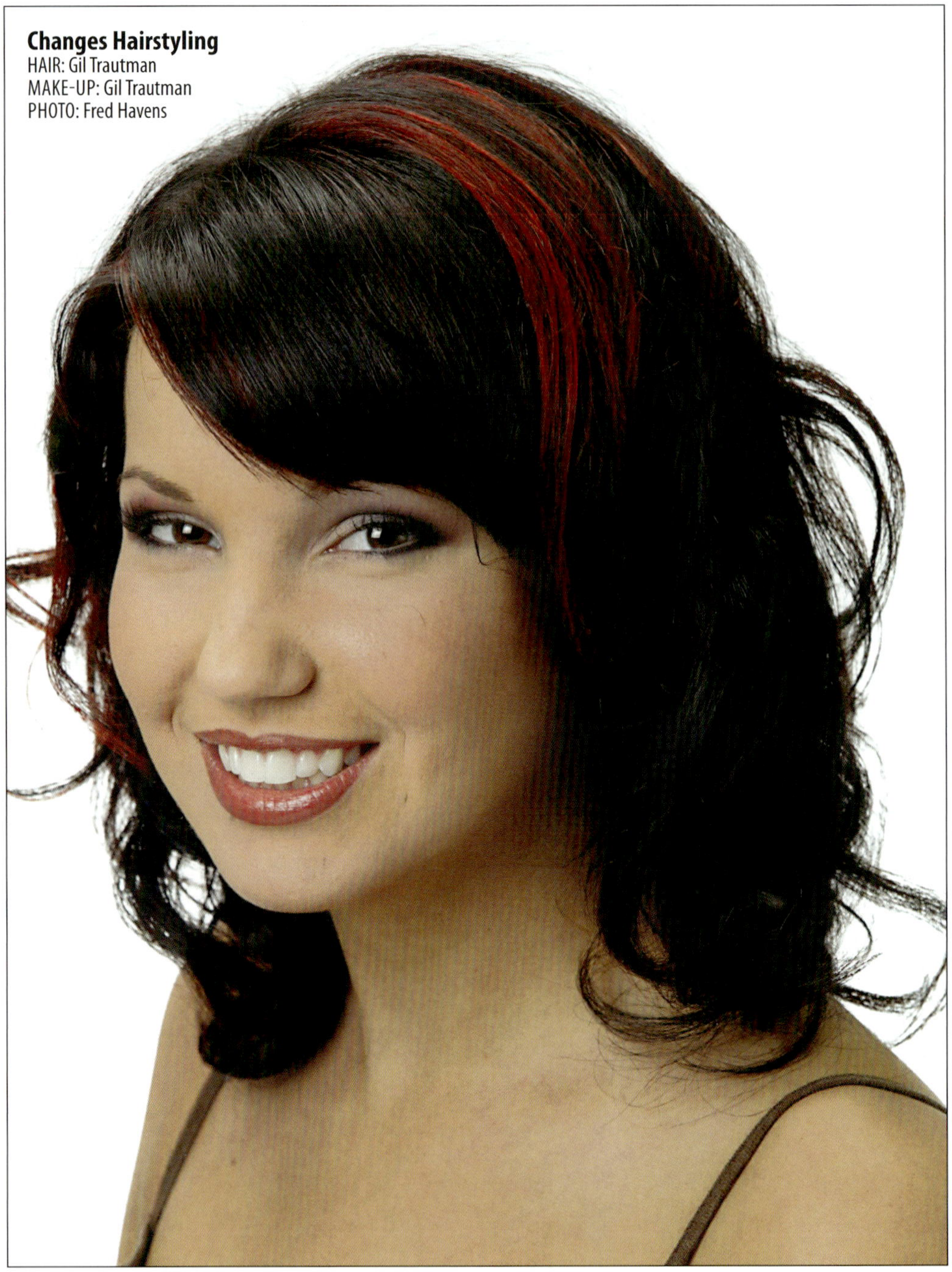

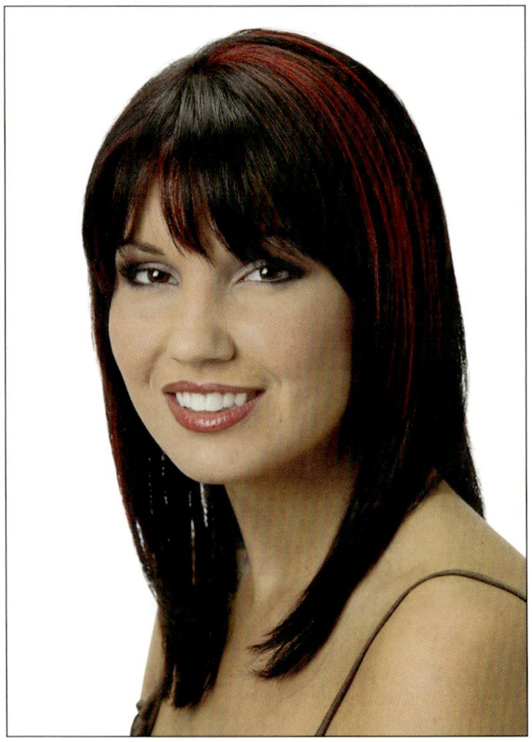

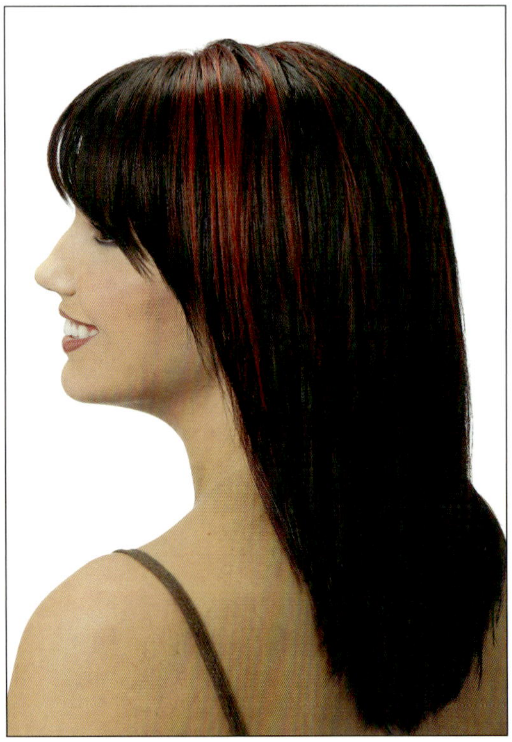

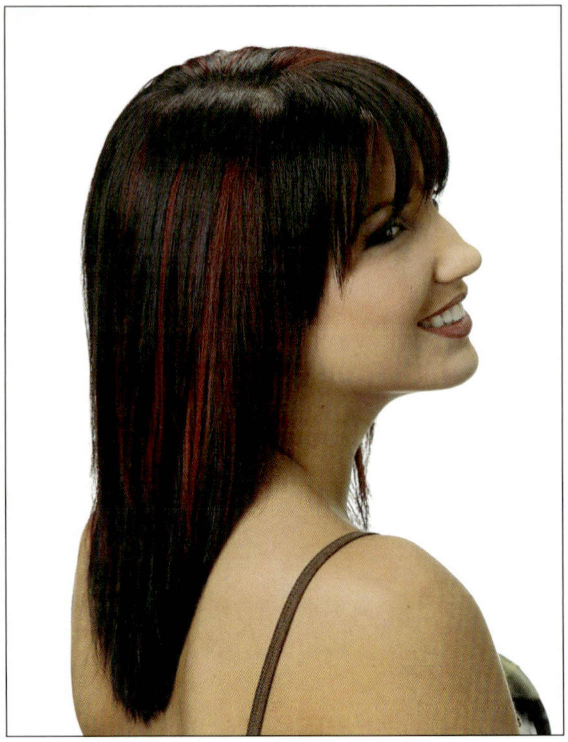

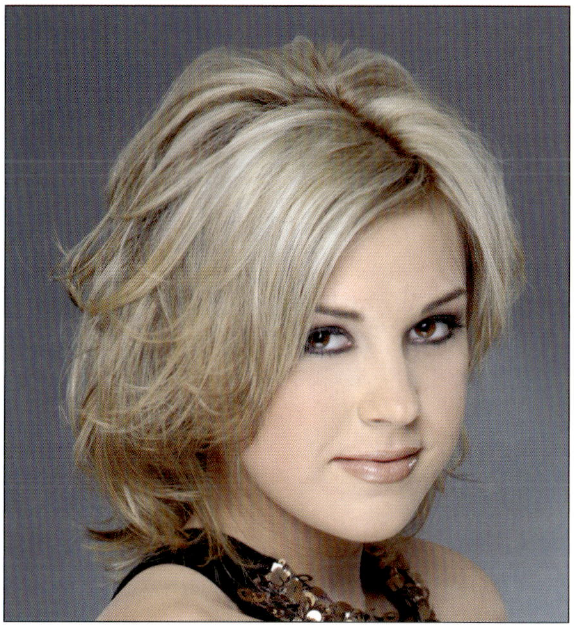

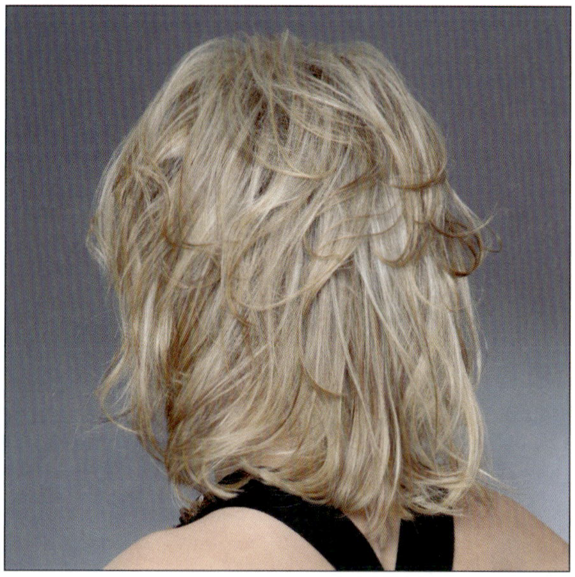

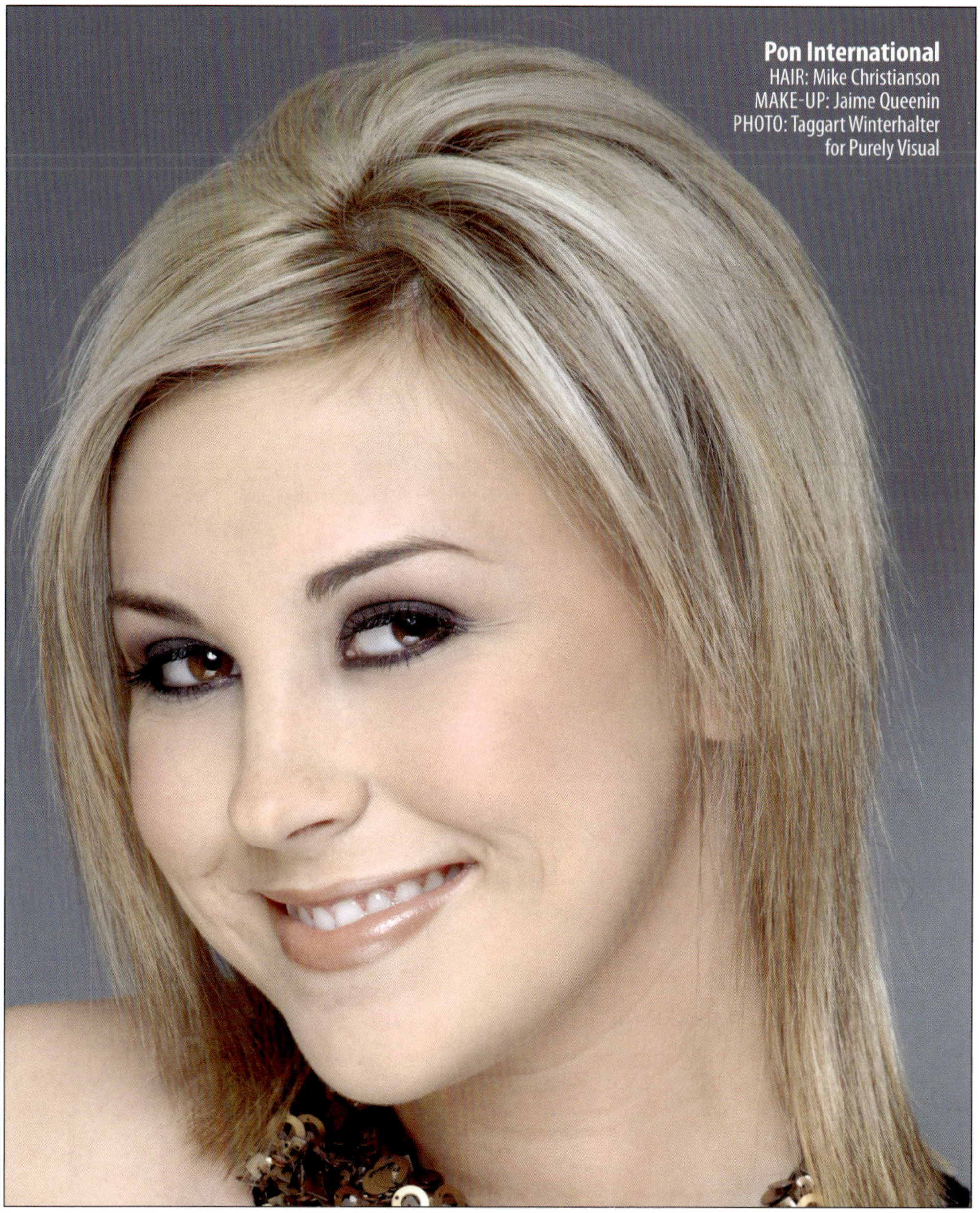

**Pon International**
HAIR: Mike Christianson
MAKE-UP: Jaime Queenin
PHOTO: Taggart Winterhalter
for Purely Visual

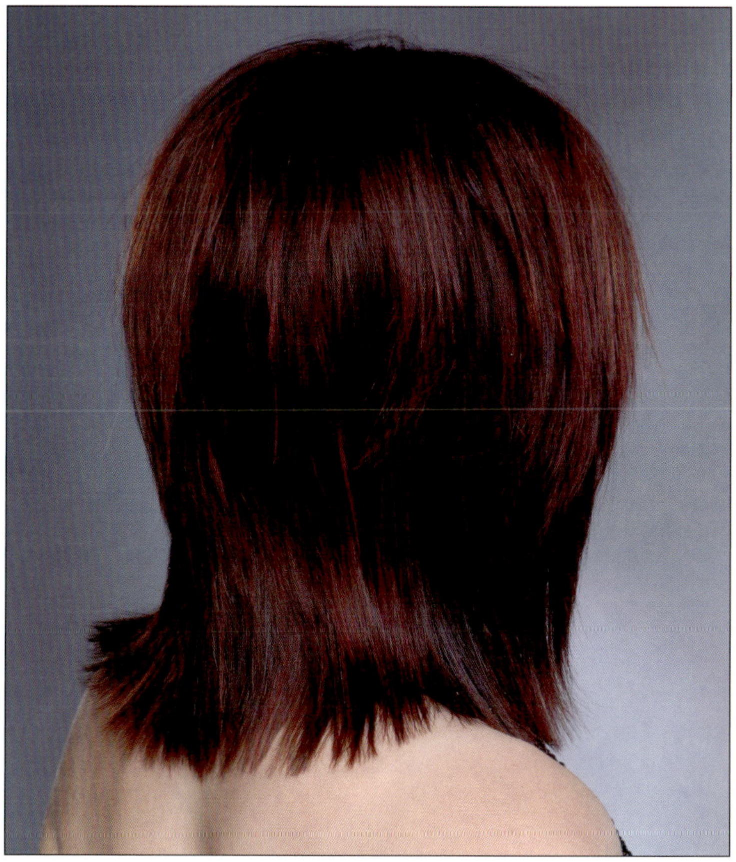

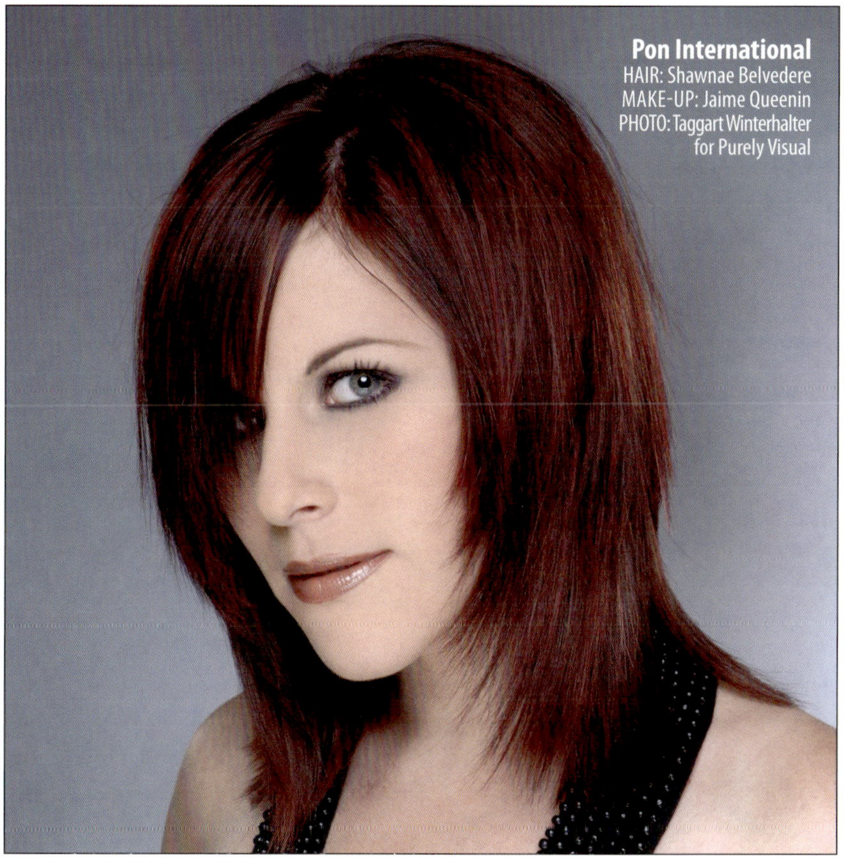

**Pon International**
HAIR: Shawnae Belvedere
MAKE-UP: Jaime Queenin
PHOTO: Taggart Winterhalter
for Purely Visual

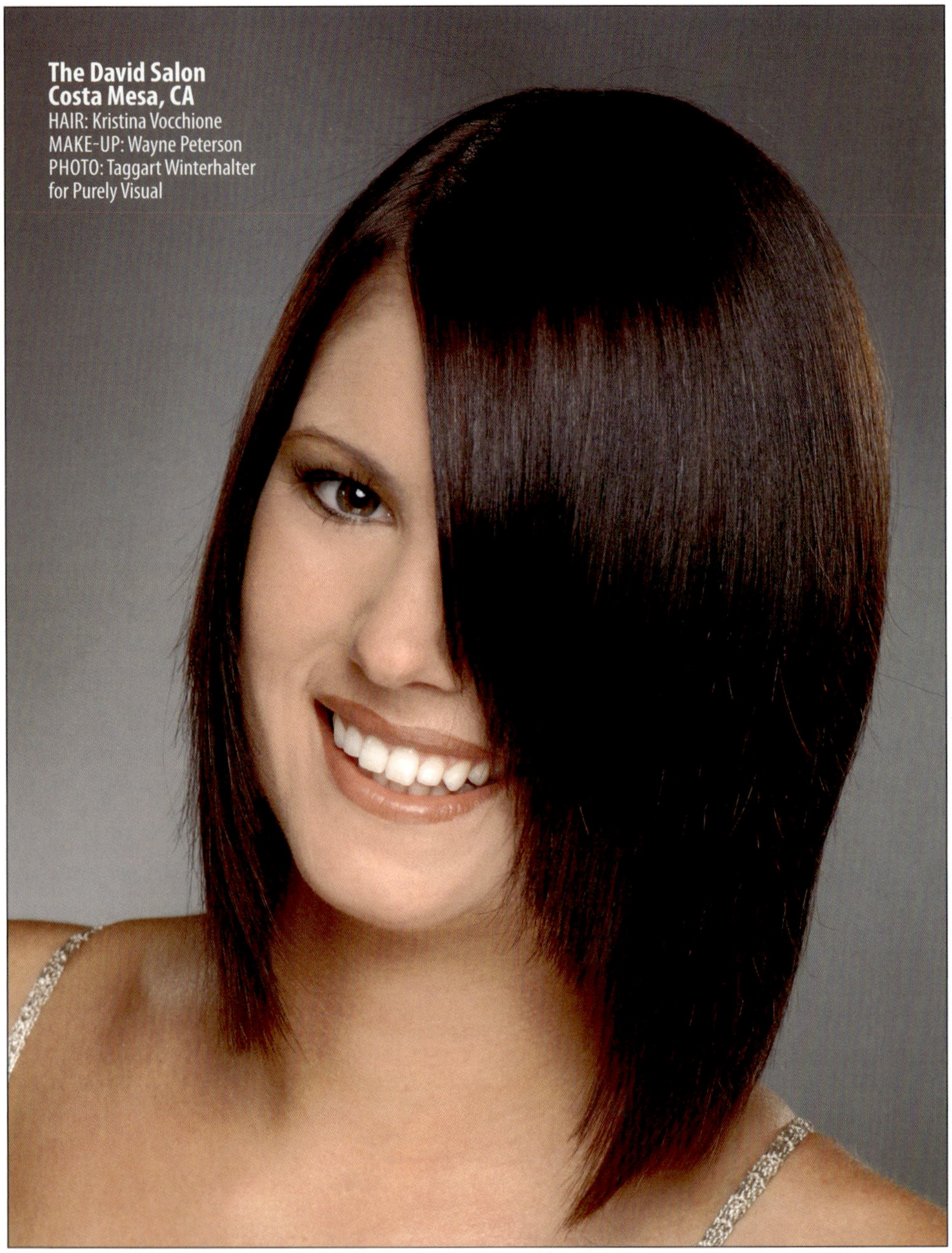

**The David Salon**
**Costa Mesa, CA**
HAIR: Kristina Vocchione
MAKE-UP: Wayne Peterson
PHOTO: Taggart Winterhalter for Purely Visual

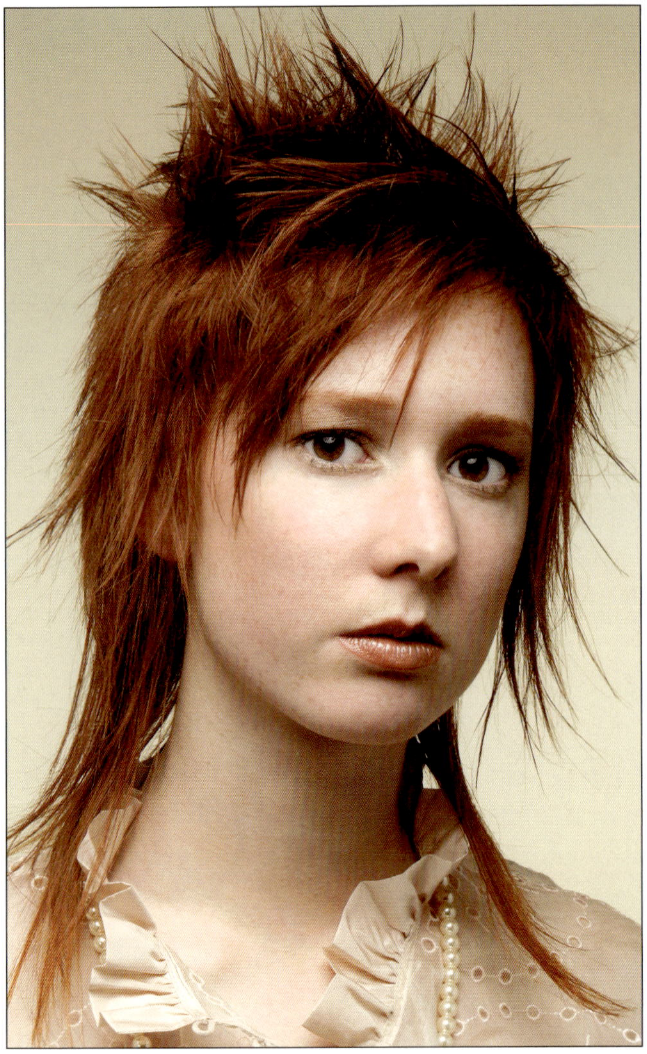

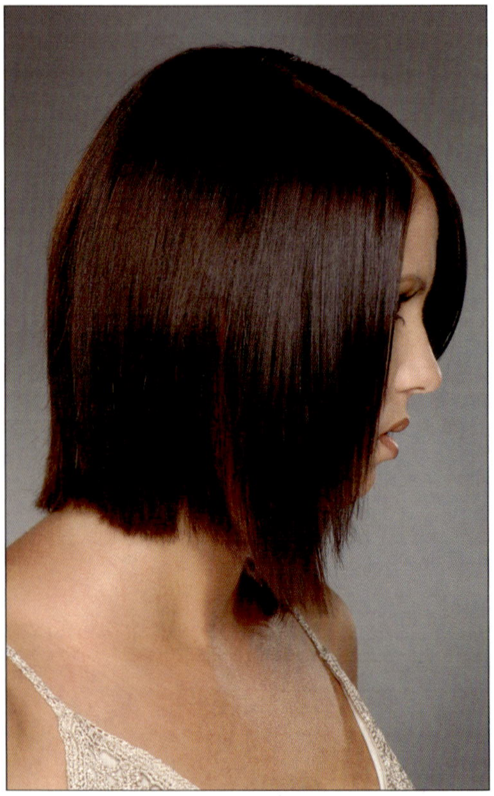

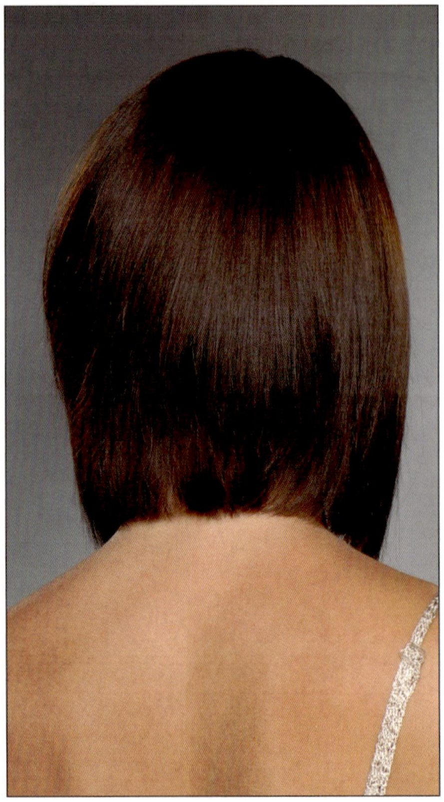

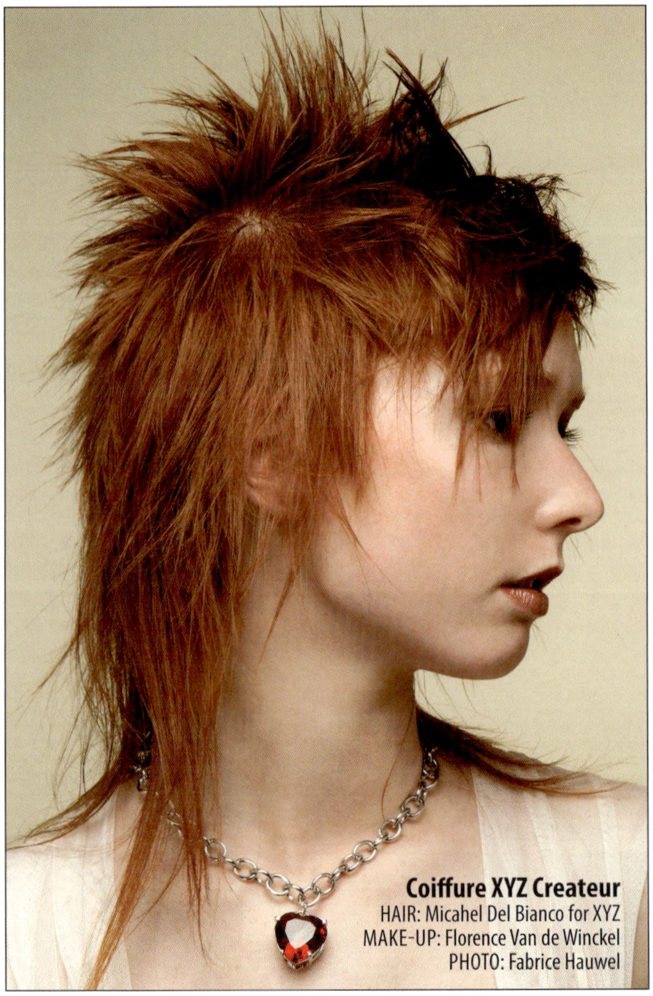

**Coiffure XYZ Createur**
HAIR: Micahel Del Bianco for XYZ
MAKE-UP: Florence Van de Winckel
PHOTO: Fabrice Hauwel

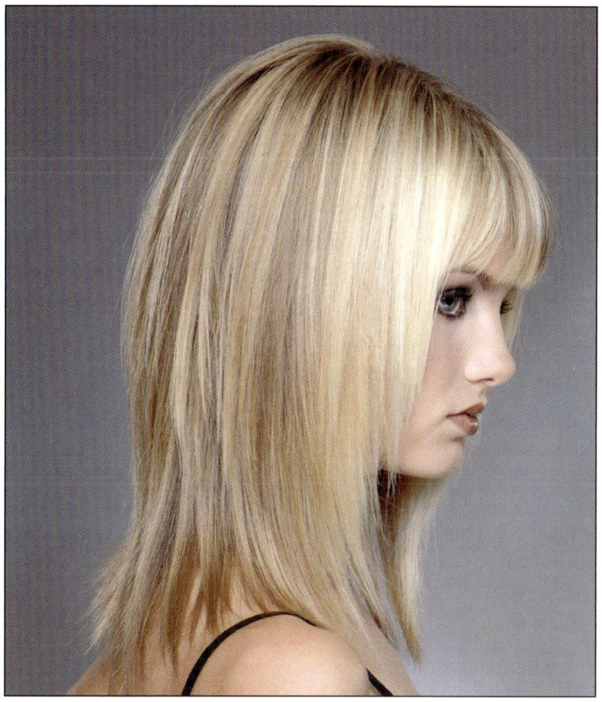

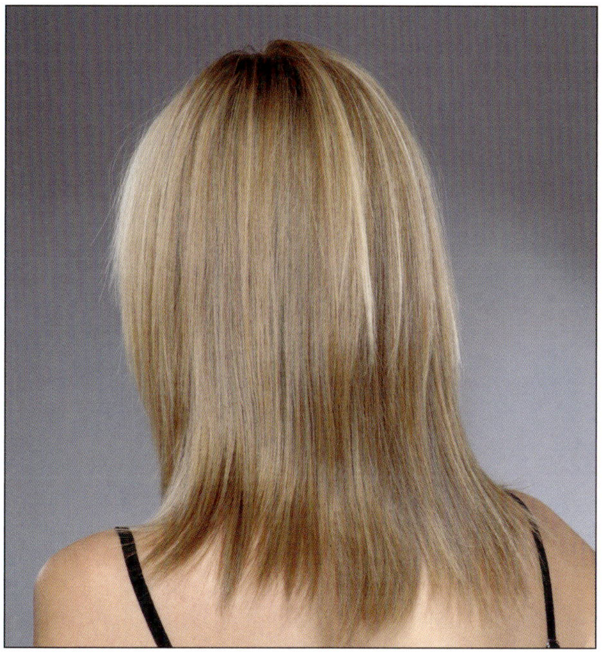

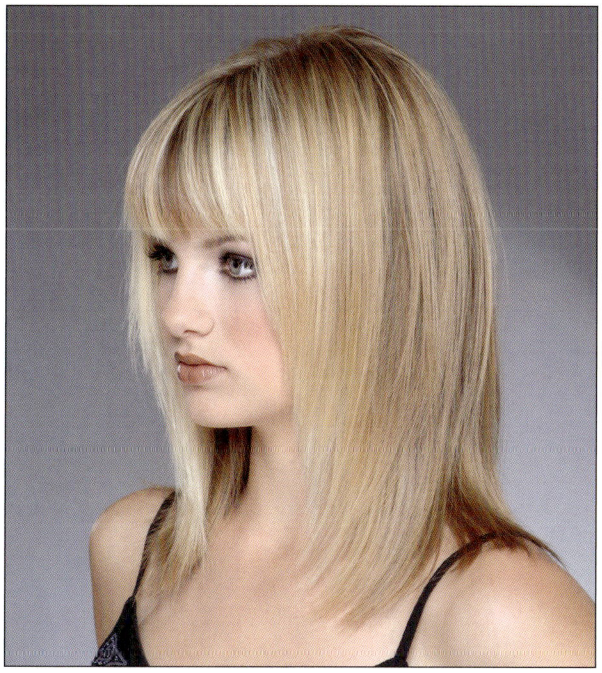

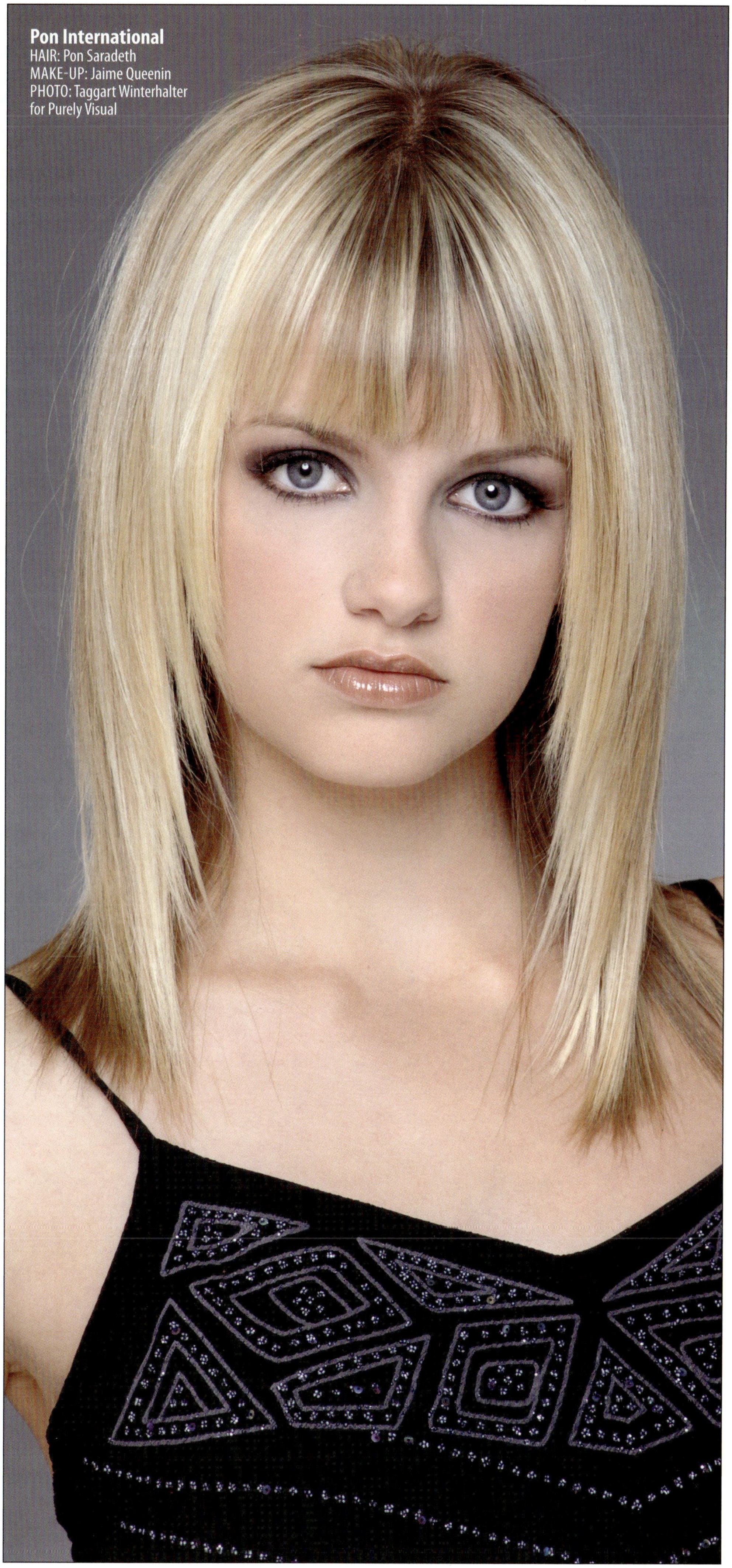

**Pon International**
HAIR: Pon Saradeth
MAKE-UP: Jaime Queenin
PHOTO: Taggart Winterhalter for Purely Visual

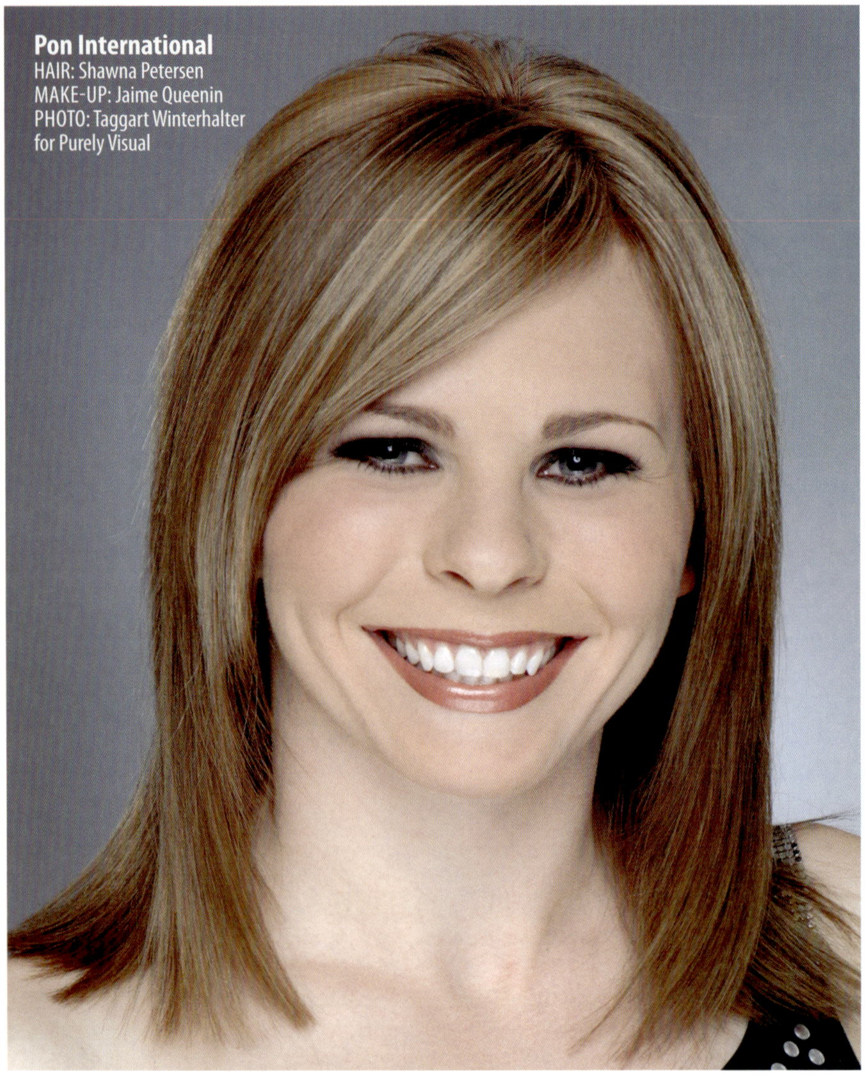
**Pon International**
HAIR: Shawna Petersen
MAKE-UP: Jaime Queenin
PHOTO: Taggart Winterhalter
for Purely Visual

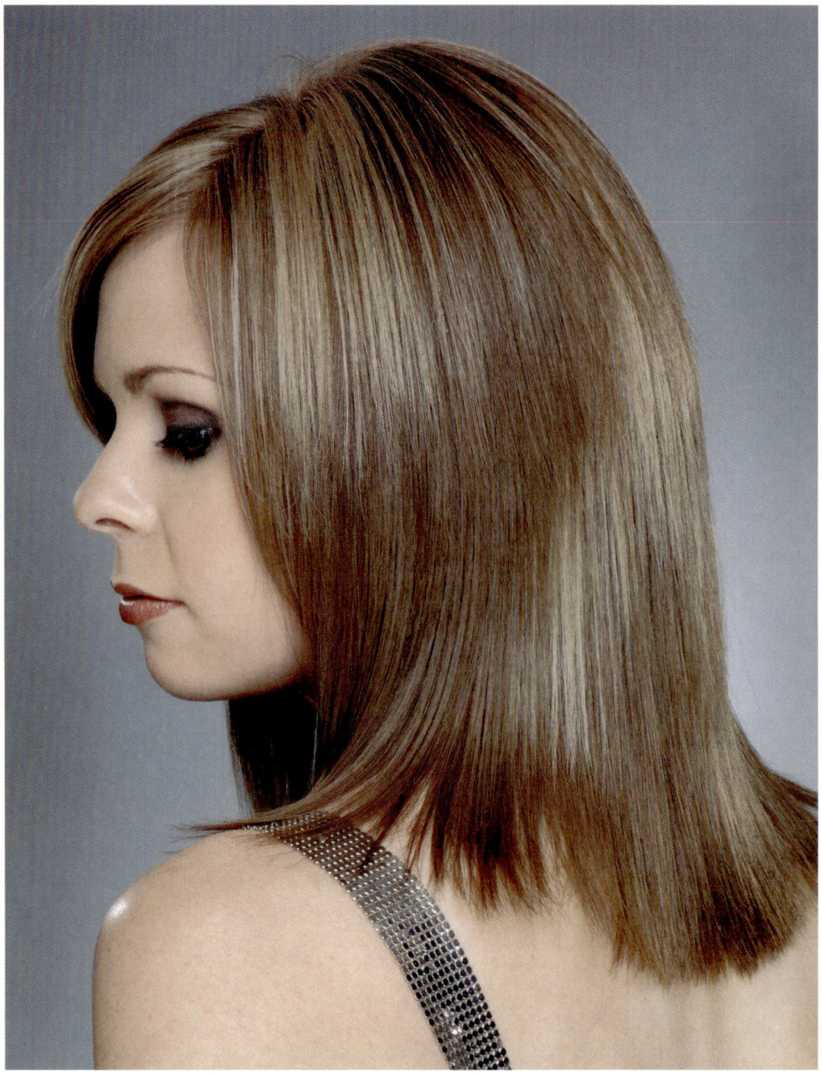

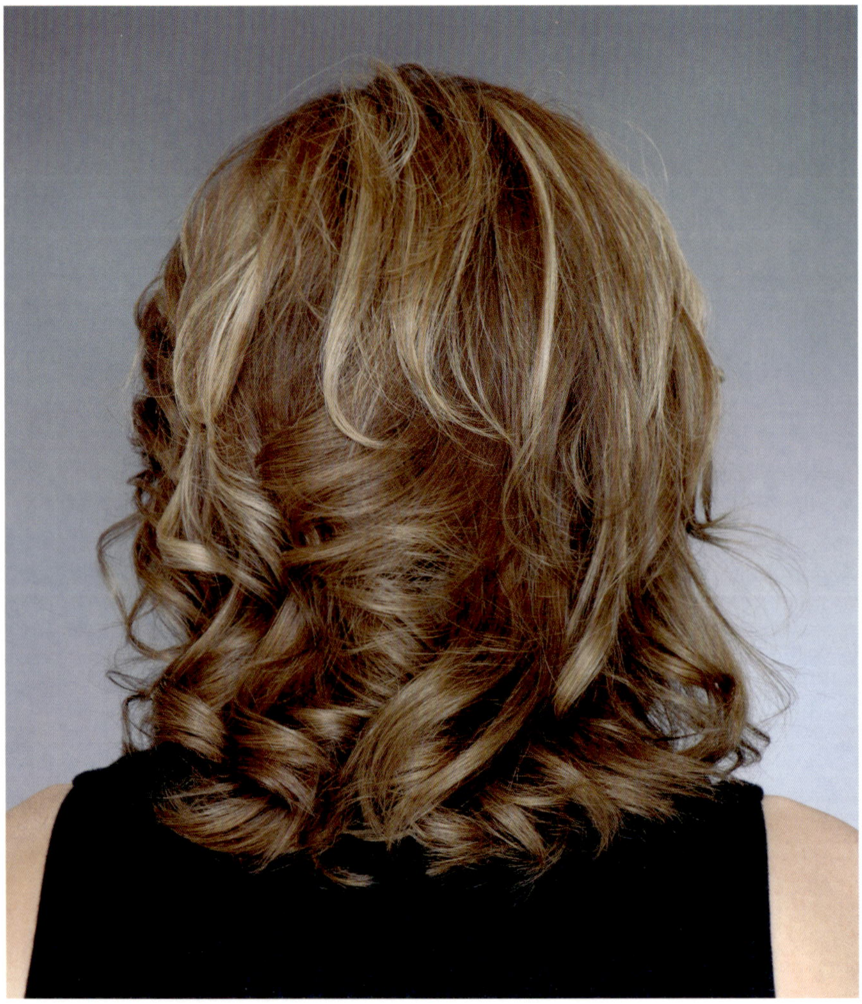

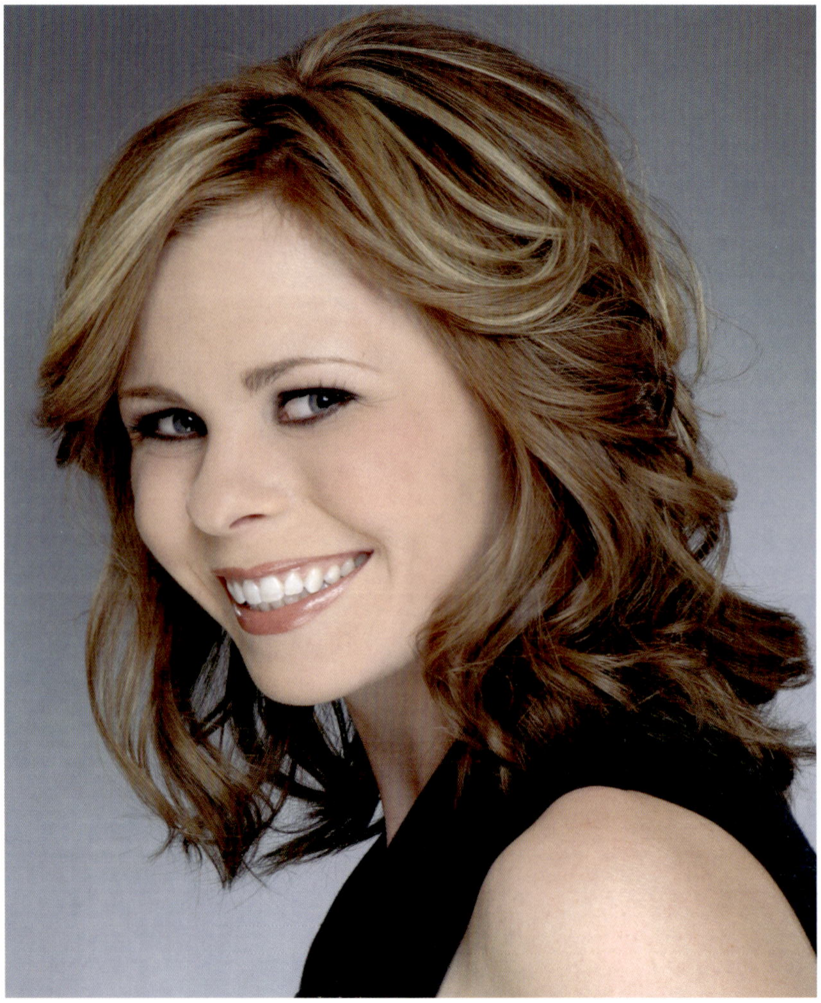

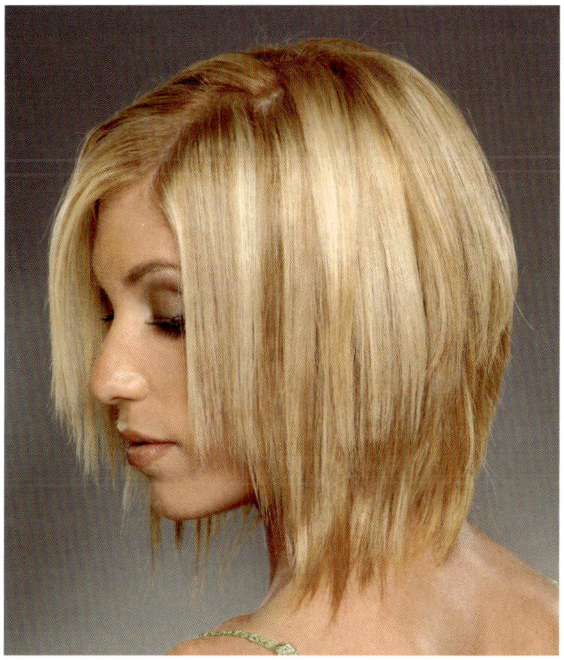

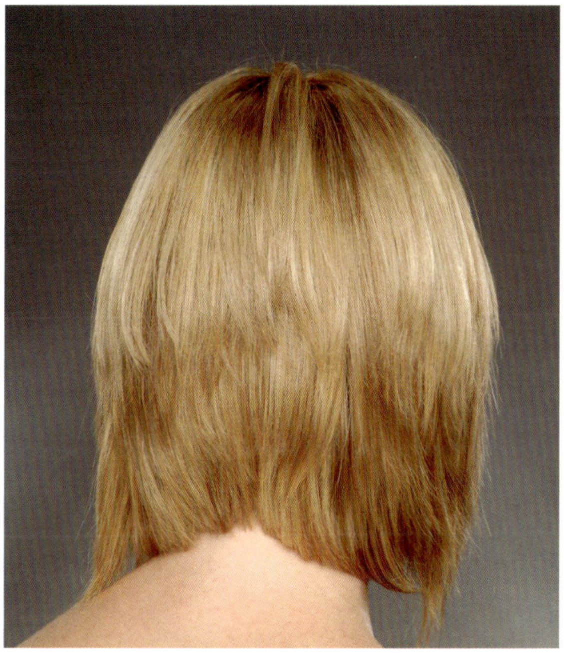

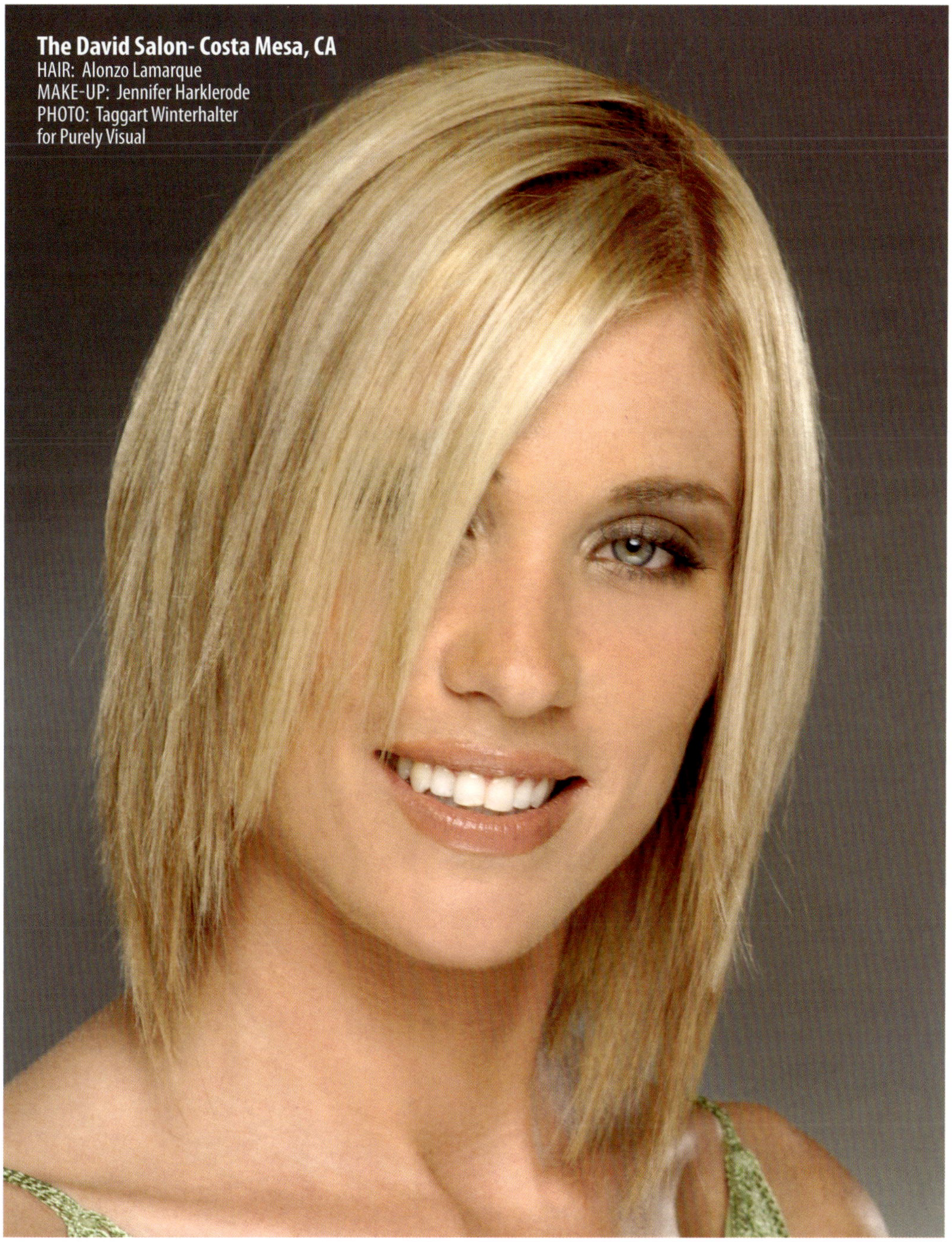

**The David Salon- Costa Mesa, CA**
HAIR: Alonzo Lamarque
MAKE-UP: Jennifer Harklerode
PHOTO: Taggart Winterhalter
for Purely Visual

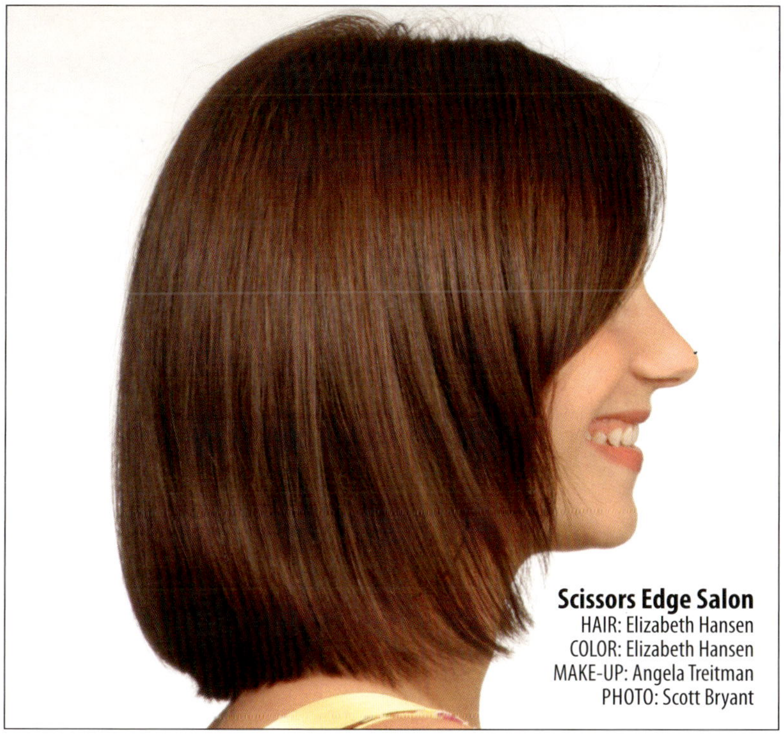

**Scissors Edge Salon**
HAIR: Elizabeth Hansen
COLOR: Elizabeth Hansen
MAKE-UP: Angela Treitman
PHOTO: Scott Bryant

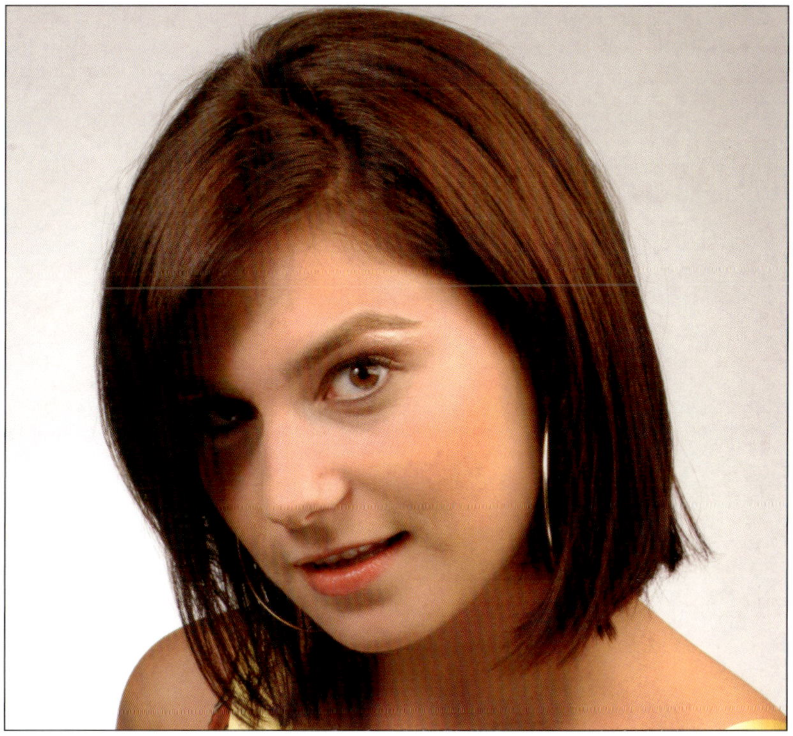

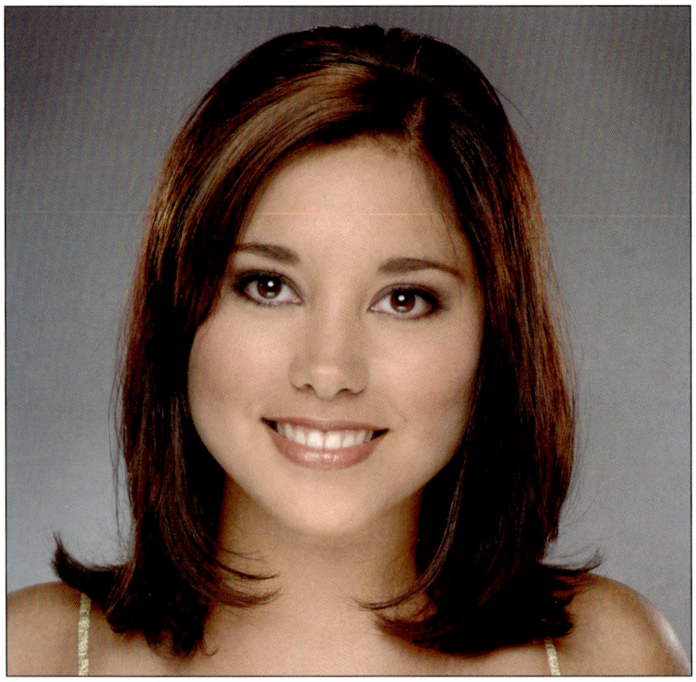

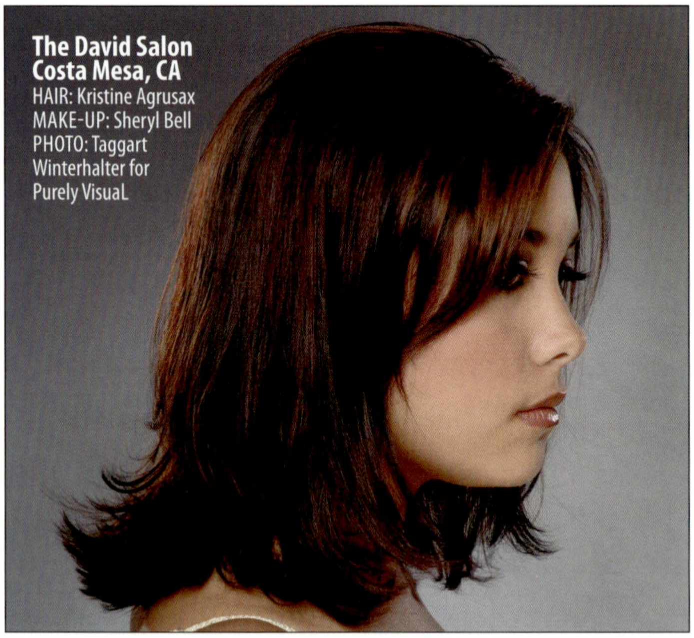

**The David Salon**
**Costa Mesa, CA**
HAIR: Kristine Agrusax
MAKE-UP: Sheryl Bell
PHOTO: Taggart Winterhalter for Purely VisuaL

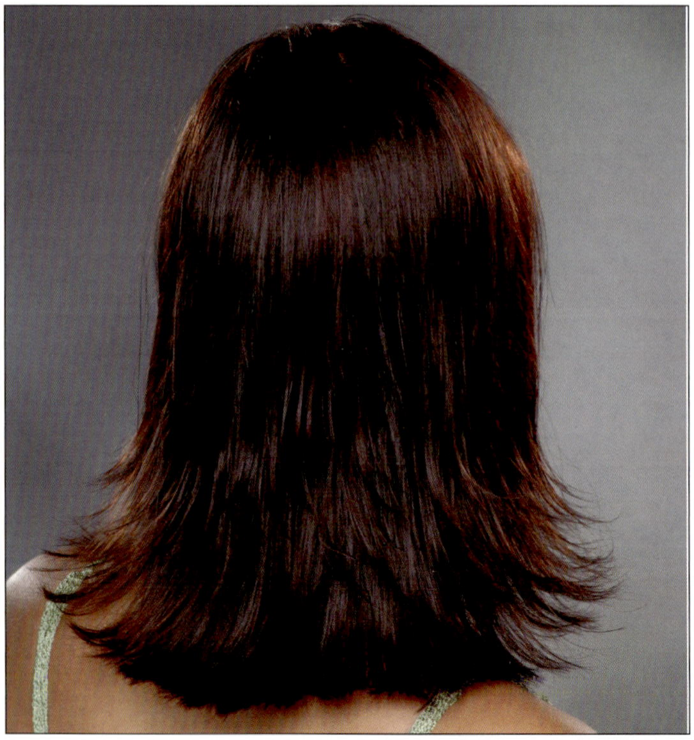

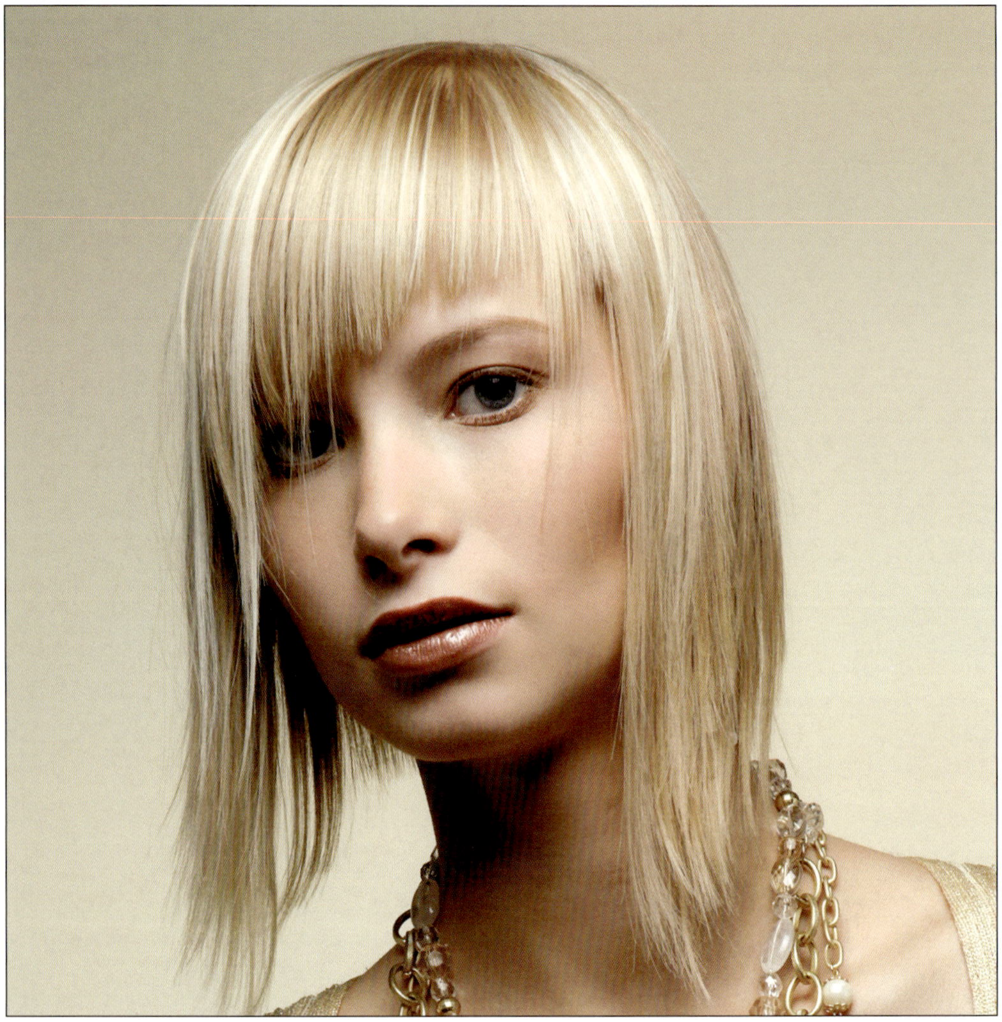

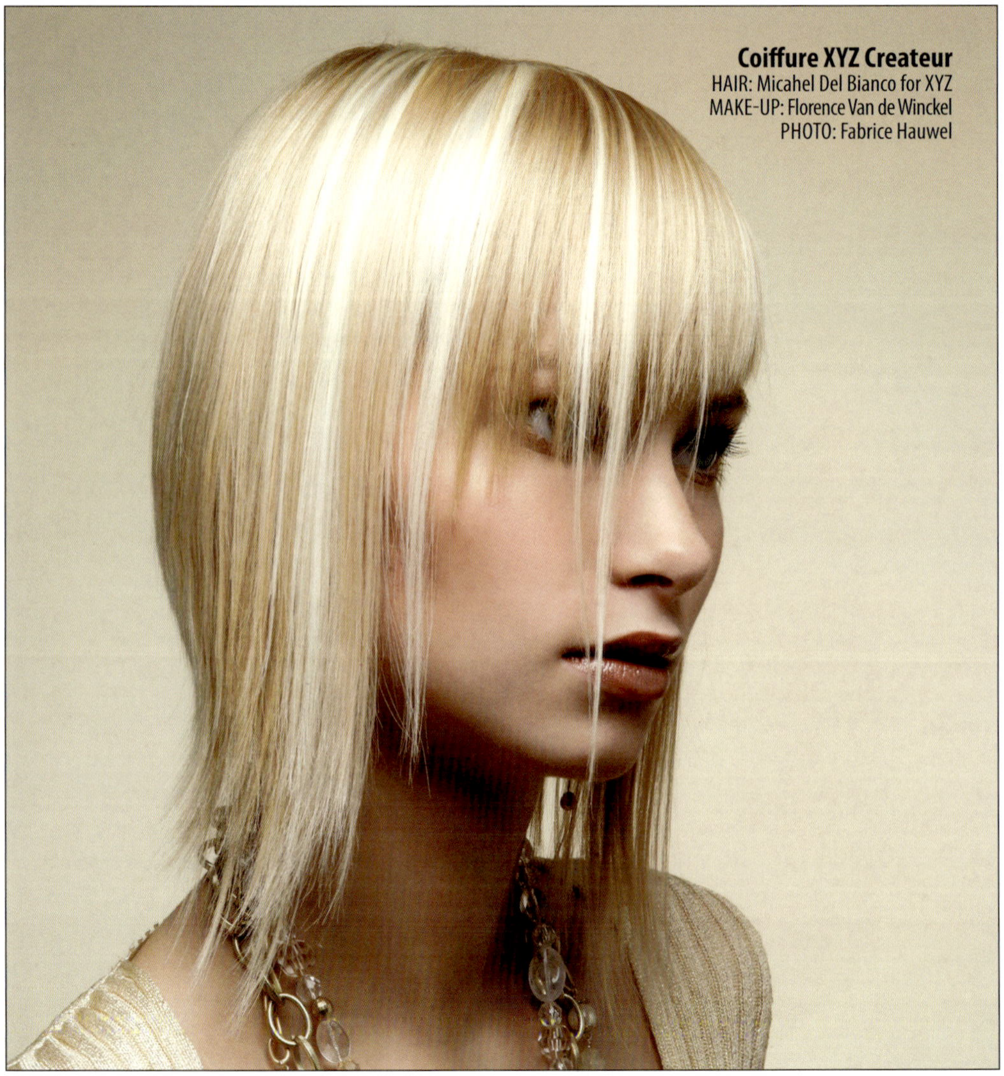

**Coiffure XYZ Createur**
HAIR: Micahel Del Bianco for XYZ
MAKE-UP: Florence Van de Winckel
PHOTO: Fabrice Hauwel

**Coiffure XYZ Createur**
HAIR: Micahel Del Bianco for XYZ
MAKE-UP: Florence Van de Winckel
PHOTO: Fabrice Hauwel



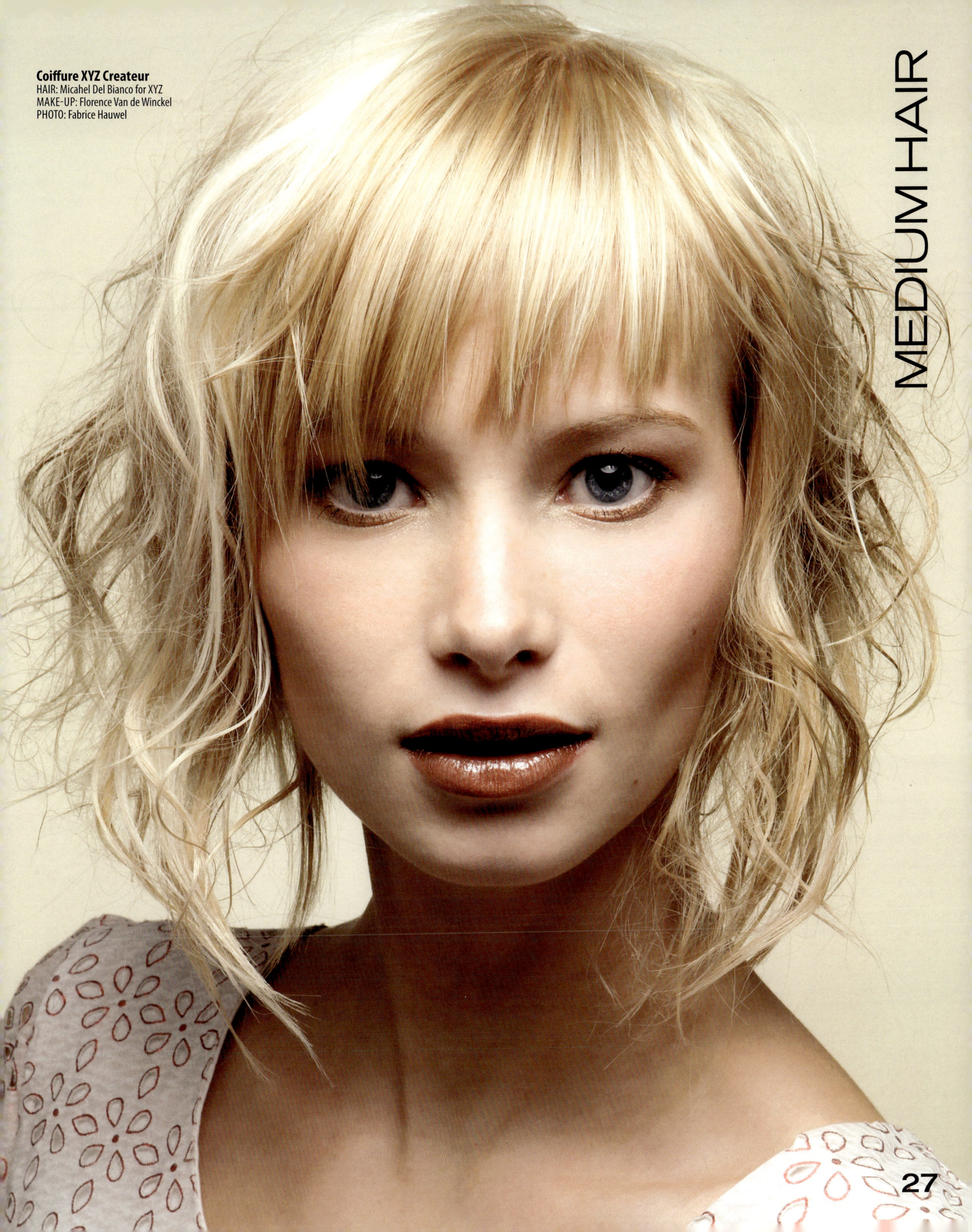

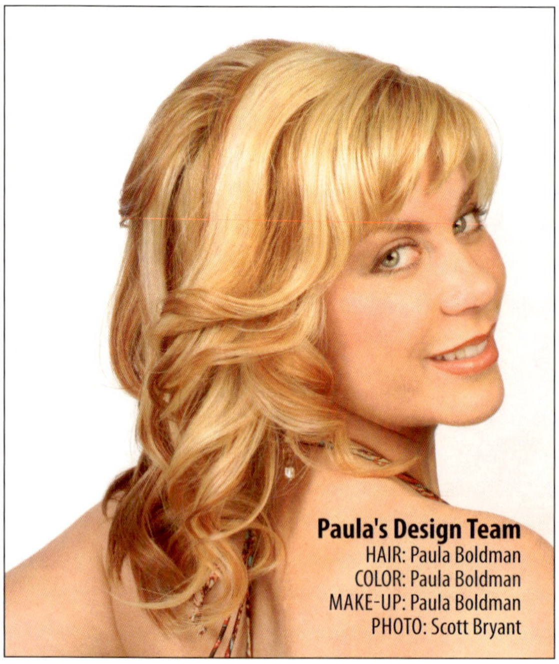

**Paula's Design Team**
HAIR: Paula Boldman
COLOR: Paula Boldman
MAKE-UP: Paula Boldman
PHOTO: Scott Bryant

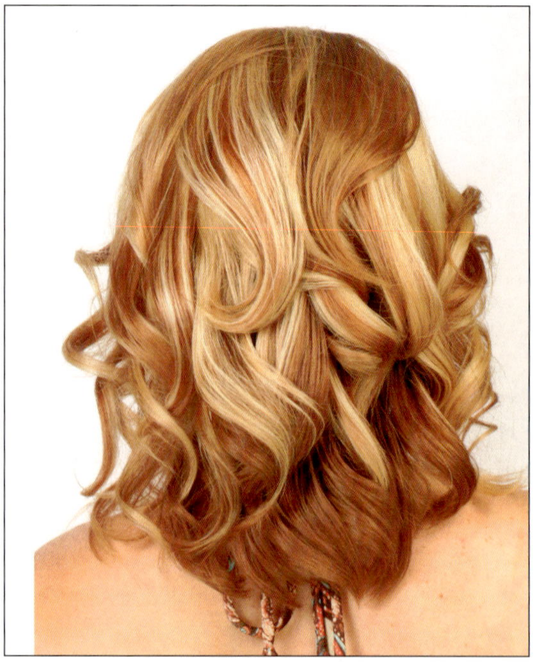

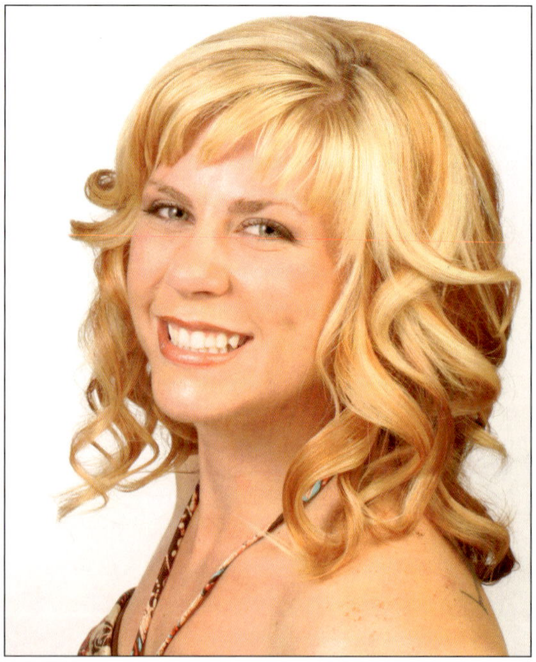

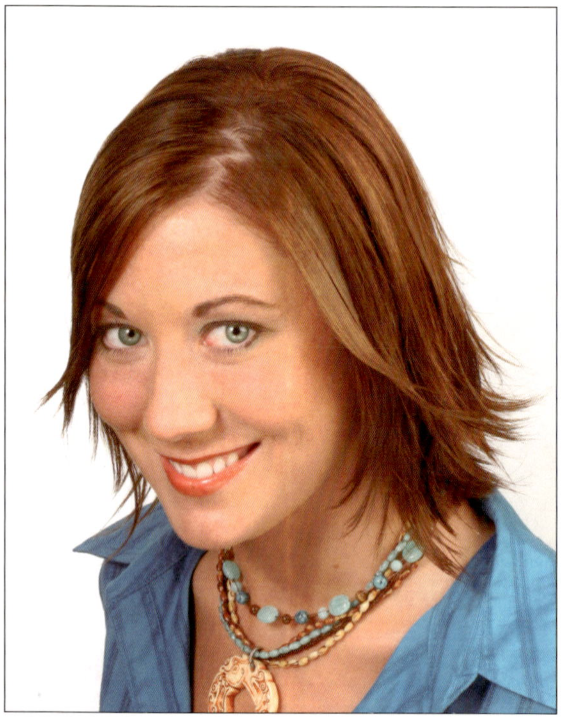

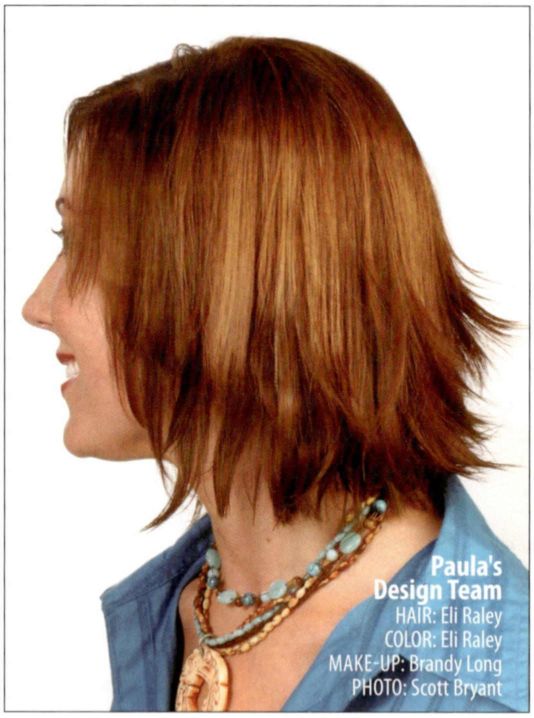

**Paula's Design Team**
HAIR: Eli Raley
COLOR: Eli Raley
MAKE-UP: Brandy Long
PHOTO: Scott Bryant

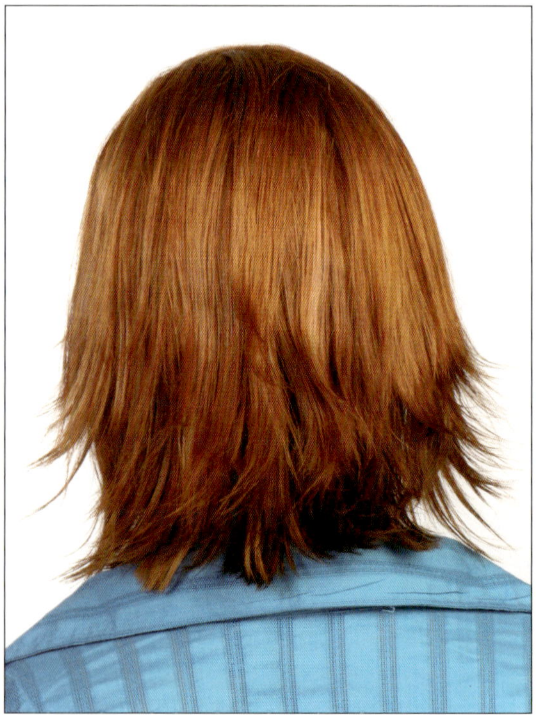

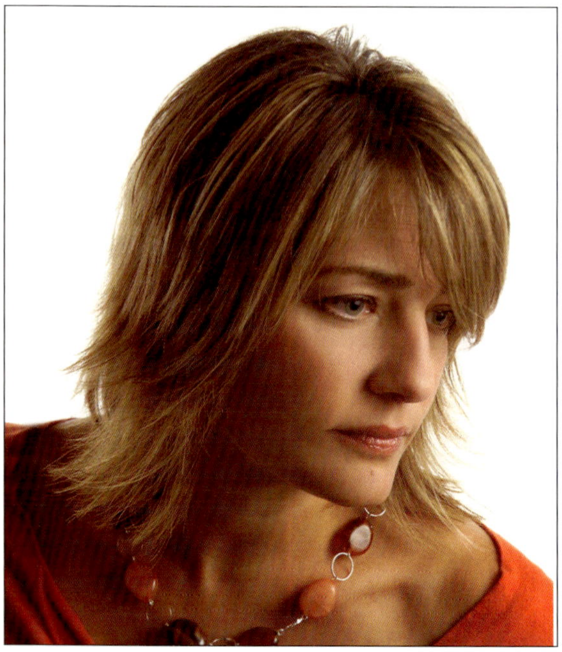

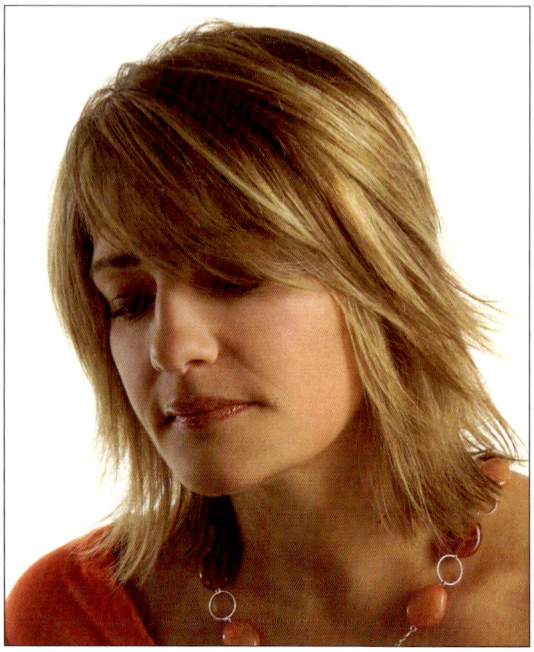

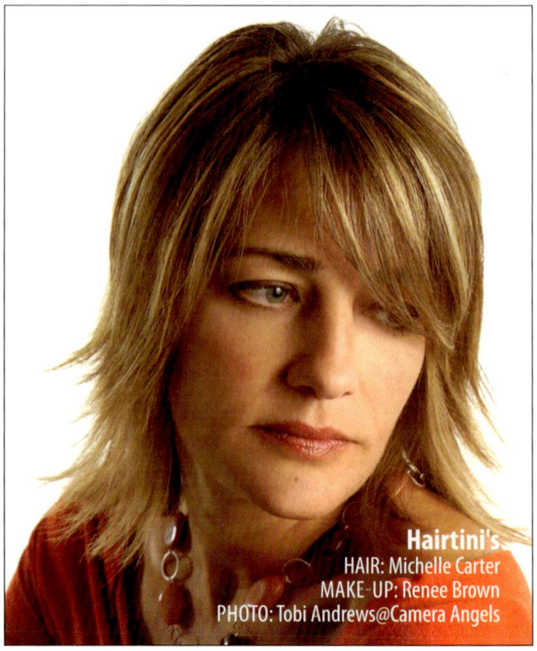

**Hairtini's**
HAIR: Michelle Carter
MAKE-UP: Renee Brown
PHOTO: Tobi Andrews@Camera Angels

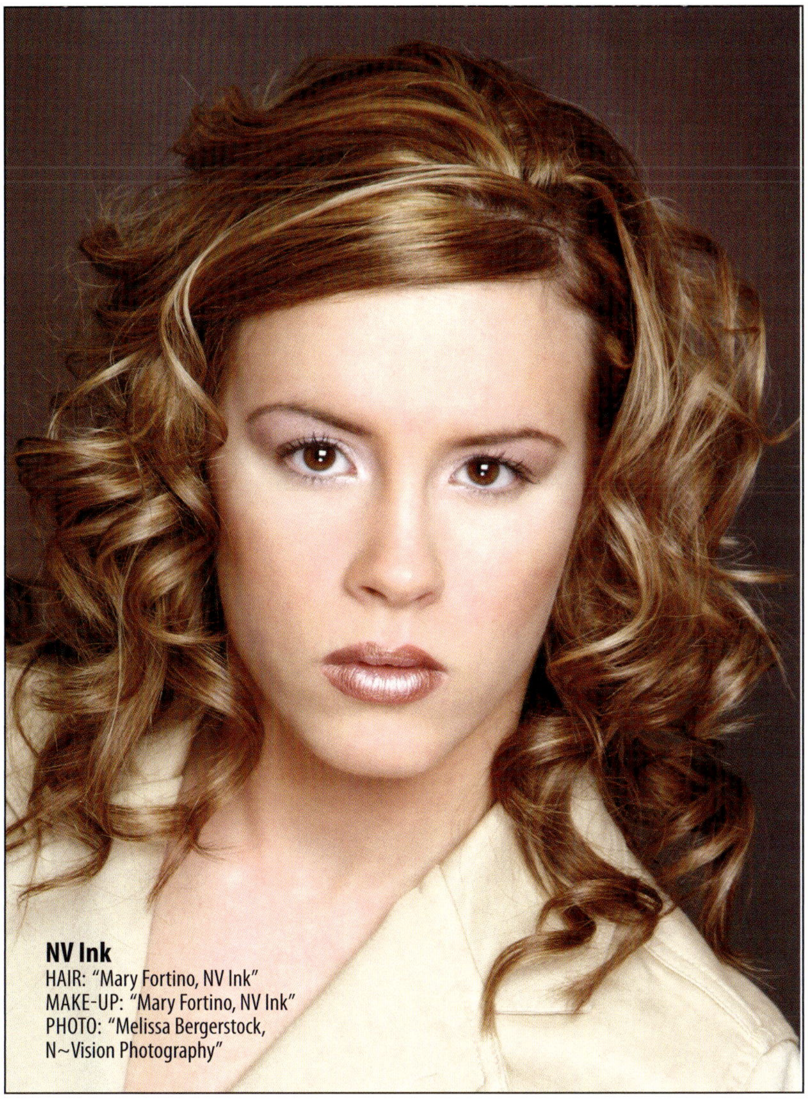

**NV Ink**
HAIR: "Mary Fortino, NV Ink"
MAKE-UP: "Mary Fortino, NV Ink"
PHOTO: "Melissa Bergerstock, N~Vision Photography"

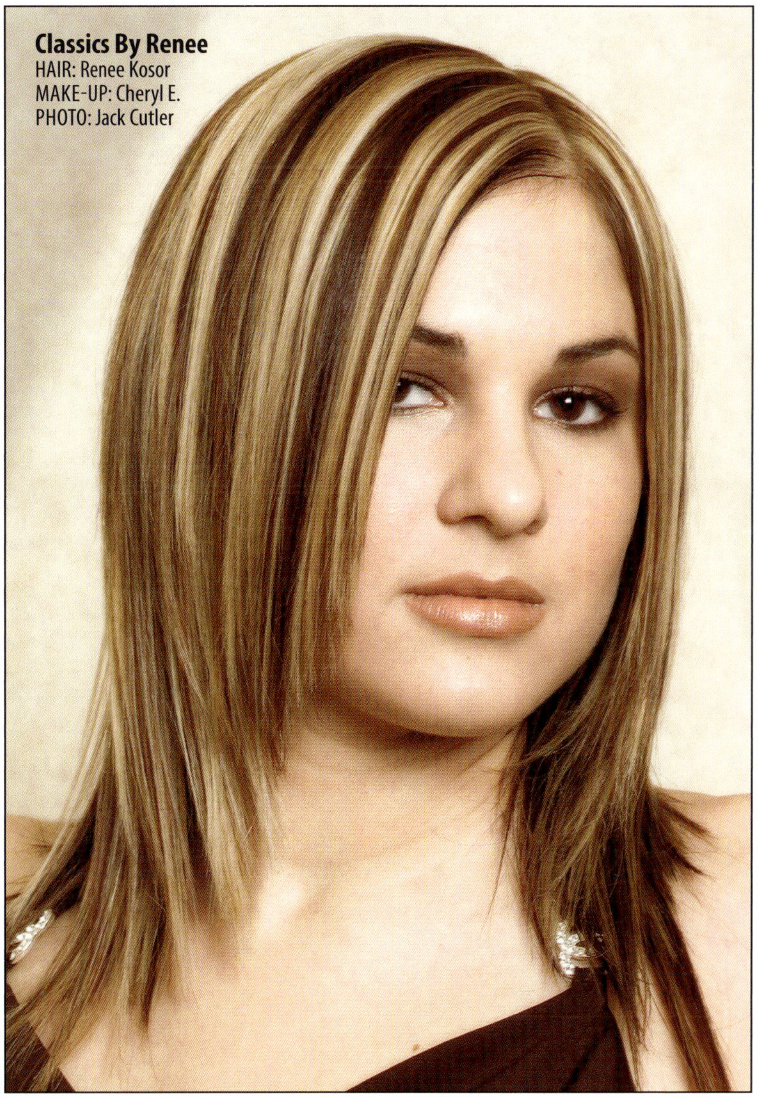

**Classics By Renee**
HAIR: Renee Kosor
MAKE-UP: Cheryl E.
PHOTO: Jack Cutler

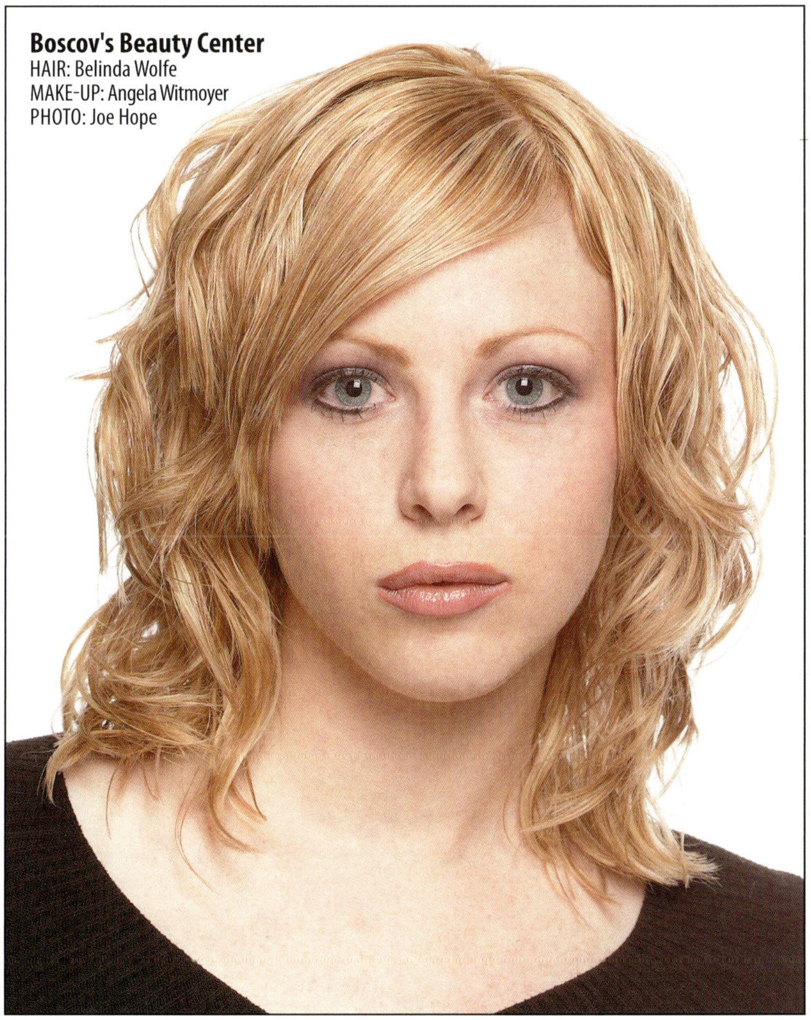

**Boscov's Beauty Center**
HAIR: Belinda Wolfe
MAKE-UP: Angela Witmoyer
PHOTO: Joe Hope

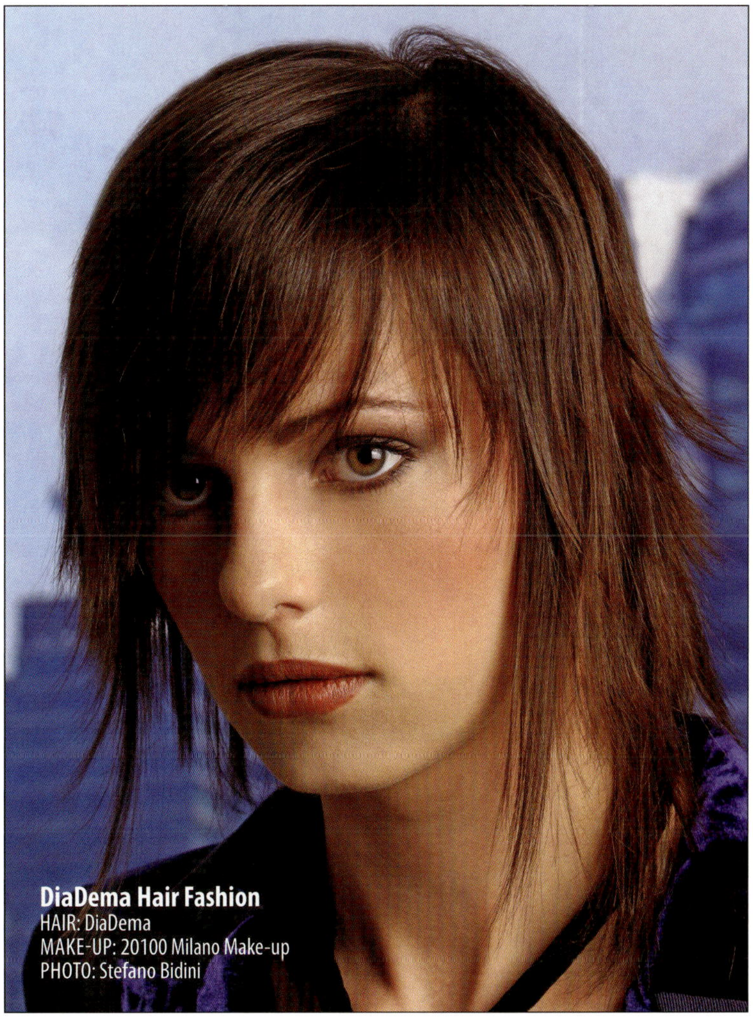

**DiaDema Hair Fashion**
HAIR: DiaDema
MAKE-UP: 20100 Milano Make-up
PHOTO: Stefano Bidini

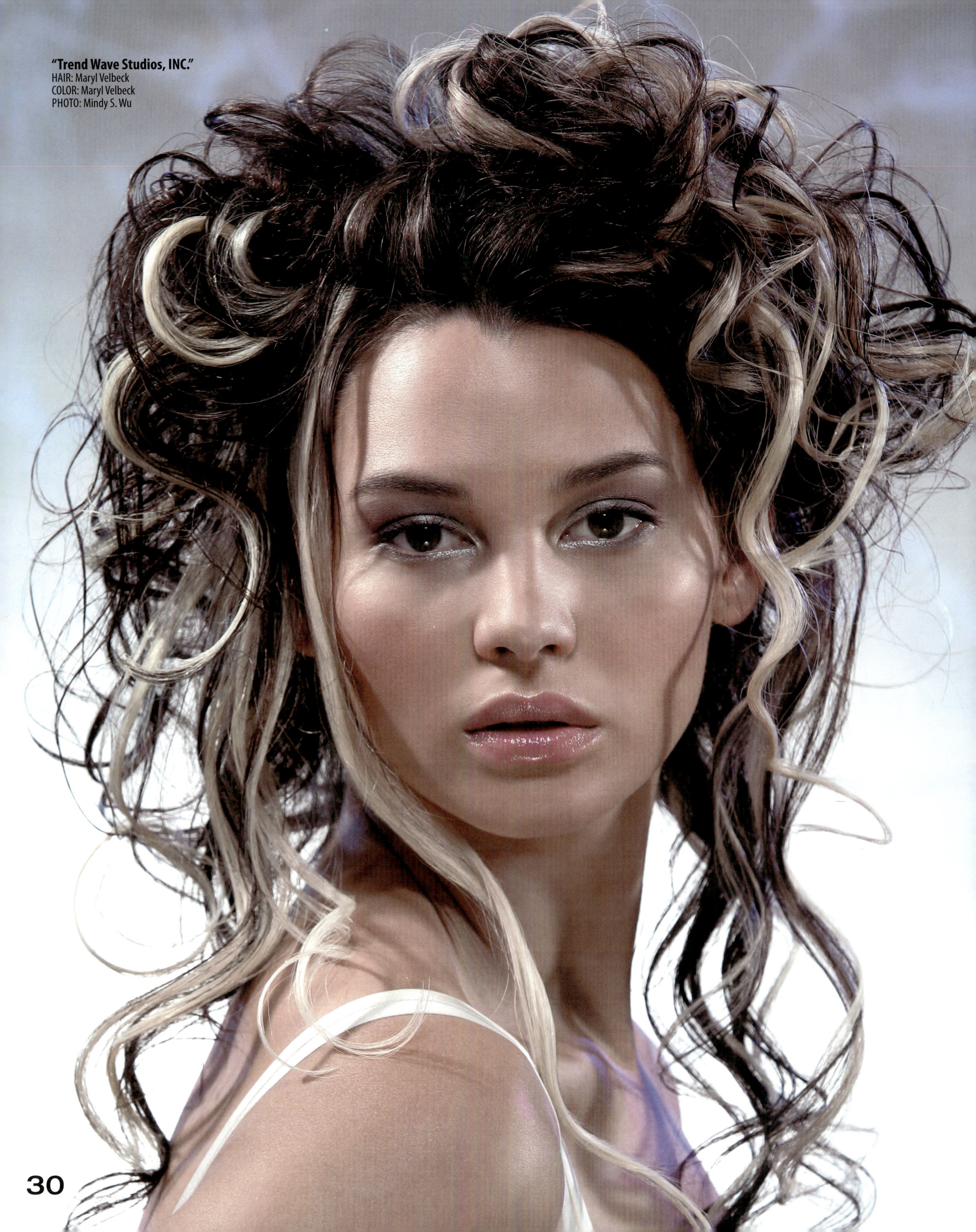

**"Trend Wave Studios, INC."**
HAIR: Maryl Velbeck
COLOR: Maryl Velbeck
PHOTO: Mindy S. Wu

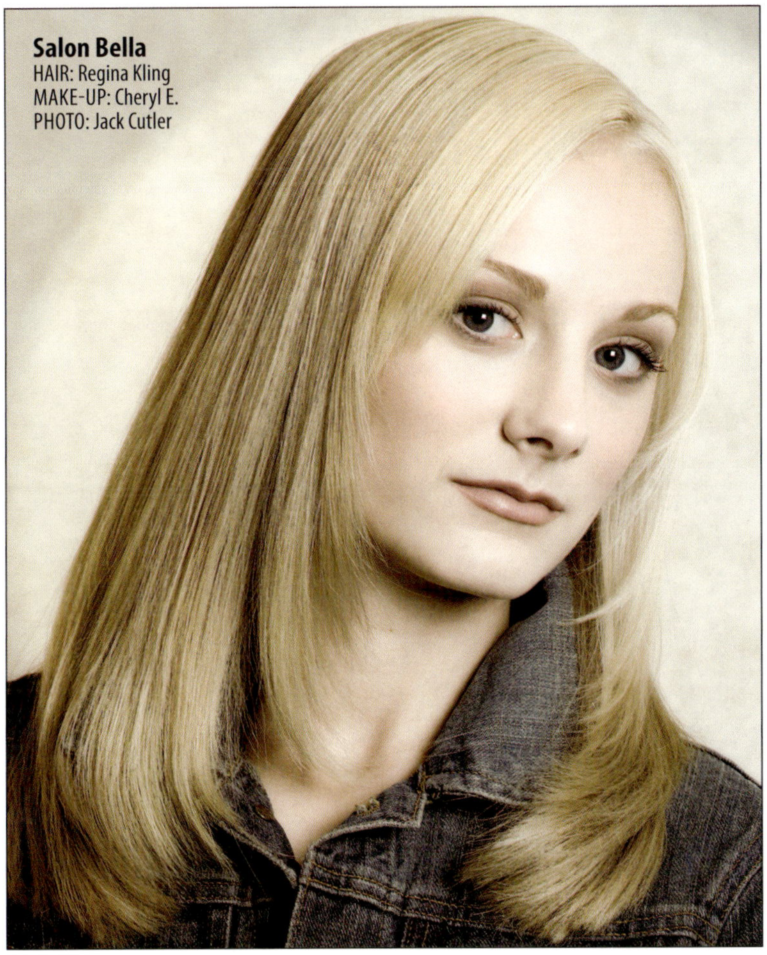

**Salon Bella**
HAIR: Regina Kling
MAKE-UP: Cheryl E.
PHOTO: Jack Cutler

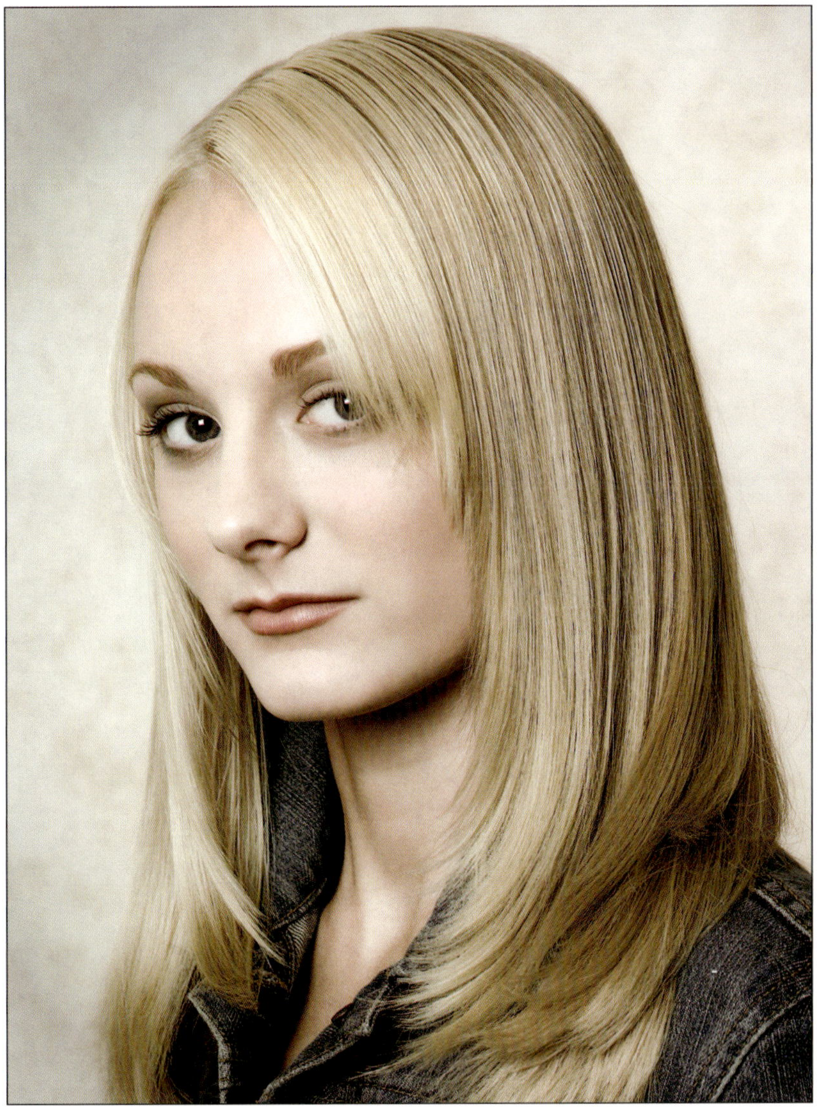

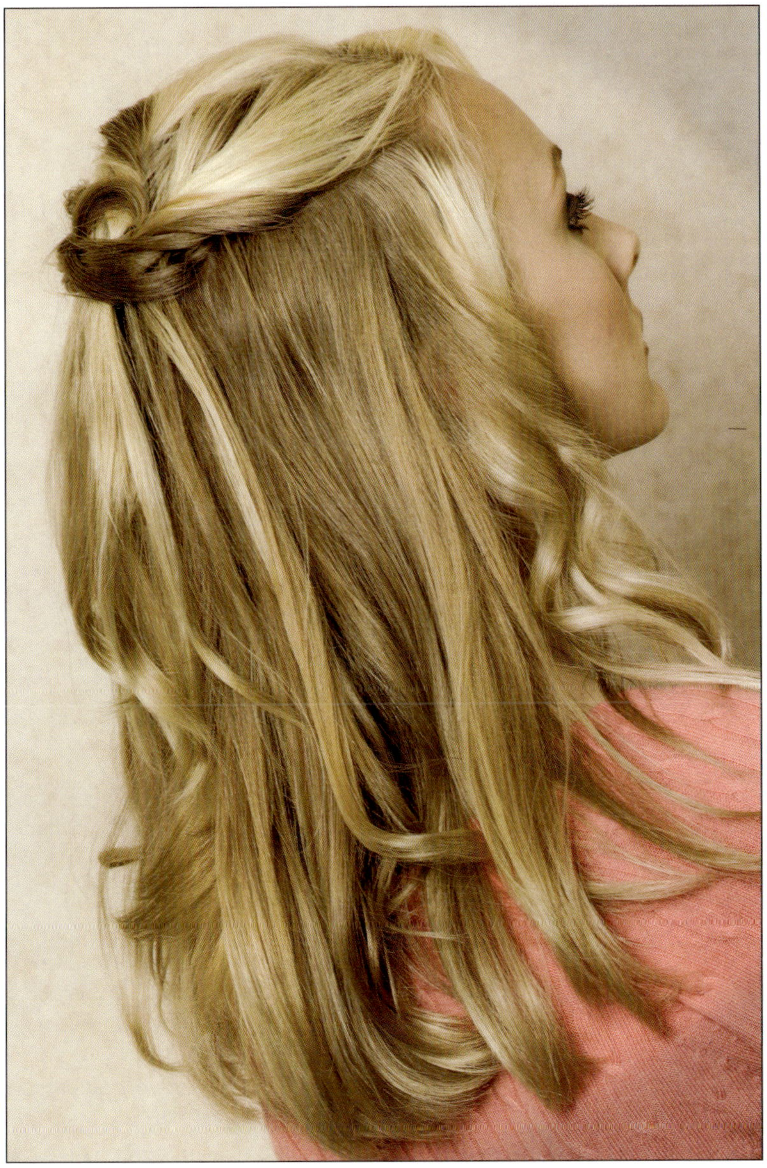

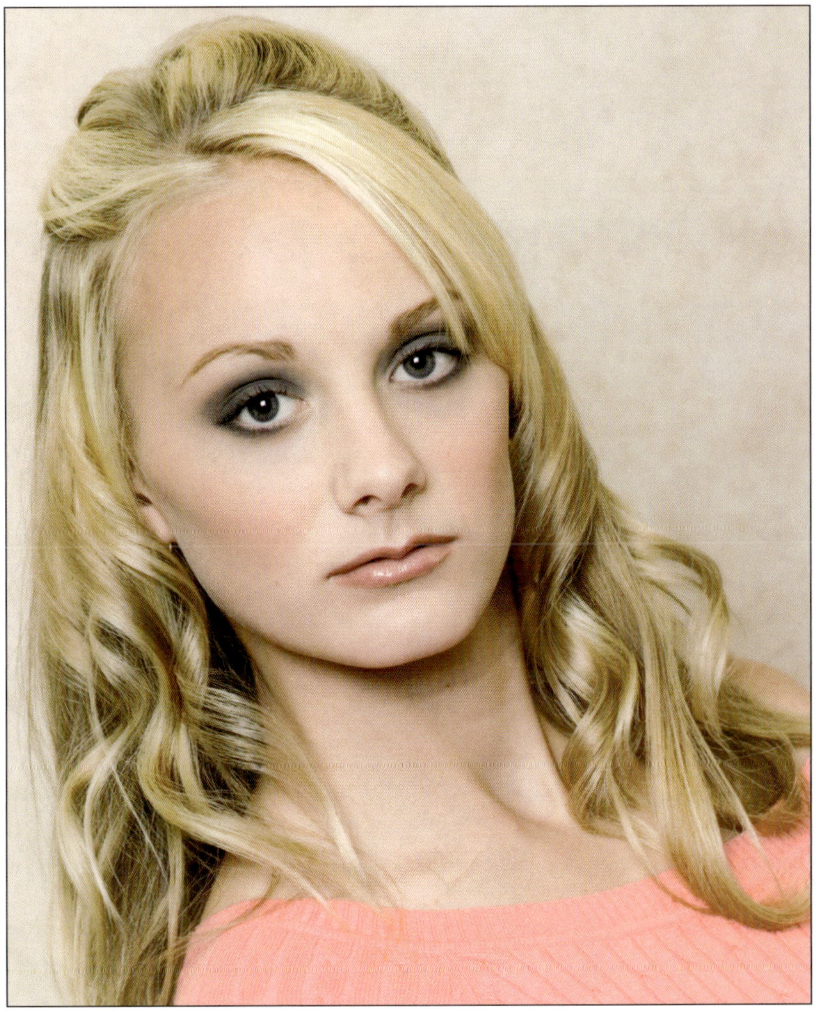

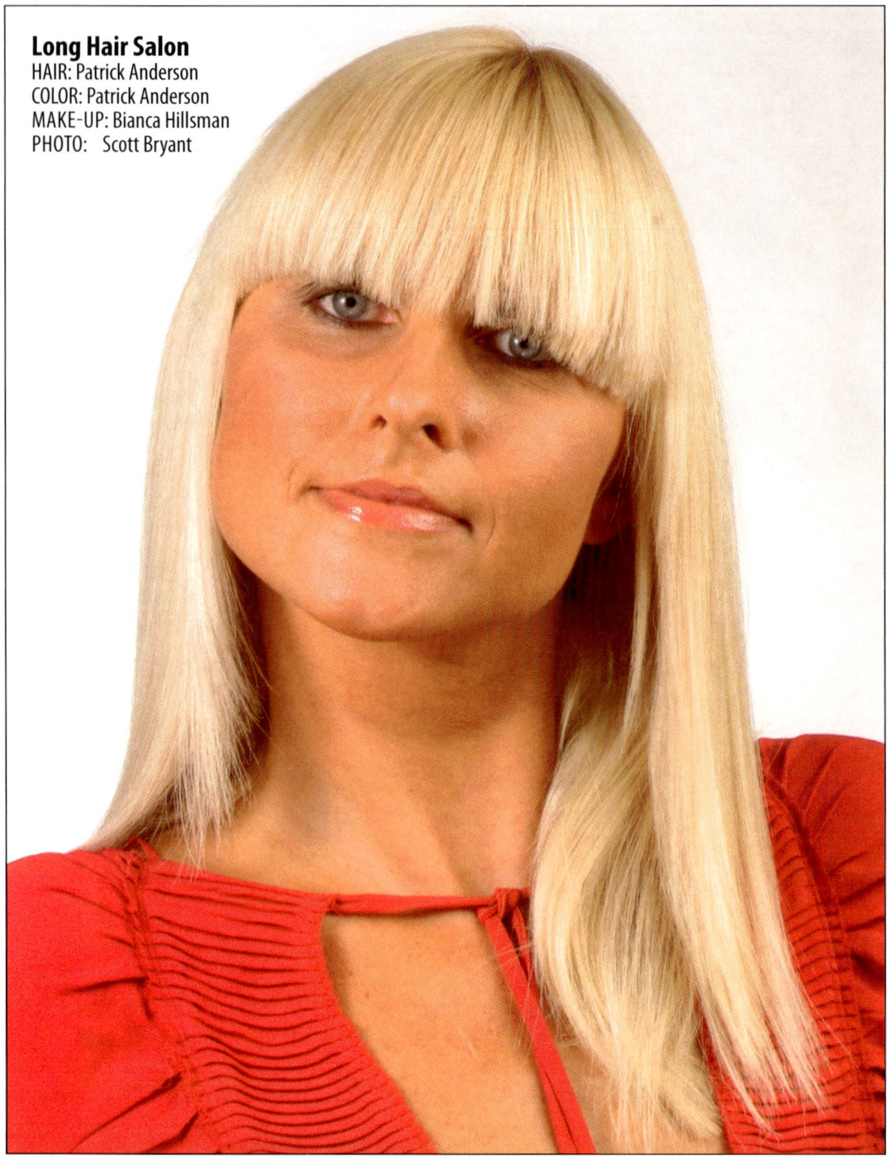

**Long Hair Salon**
HAIR: Patrick Anderson
COLOR: Patrick Anderson
MAKE-UP: Bianca Hillsman
PHOTO: Scott Bryant

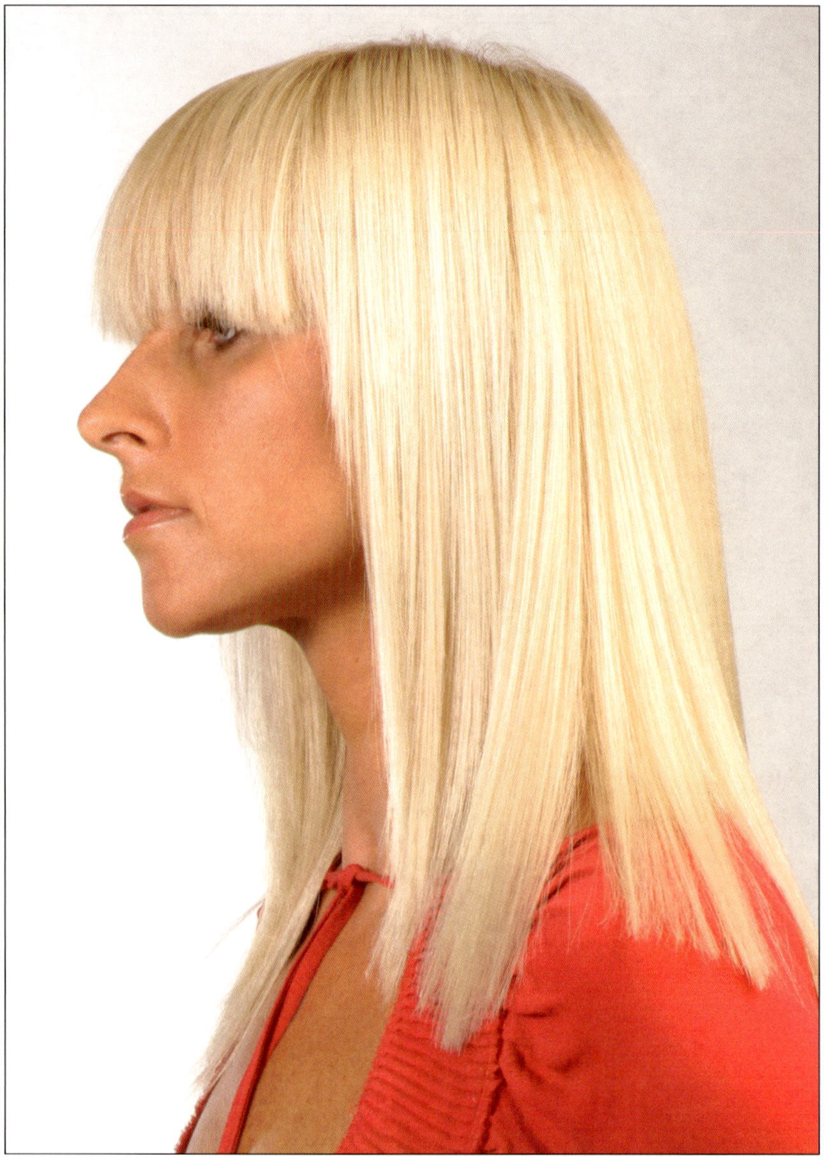

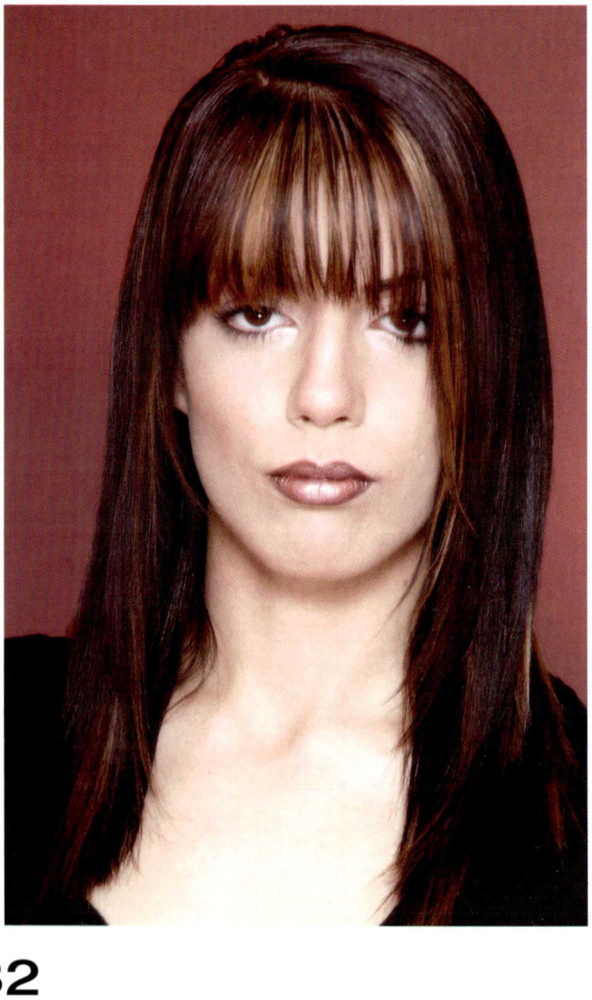

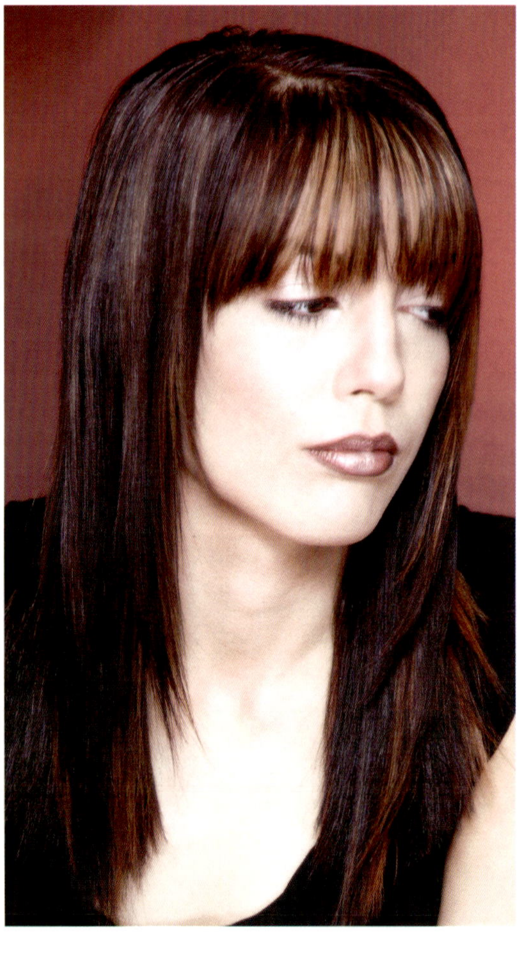

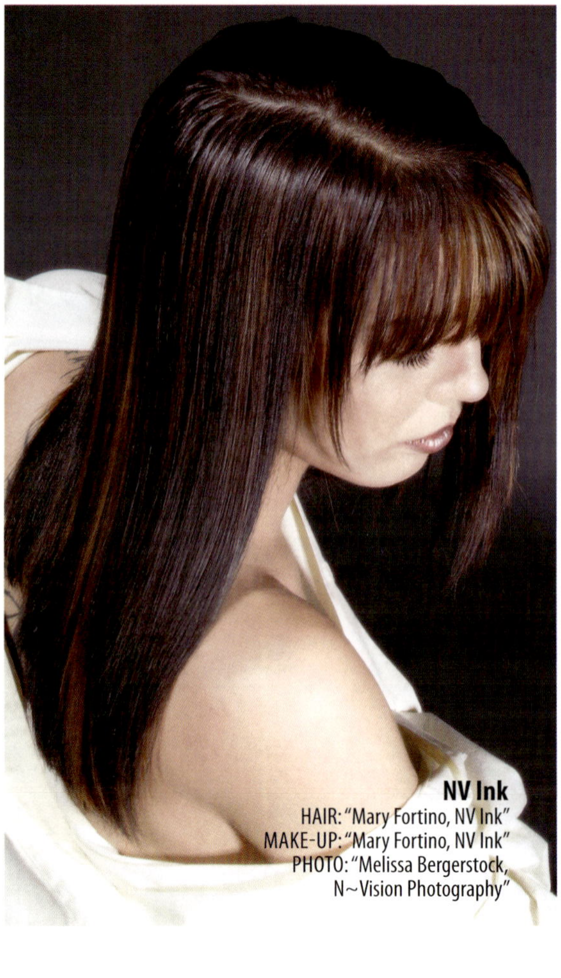

**NV Ink**
HAIR: "Mary Fortino, NV Ink"
MAKE-UP: "Mary Fortino, NV Ink"
PHOTO: "Melissa Bergerstock, N~Vision Photography"

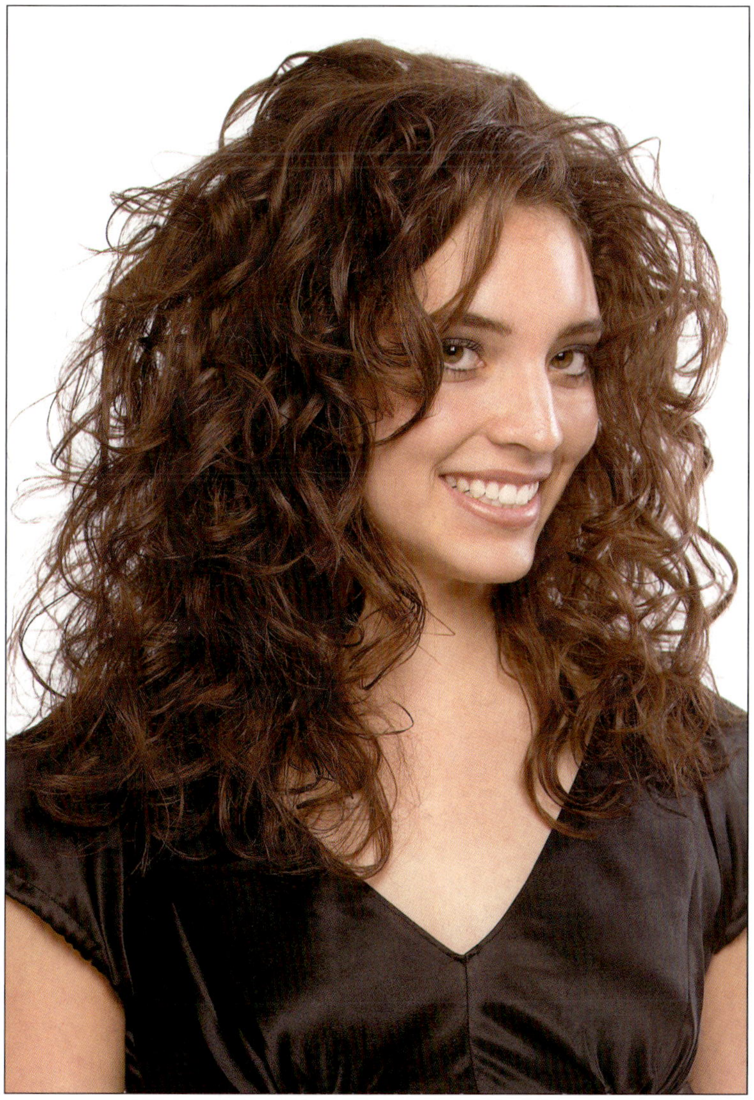

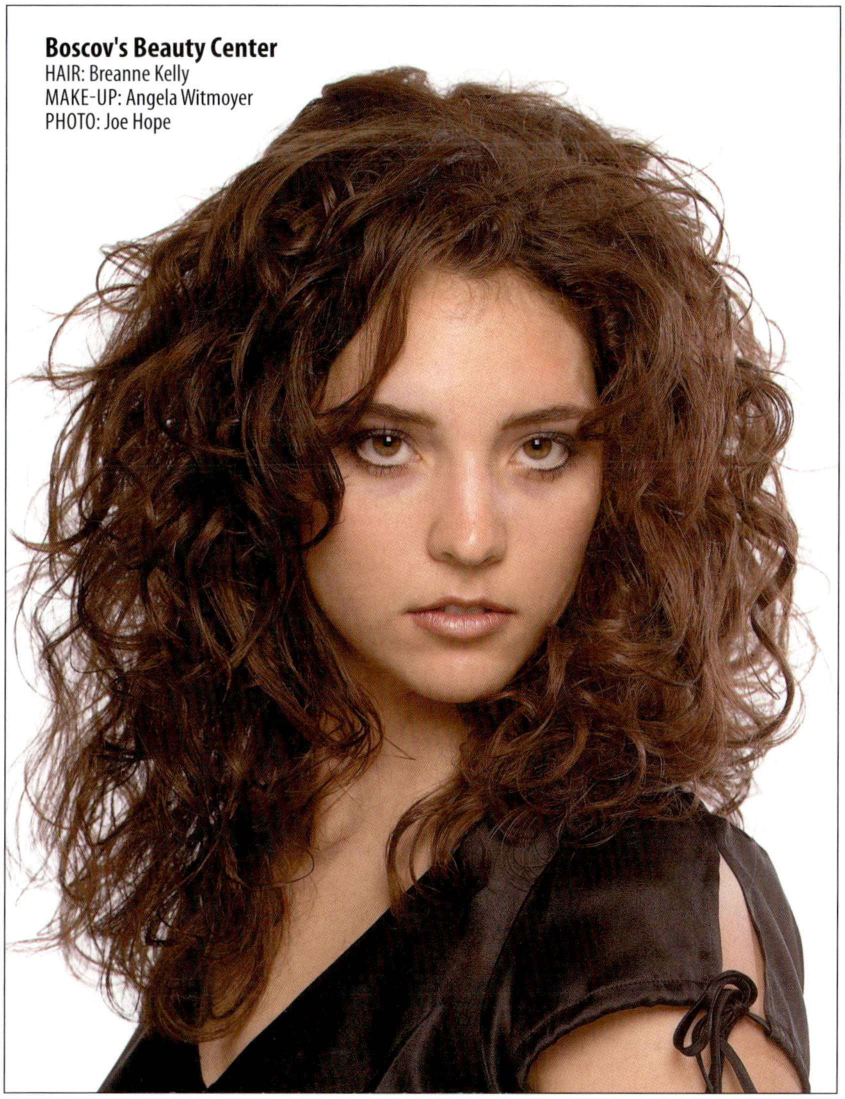

**Boscov's Beauty Center**
HAIR: Breanne Kelly
MAKE-UP: Angela Witmoyer
PHOTO: Joe Hope

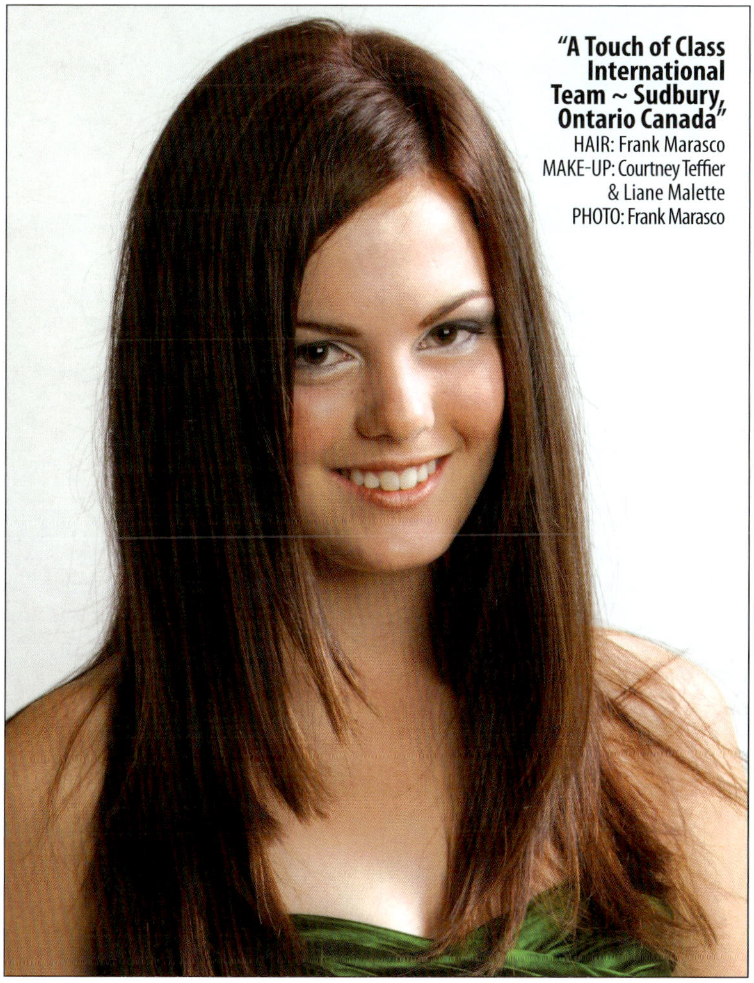

**"A Touch of Class International Team ~ Sudbury, Ontario Canada"**
HAIR: Frank Marasco
MAKE-UP: Courtney Teffier & Liane Malette
PHOTO: Frank Marasco

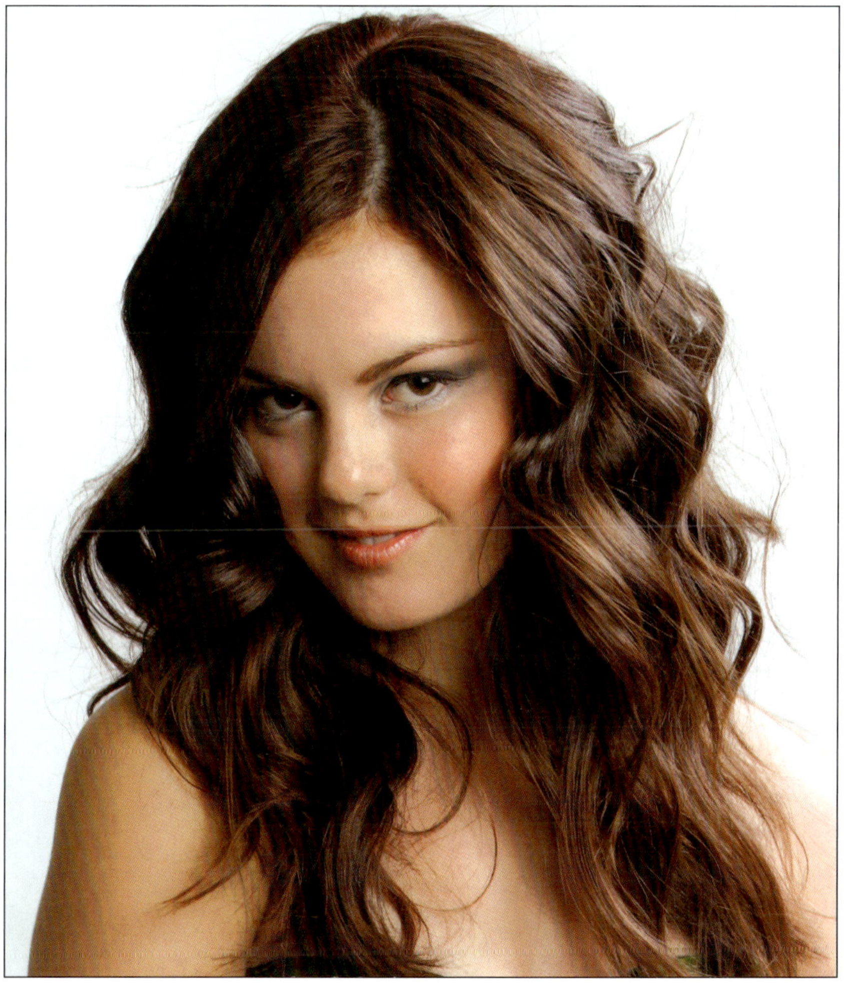

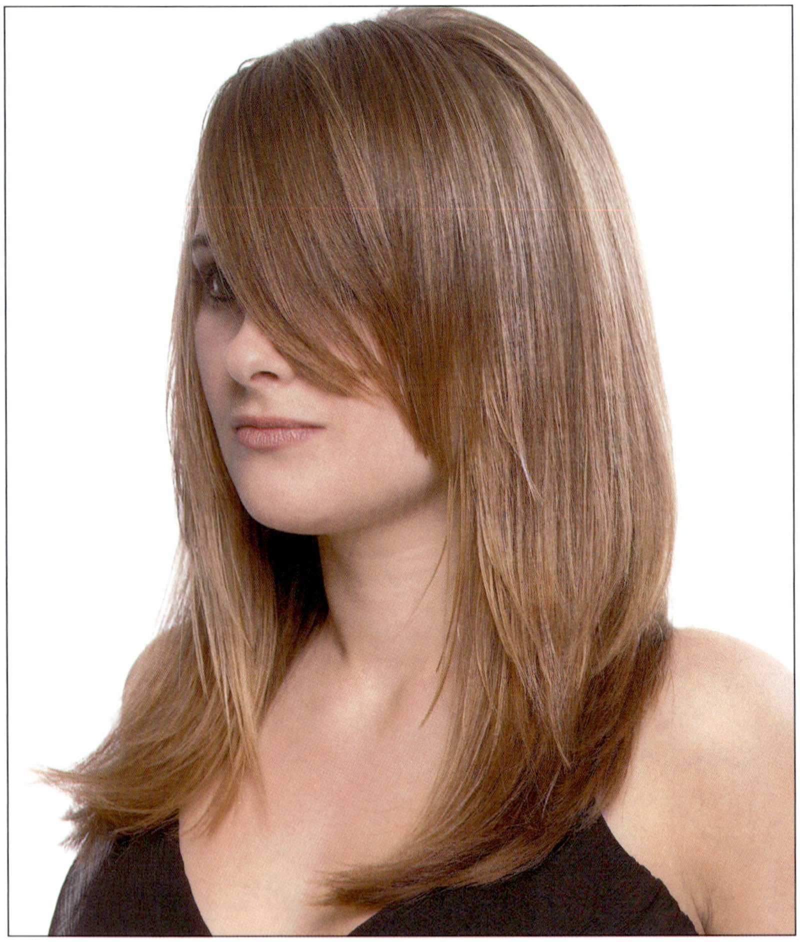

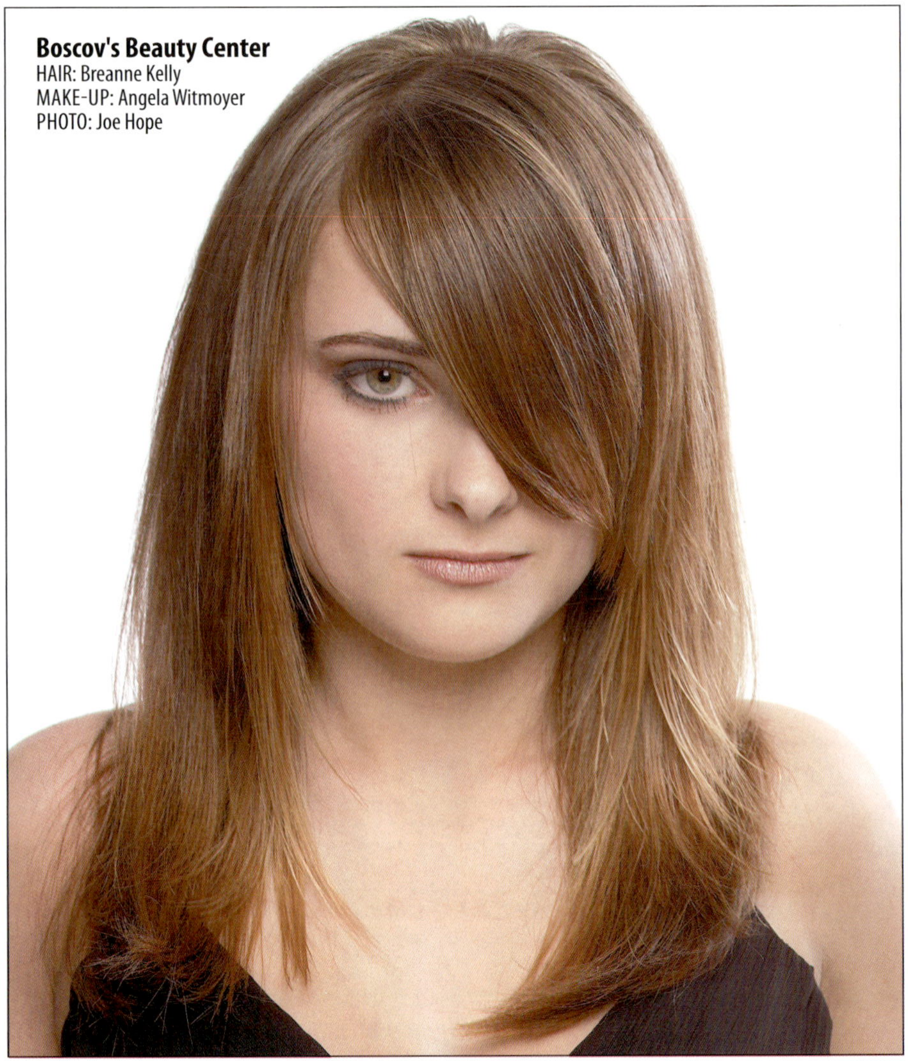

**Boscov's Beauty Center**
HAIR: Breanne Kelly
MAKE-UP: Angela Witmoyer
PHOTO: Joe Hope

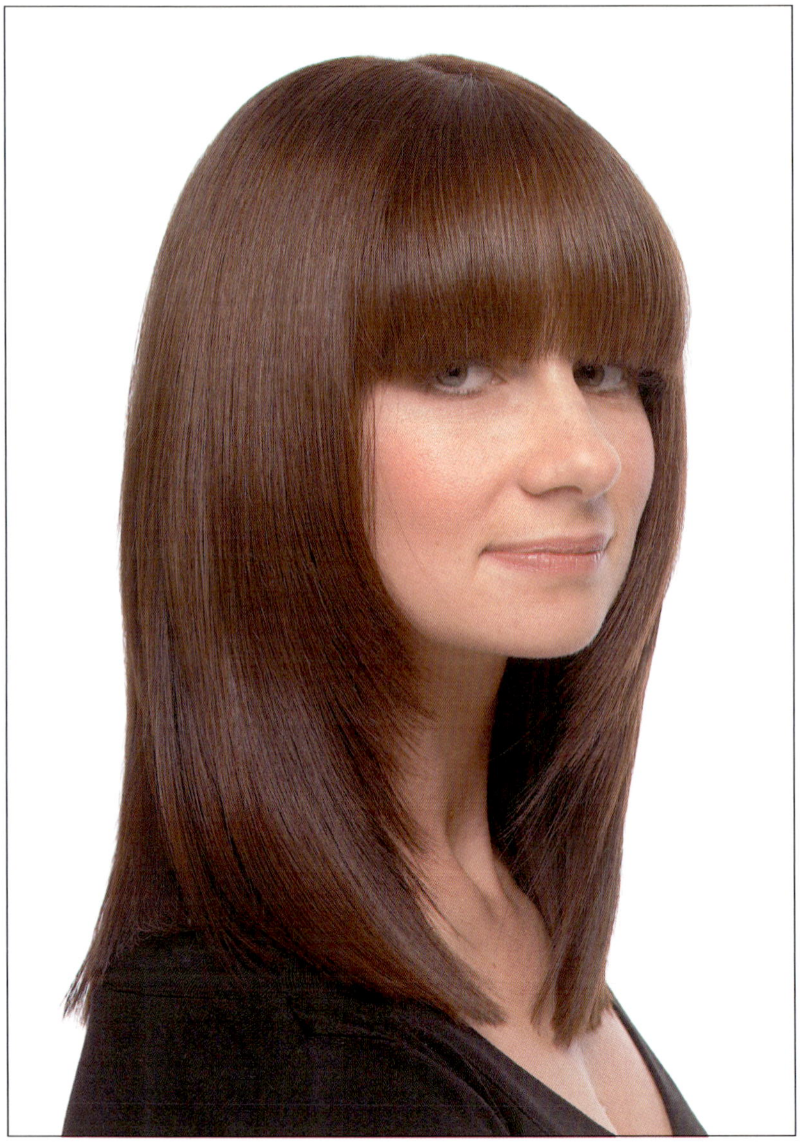

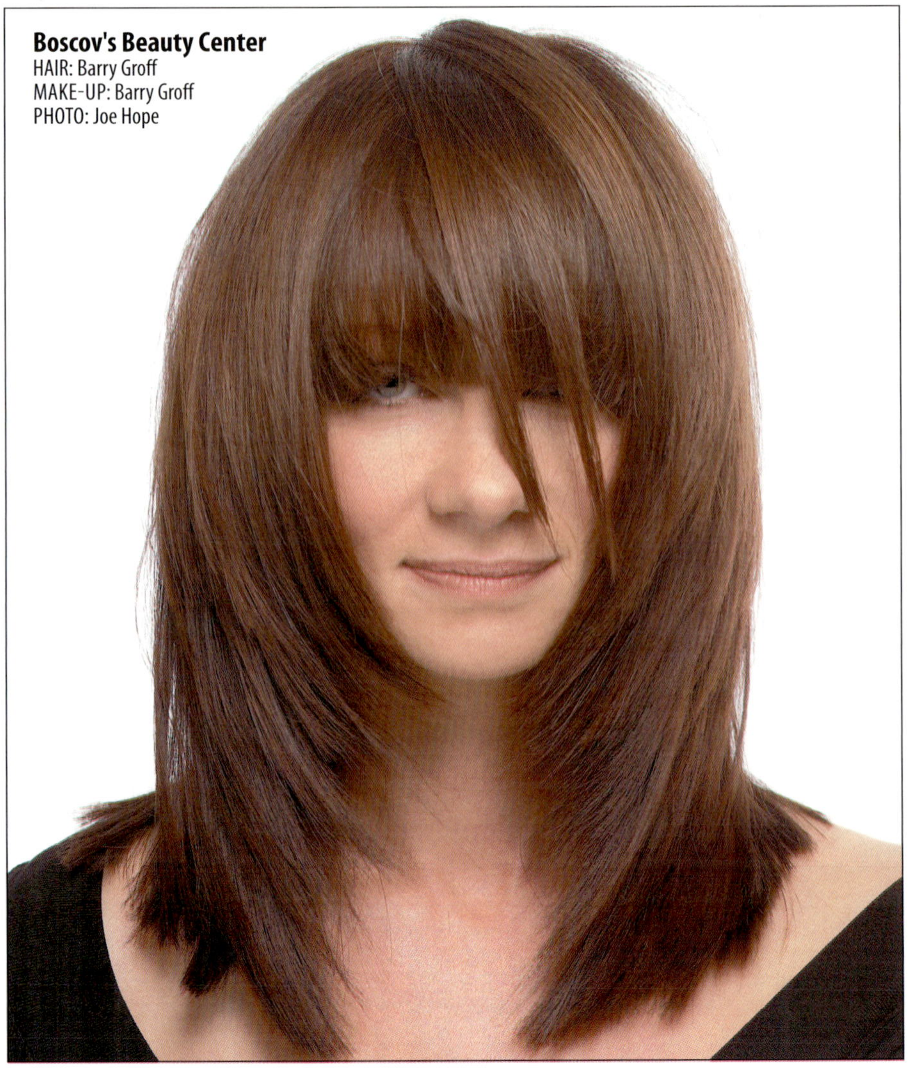

**Boscov's Beauty Center**
HAIR: Barry Groff
MAKE-UP: Barry Groff
PHOTO: Joe Hope

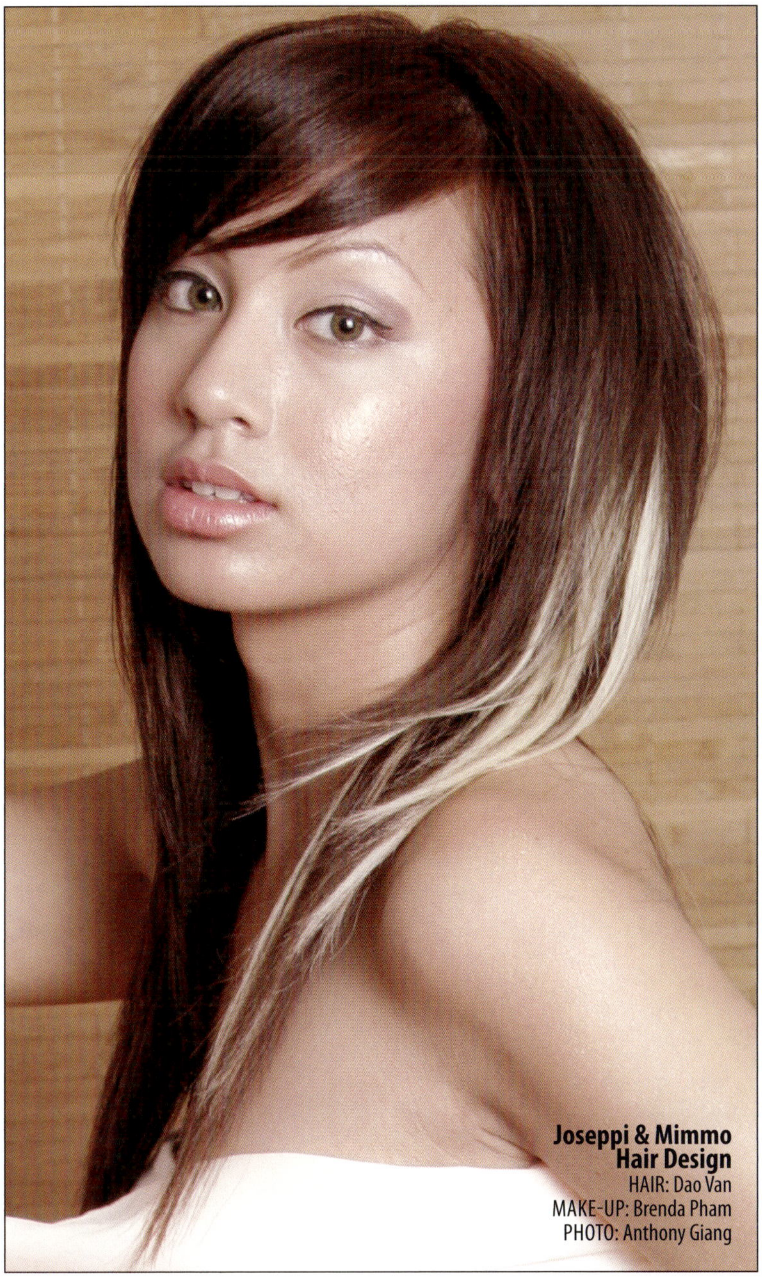

**Joseppi & Mimmo Hair Design**
HAIR: Dao Van
MAKE-UP: Brenda Pham
PHOTO: Anthony Giang

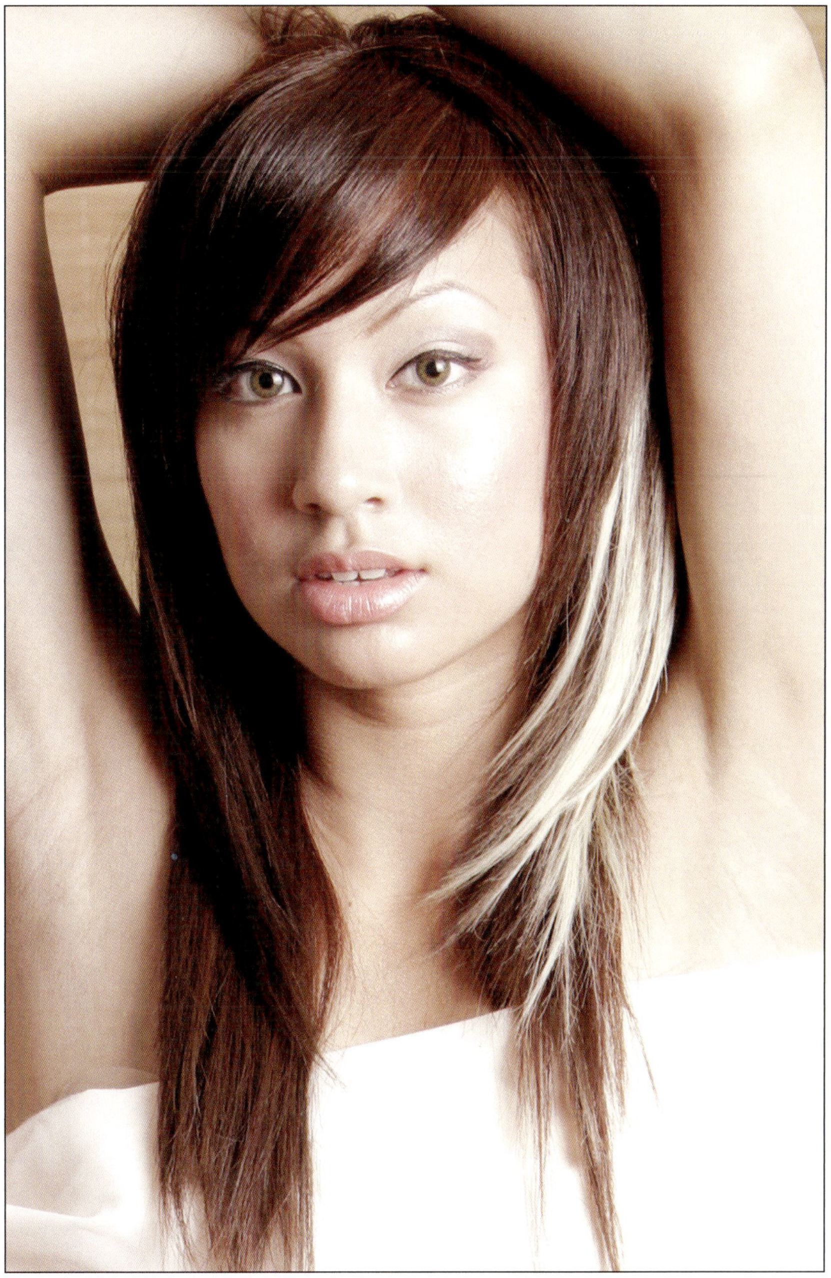

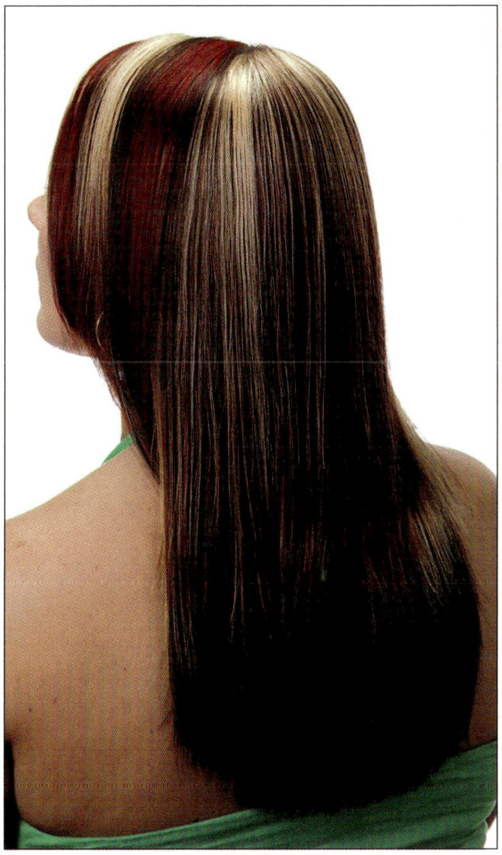

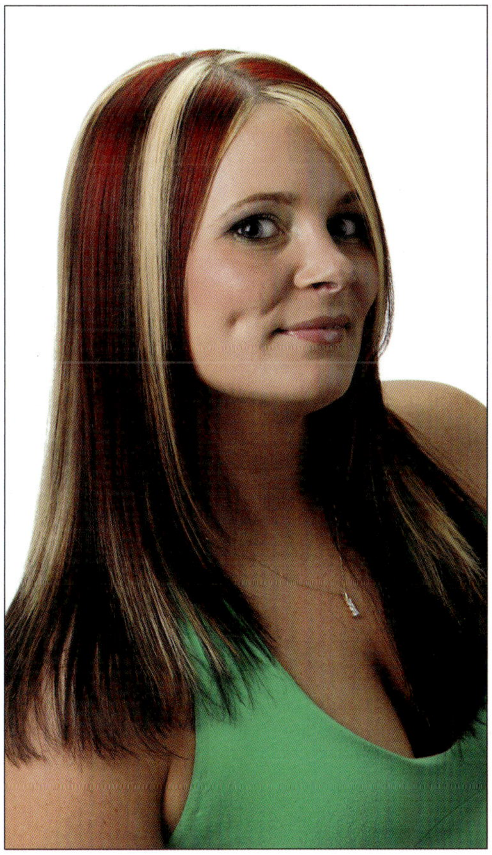

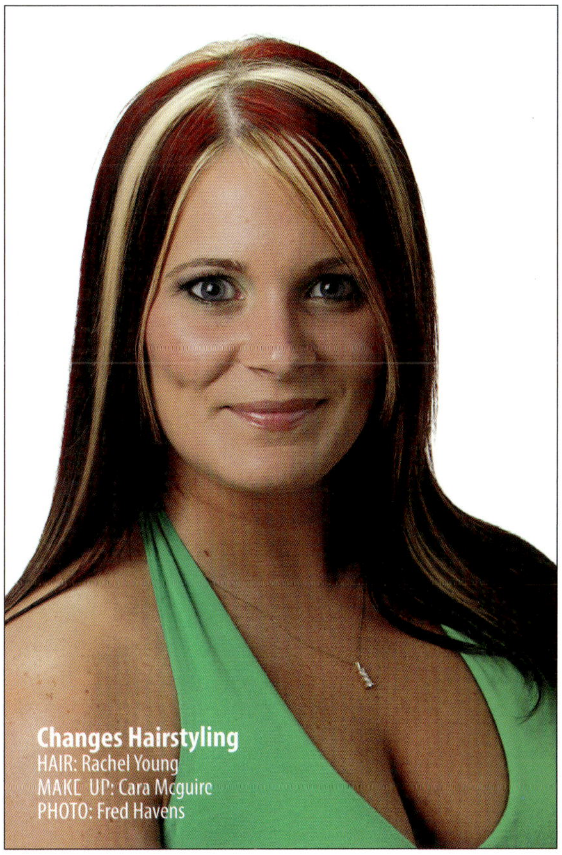

**Changes Hairstyling**
HAIR: Rachel Young
MAKE-UP: Cara Mcguire
PHOTO: Fred Havens

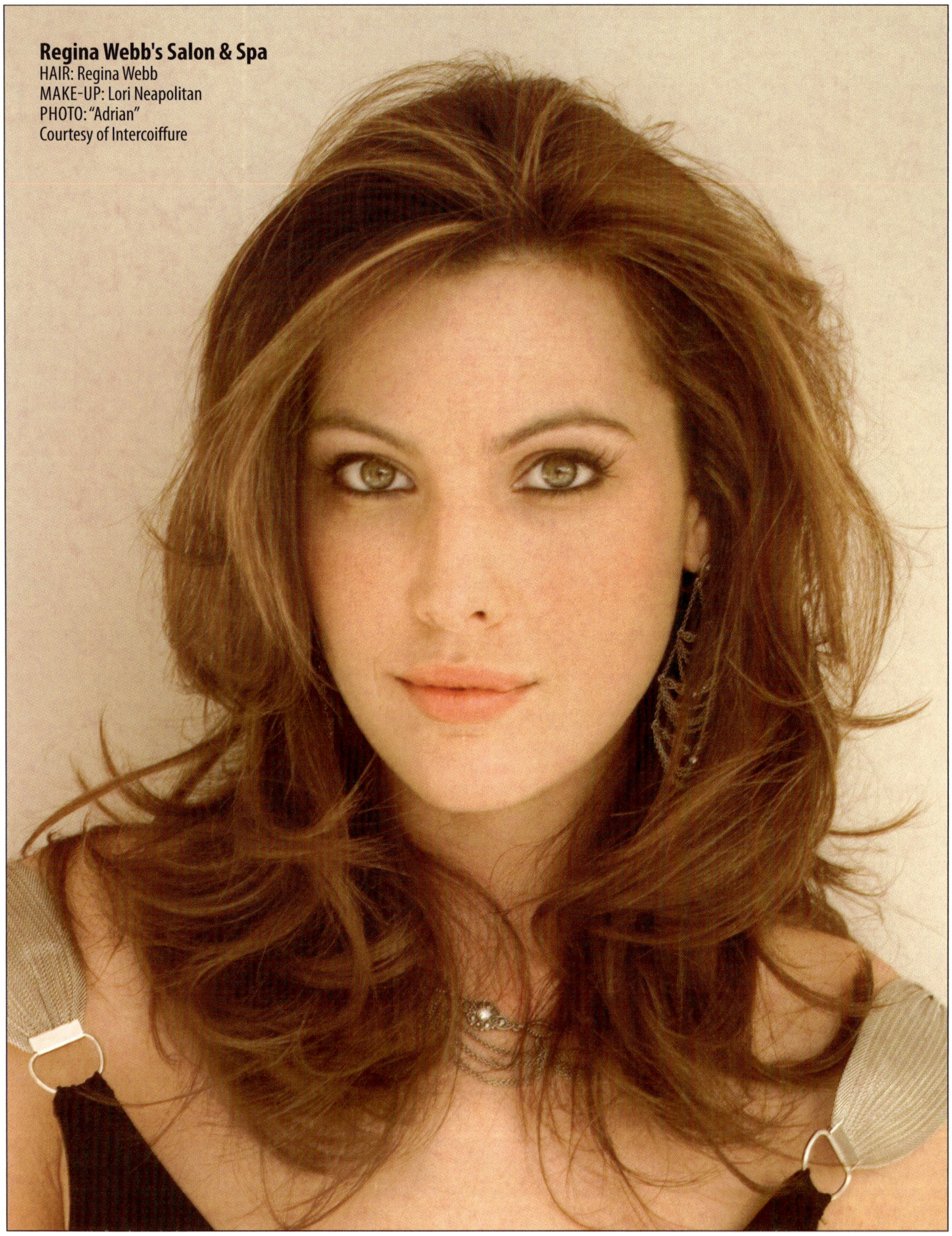
**Regina Webb's Salon & Spa**
HAIR: Regina Webb
MAKE-UP: Lori Neapolitan
PHOTO: "Adrian"
Courtesy of Intercoiffure

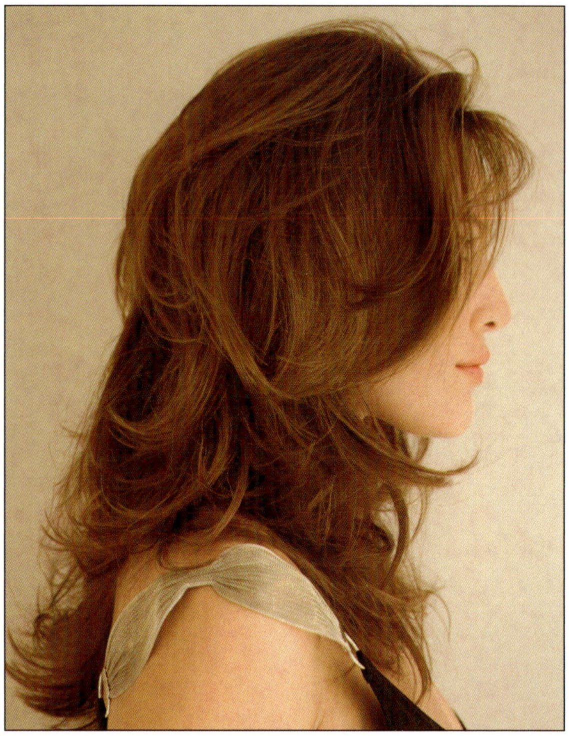

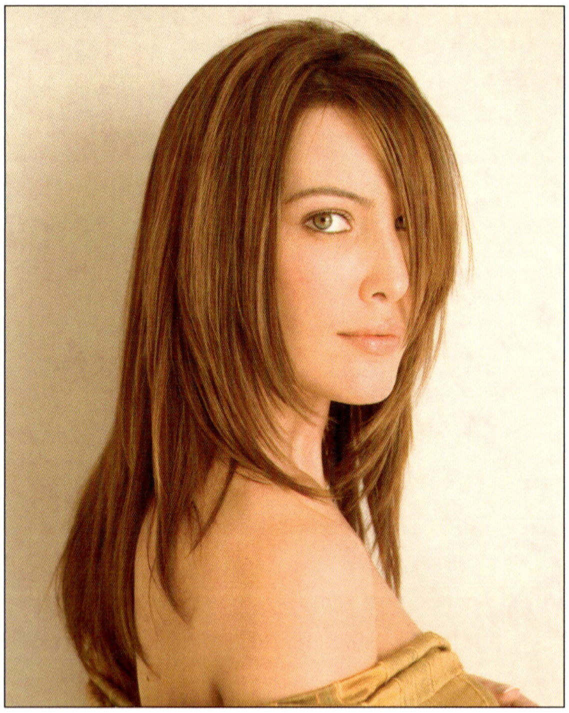

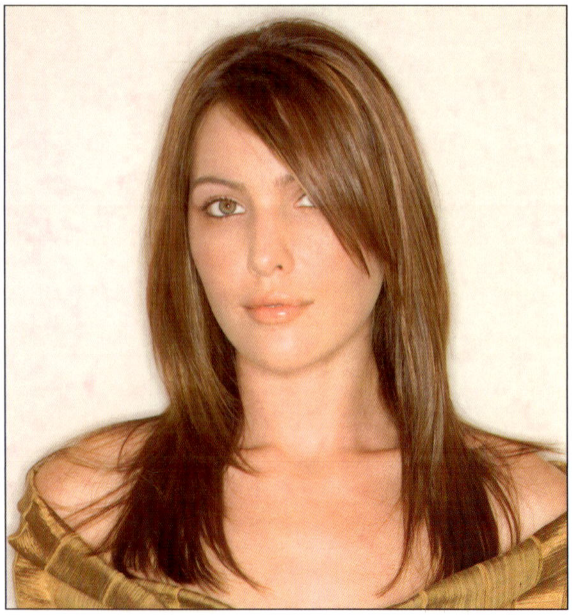

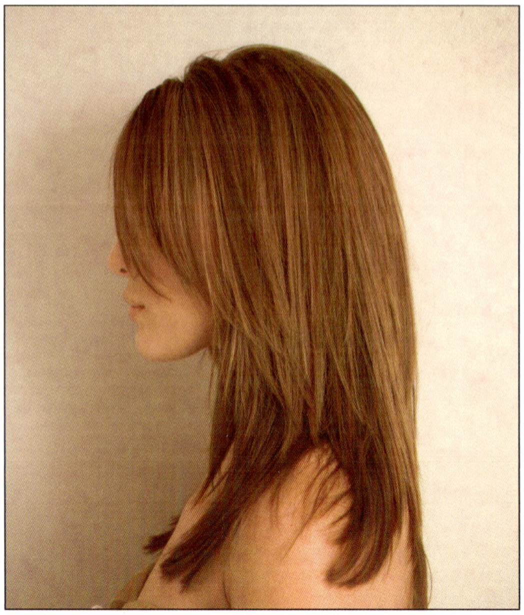

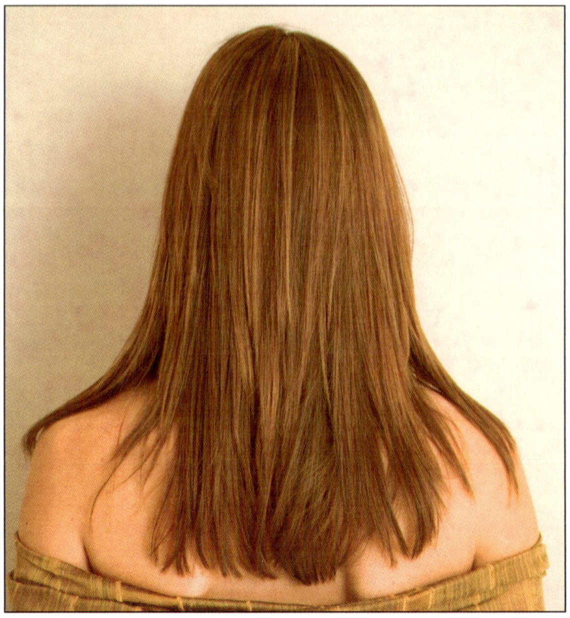

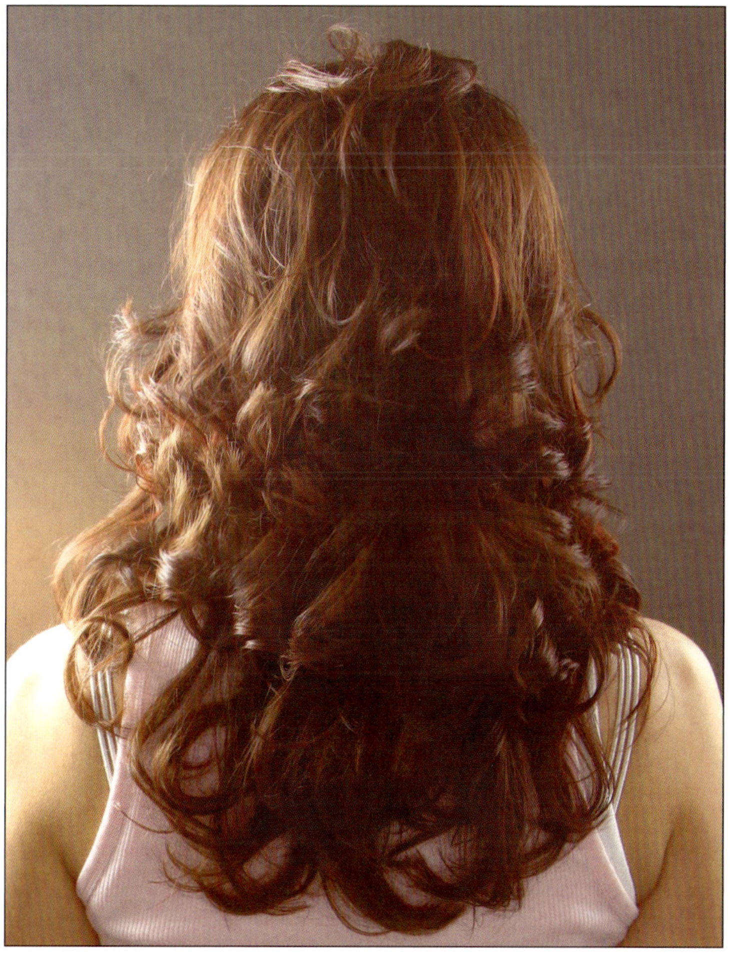

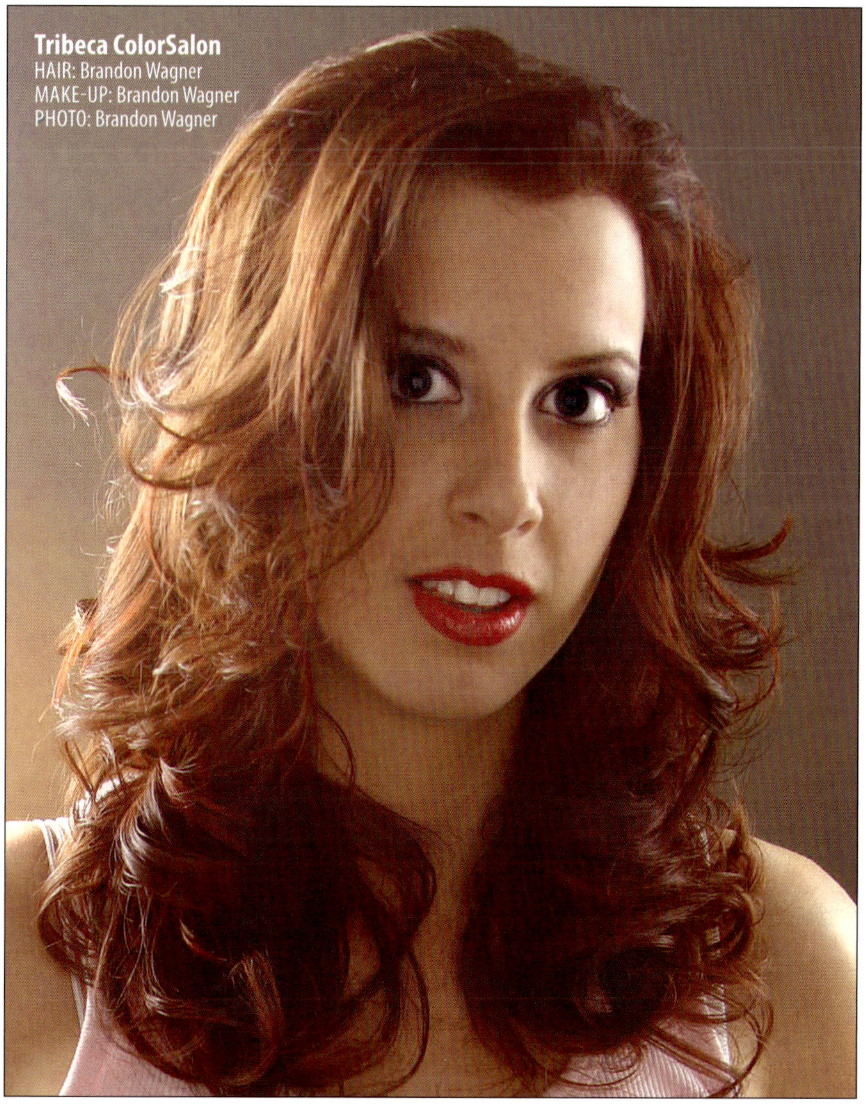

**Tribeca ColorSalon**
HAIR: Brandon Wagner
MAKE-UP: Brandon Wagner
PHOTO: Brandon Wagner

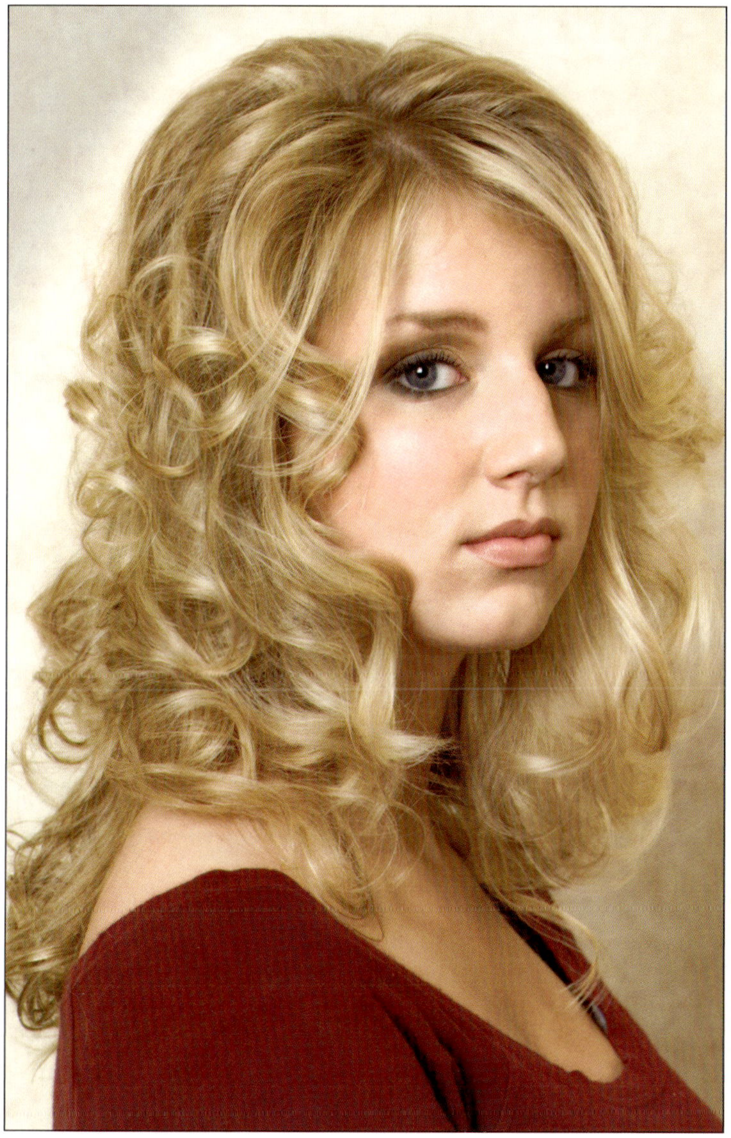

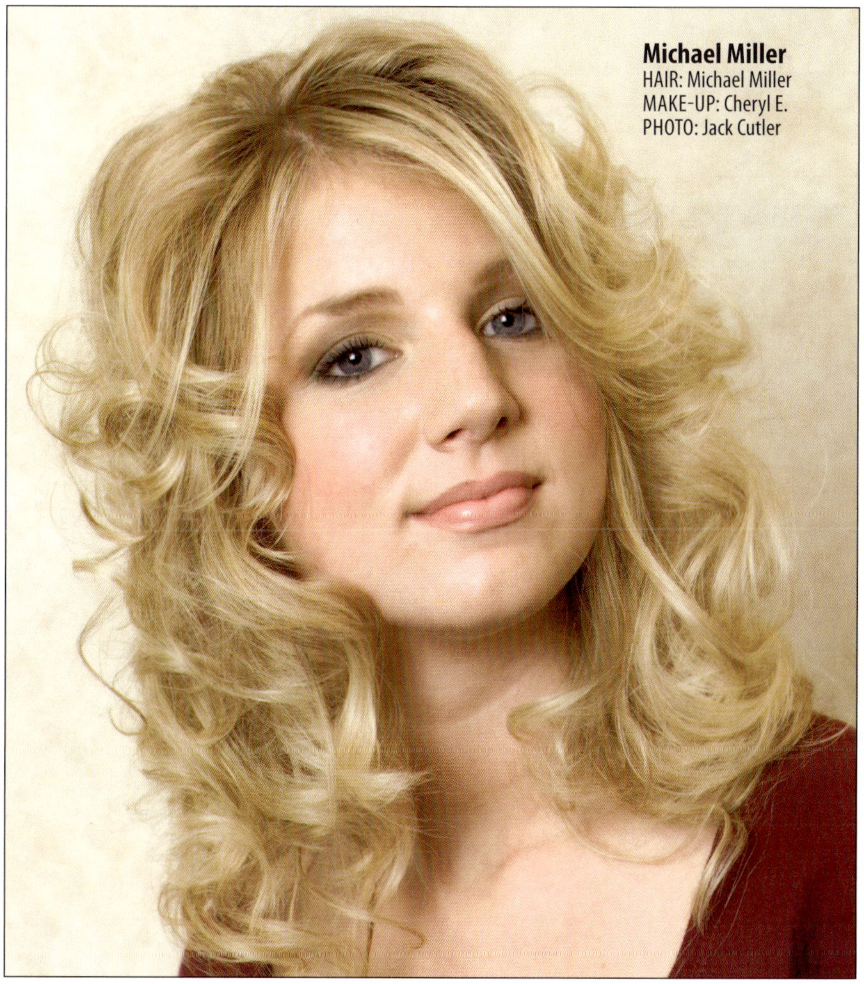

**Michael Miller**
HAIR: Michael Miller
MAKE-UP: Cheryl E.
PHOTO: Jack Cutler

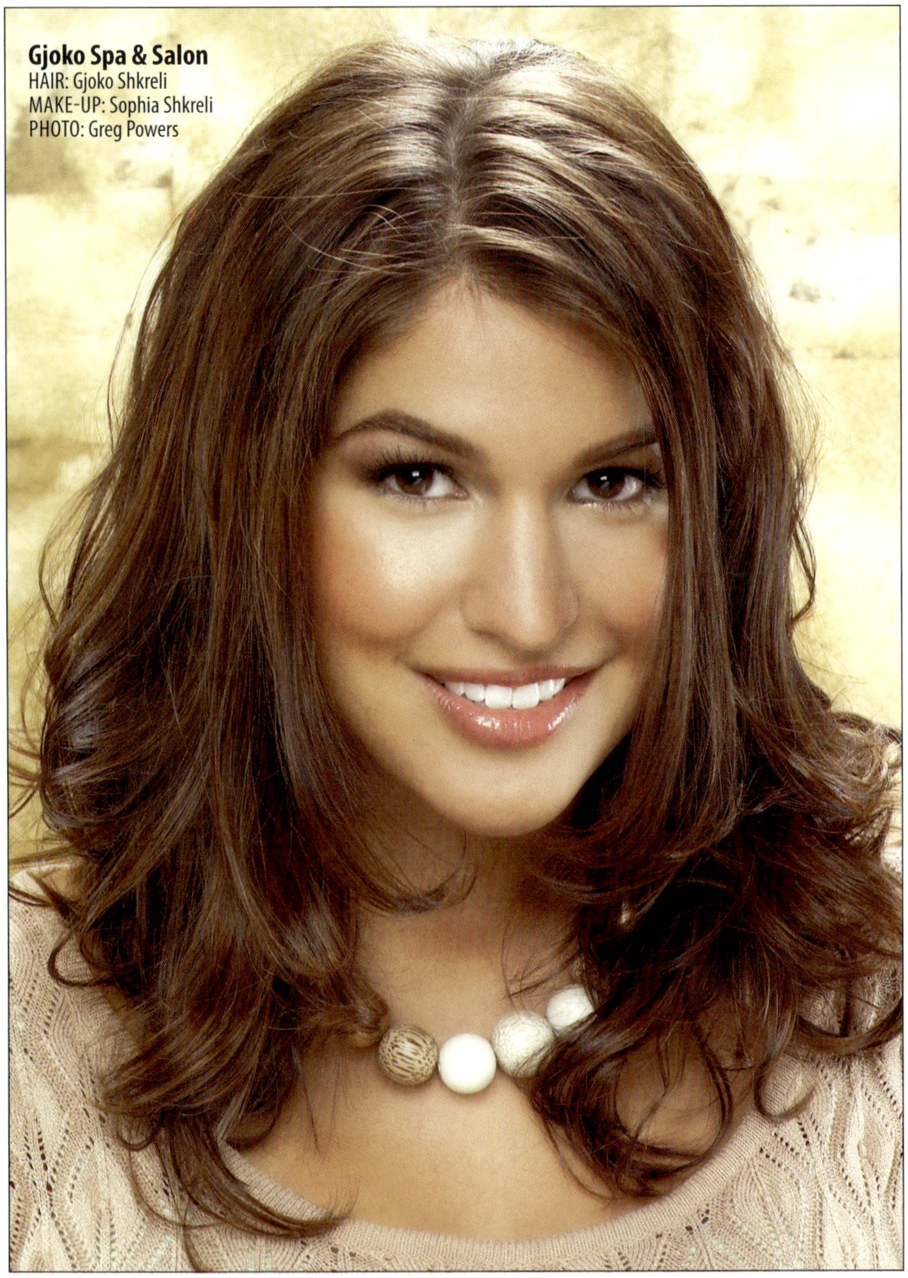

**Gjoko Spa & Salon**
HAIR: Gjoko Shkreli
MAKE-UP: Sophia Shkreli
PHOTO: Greg Powers

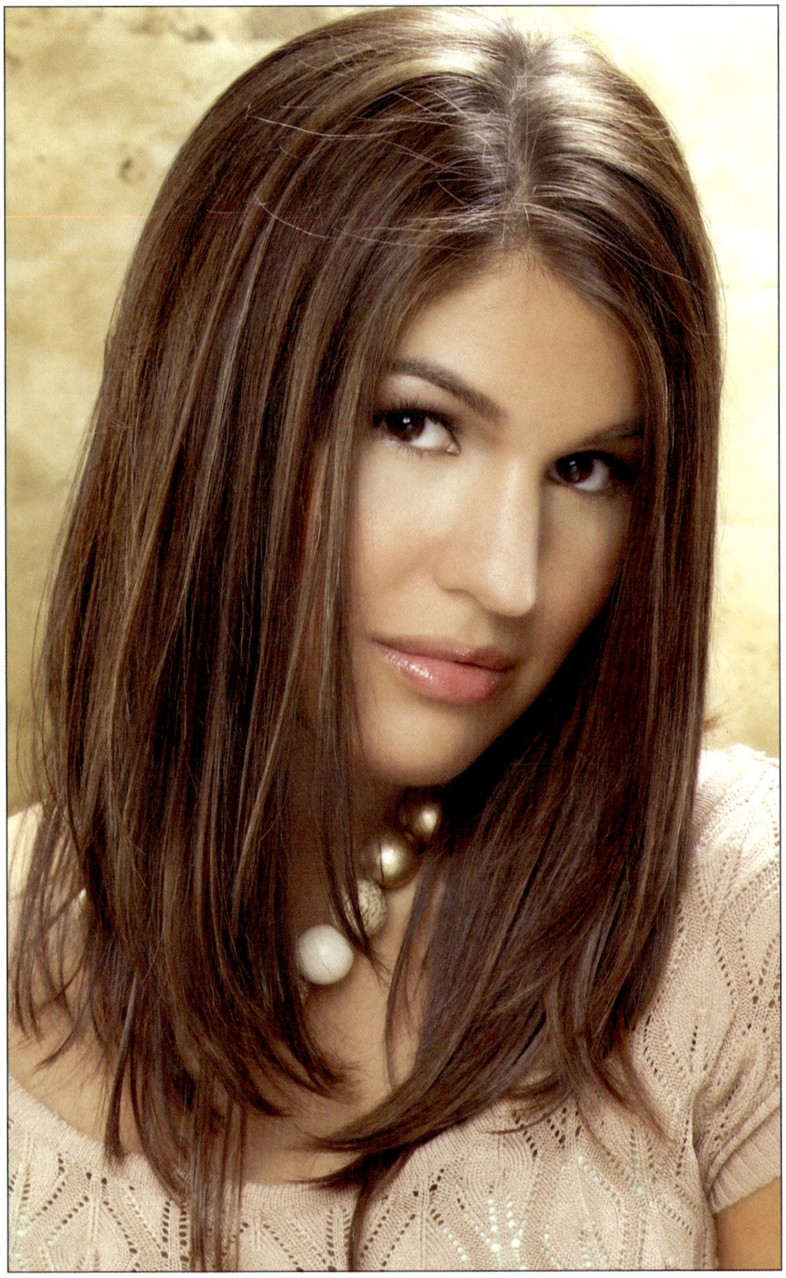

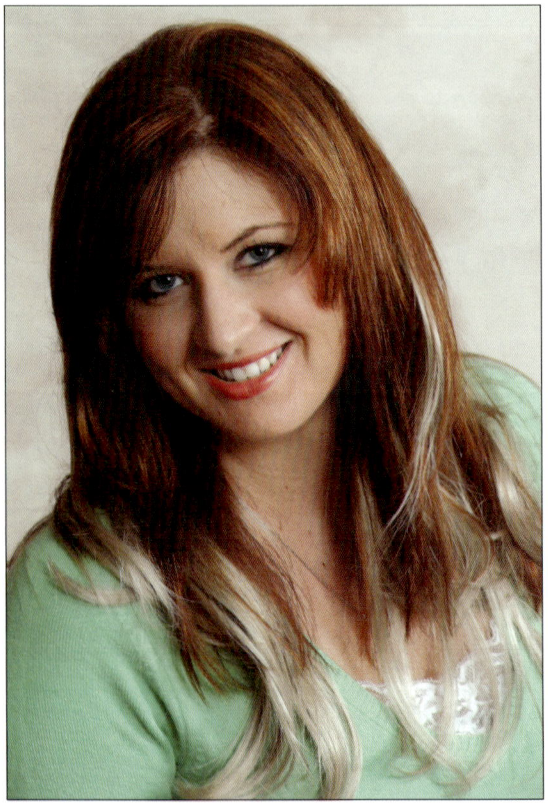

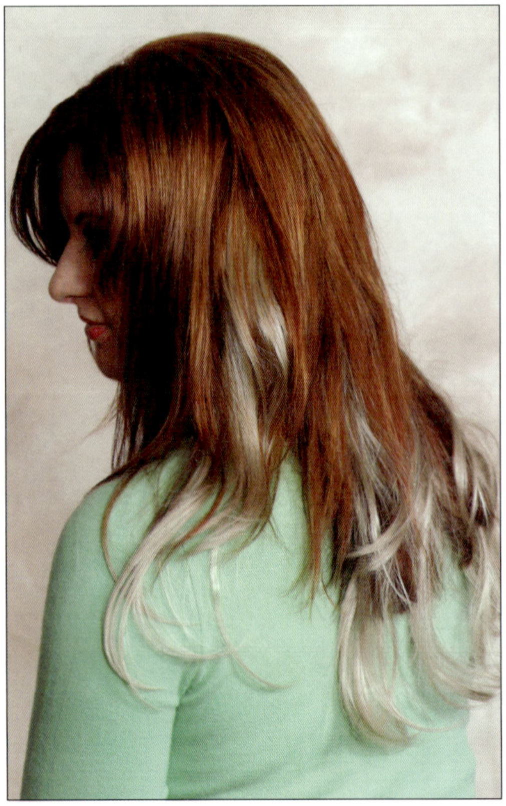

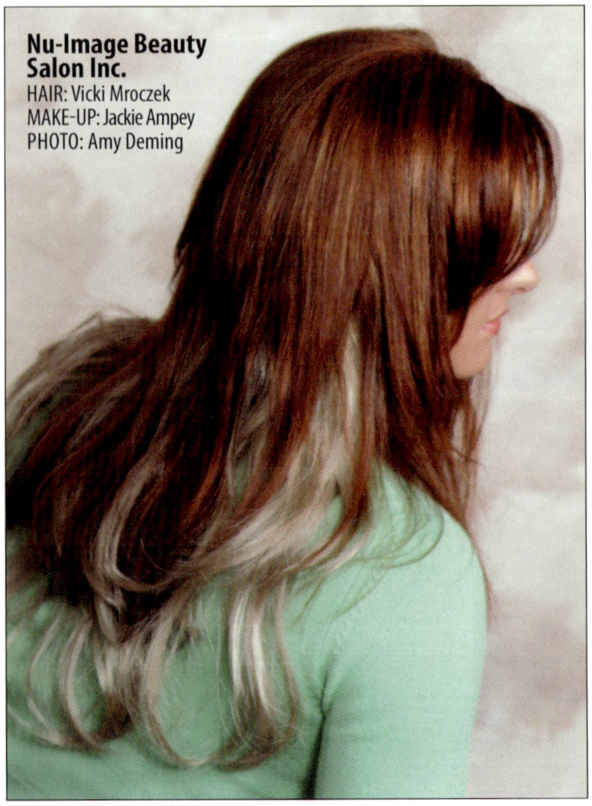

**Nu-Image Beauty Salon Inc.**
HAIR: Vicki Mroczek
MAKE-UP: Jackie Ampey
PHOTO: Amy Deming

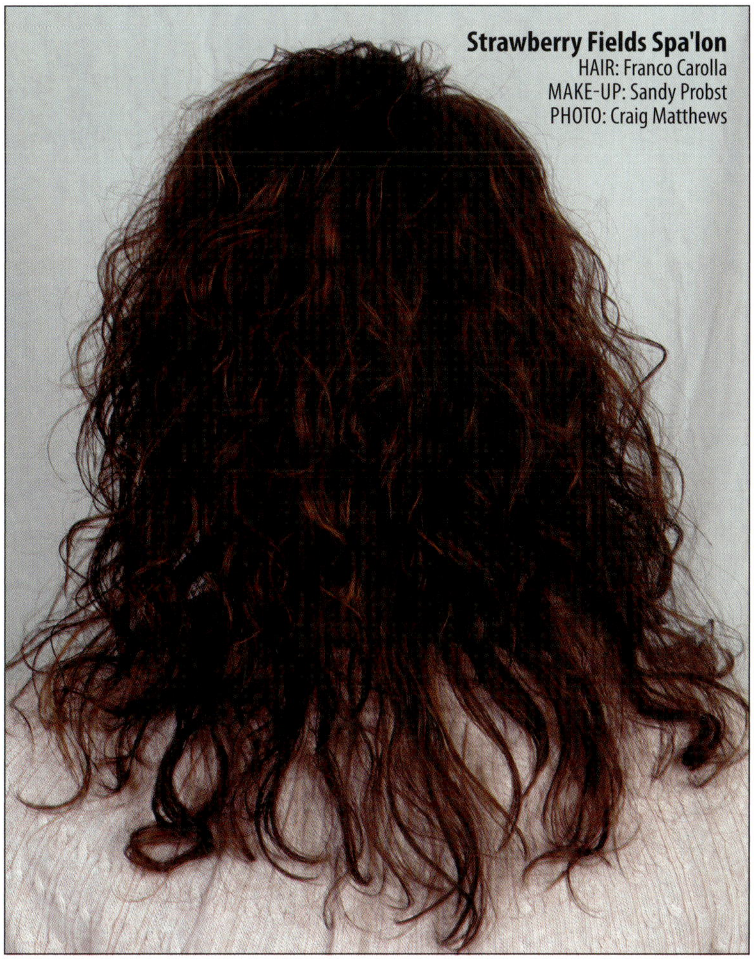

**Strawberry Fields Spa'lon**
HAIR: Franco Carolla
MAKE-UP: Sandy Probst
PHOTO: Craig Matthews

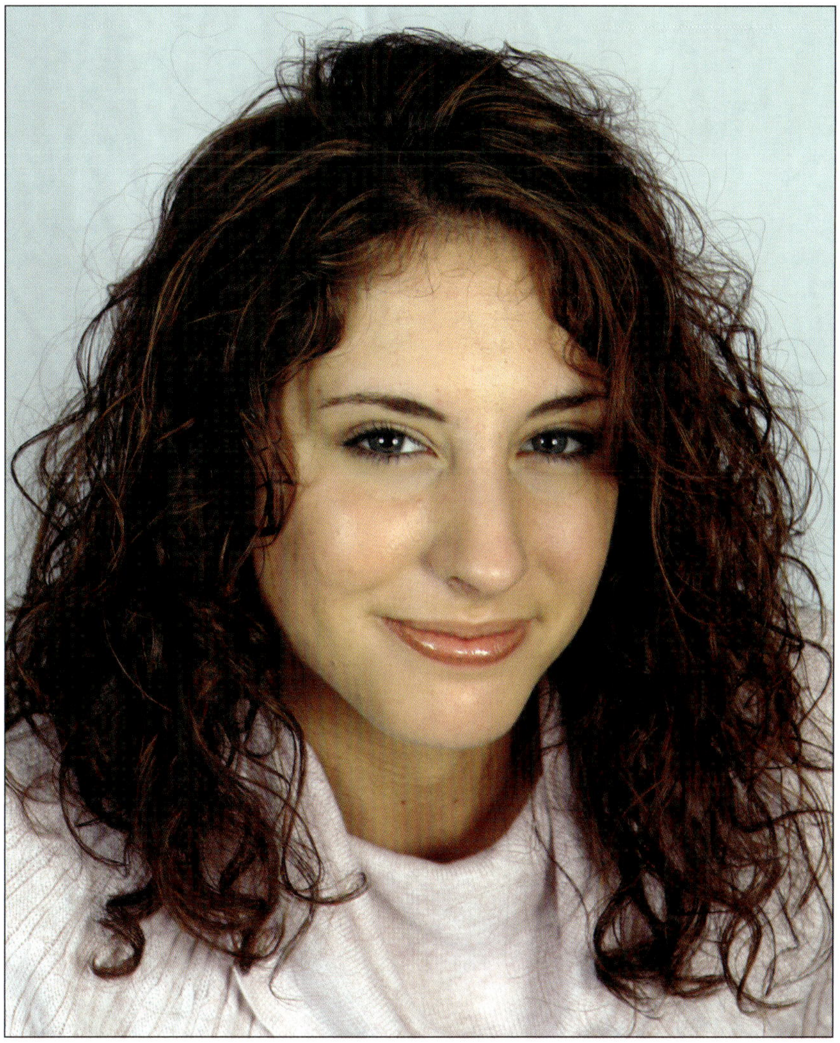

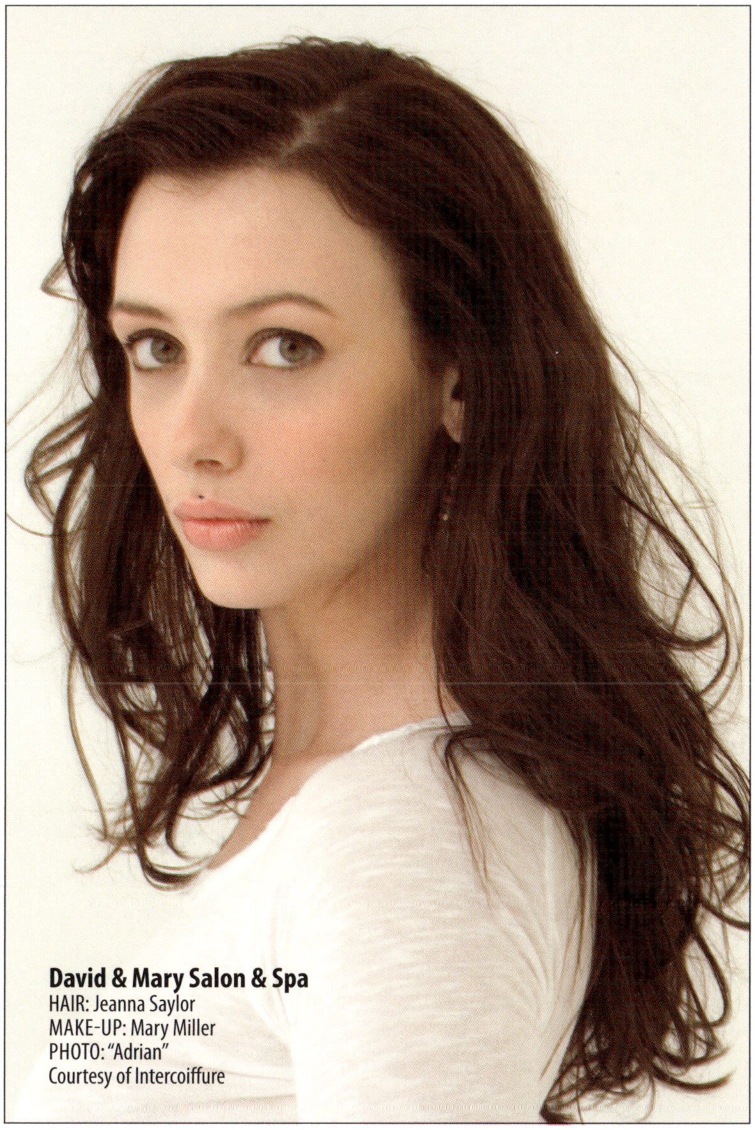

**David & Mary Salon & Spa**
HAIR: Jeanna Saylor
MAKE-UP: Mary Miller
PHOTO: "Adrian"
Courtesy of Intercoiffure

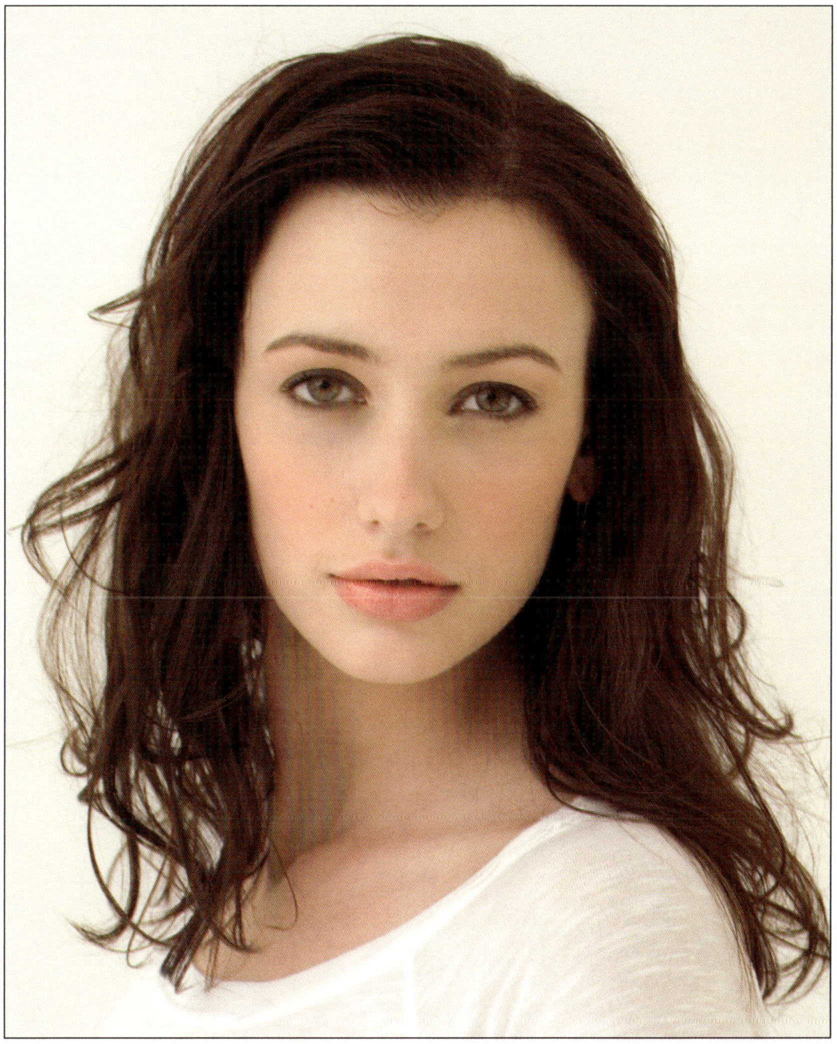

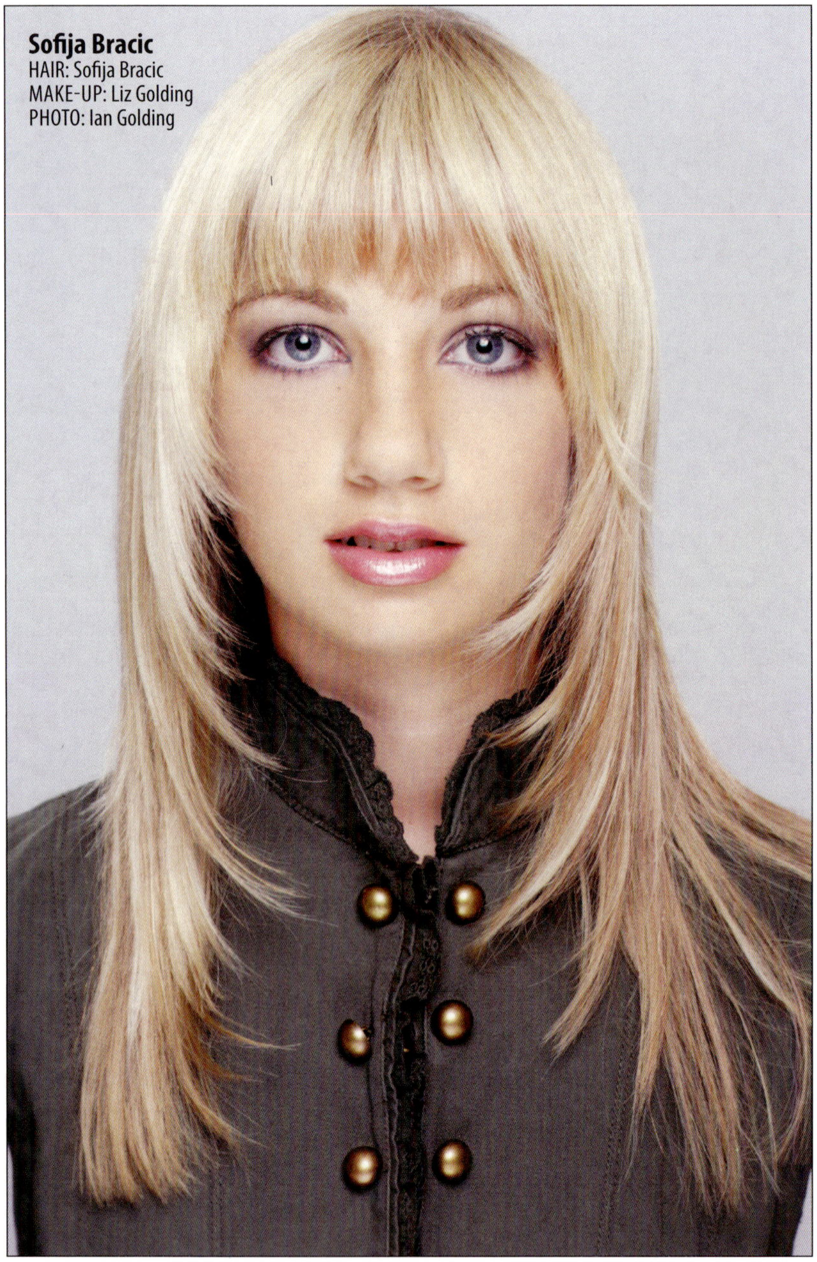

**Sofija Bracic**
HAIR: Sofija Bracic
MAKE-UP: Liz Golding
PHOTO: Ian Golding

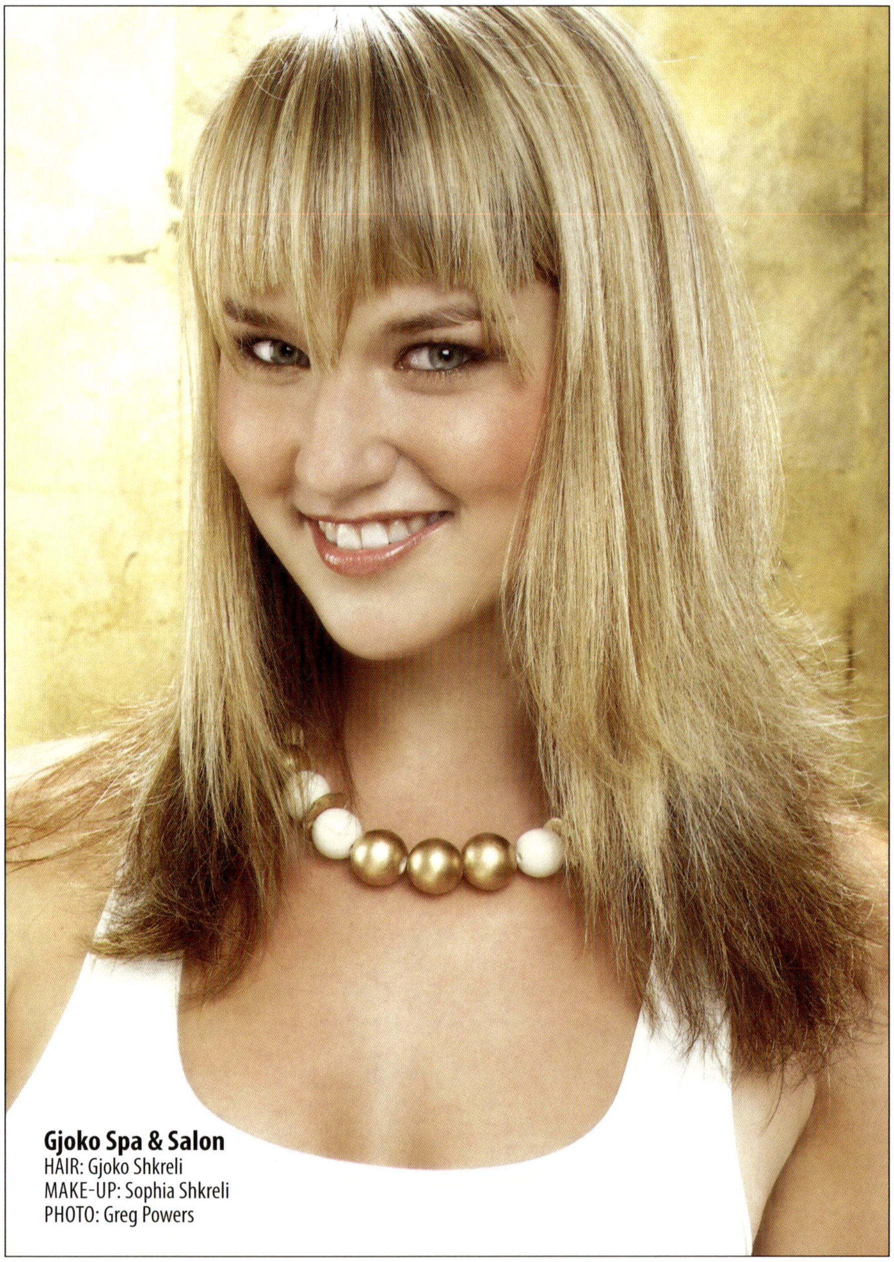

**Gjoko Spa & Salon**
HAIR: Gjoko Shkreli
MAKE-UP: Sophia Shkreli
PHOTO: Greg Powers

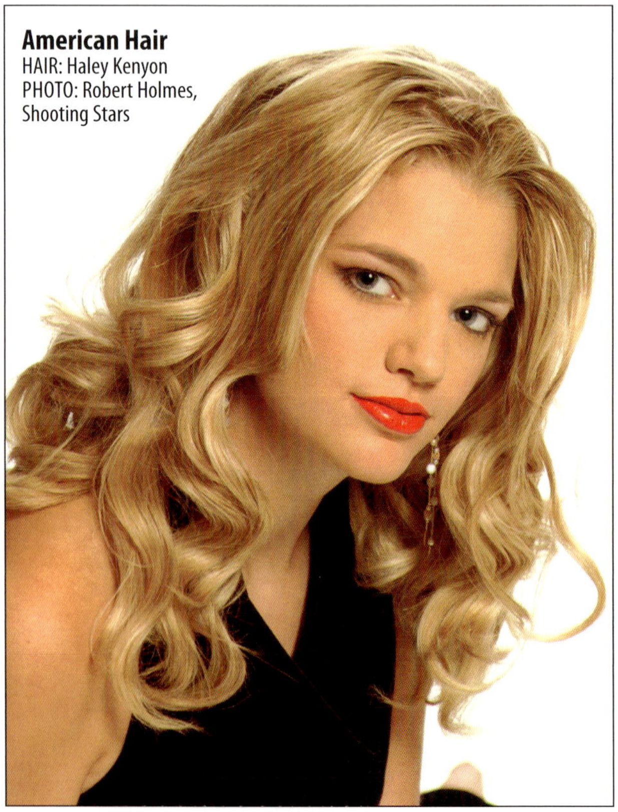

**American Hair**
HAIR: Haley Kenyon
PHOTO: Robert Holmes, Shooting Stars

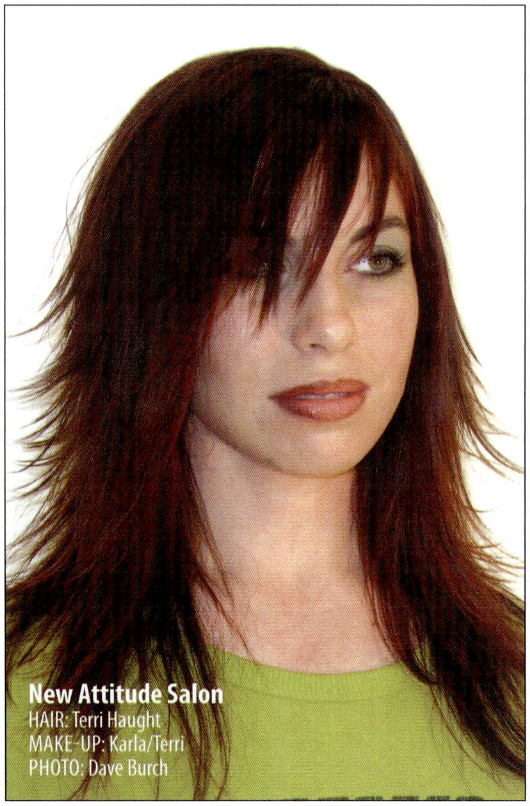

**New Attitude Salon**
HAIR: Terri Haught
MAKE-UP: Karla/Terri
PHOTO: Dave Burch

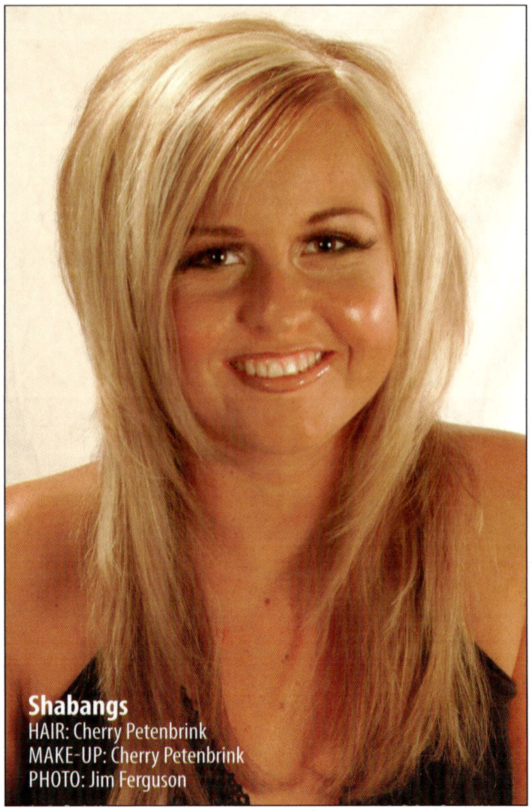

**Shabangs**
HAIR: Cherry Petenbrink
MAKE-UP: Cherry Petenbrink
PHOTO: Jim Ferguson

**Gjoko Spa & Salon**
HAIR: Gjoko Shkreli
MAKE-UP: Sophia Shkreli
PHOTO: Greg Powers

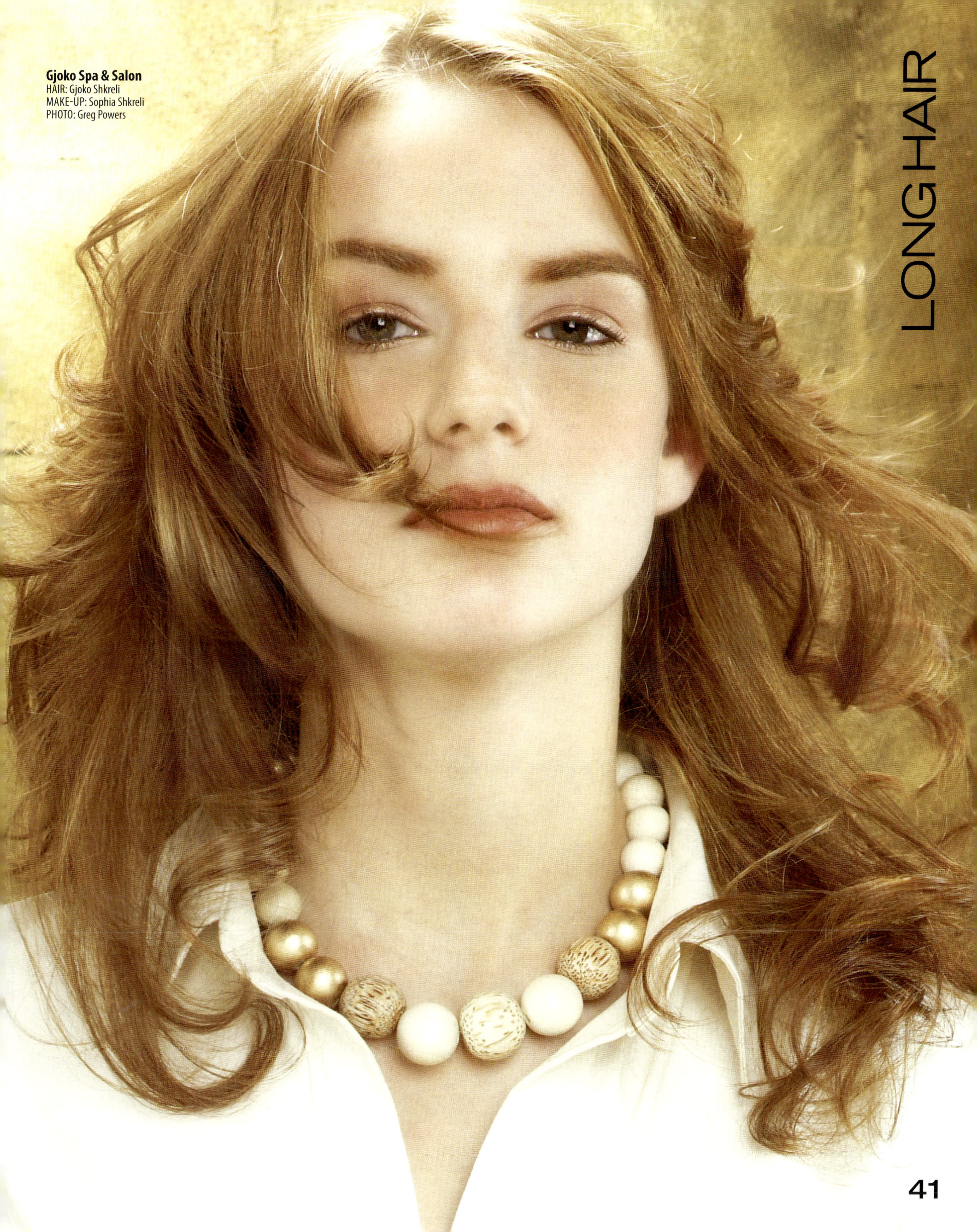

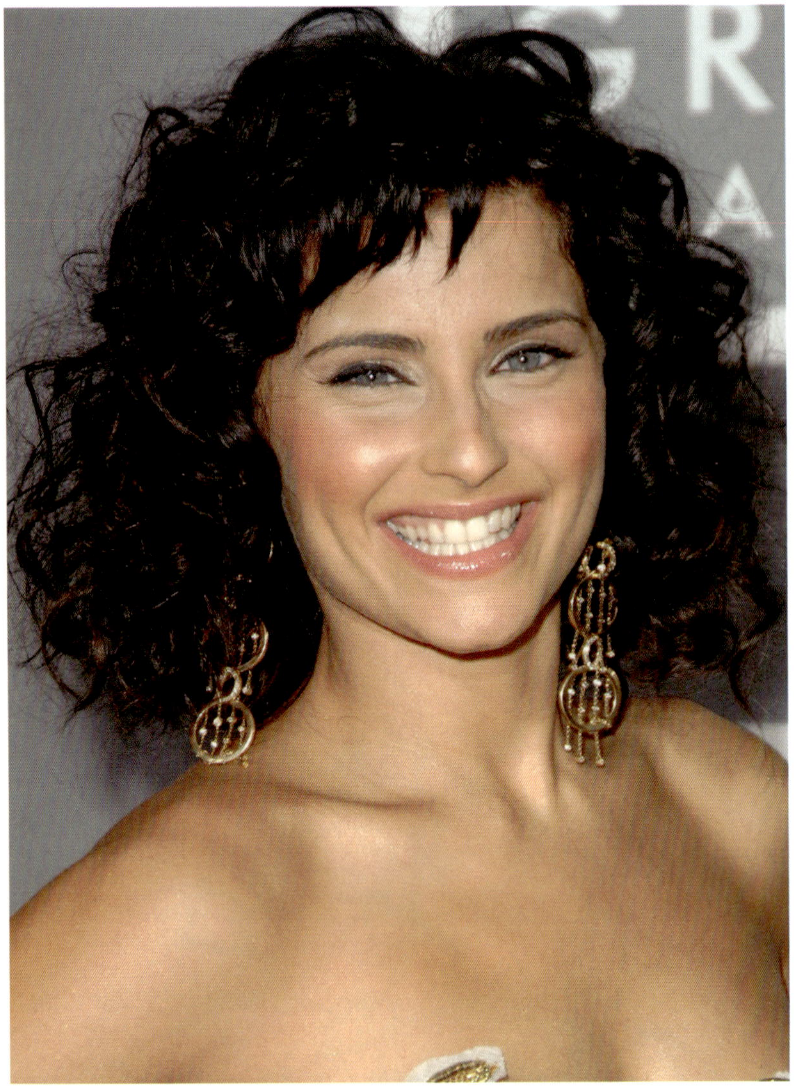

**Nelly Furtado**
PHOTO: Jon Kopaloff/FilmMagic.co

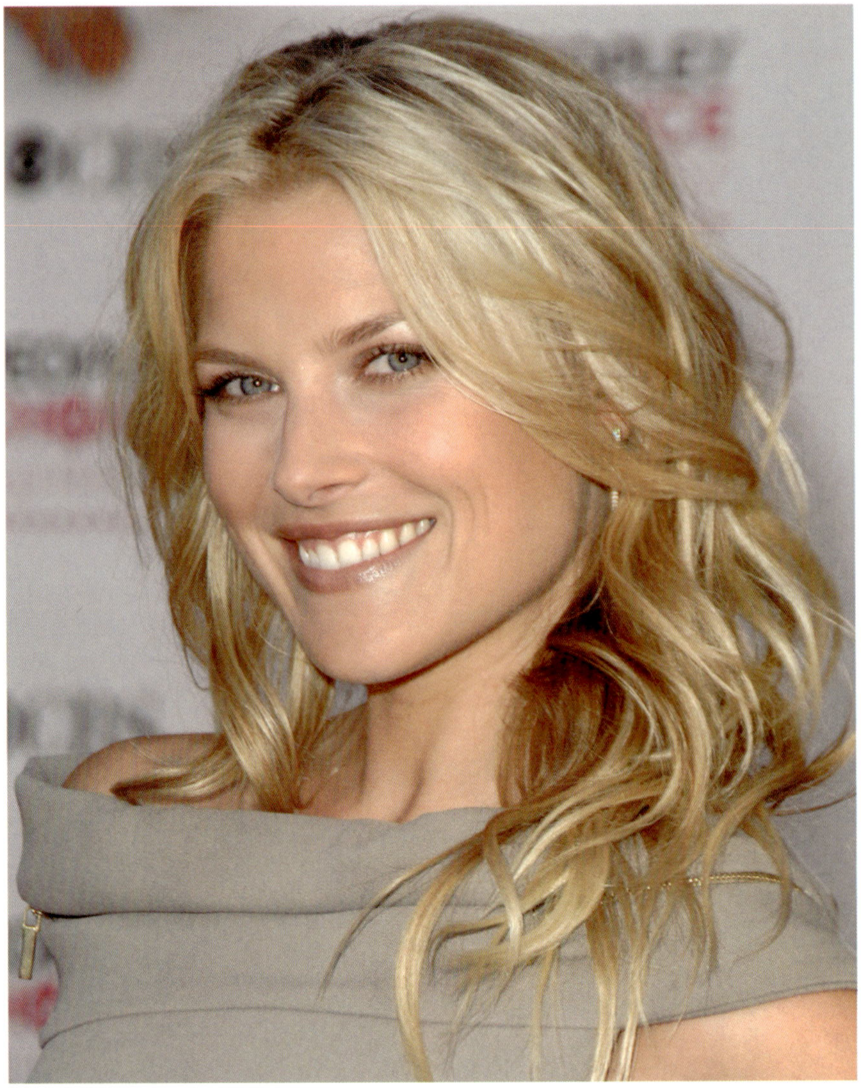

**Ali Larter**
PHOTO: Jon Kopaloff/FilmMagic.com

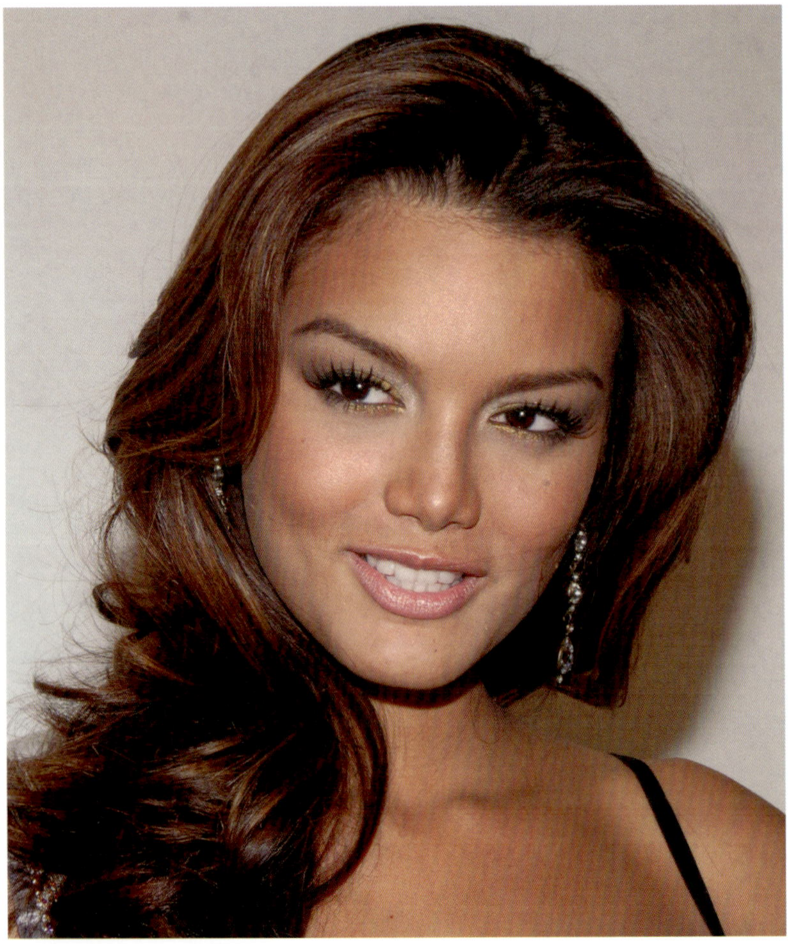

**Miss Universe Zuleyka Rivera**
PHOTO: Michael Loccisano/FilmMagic.com

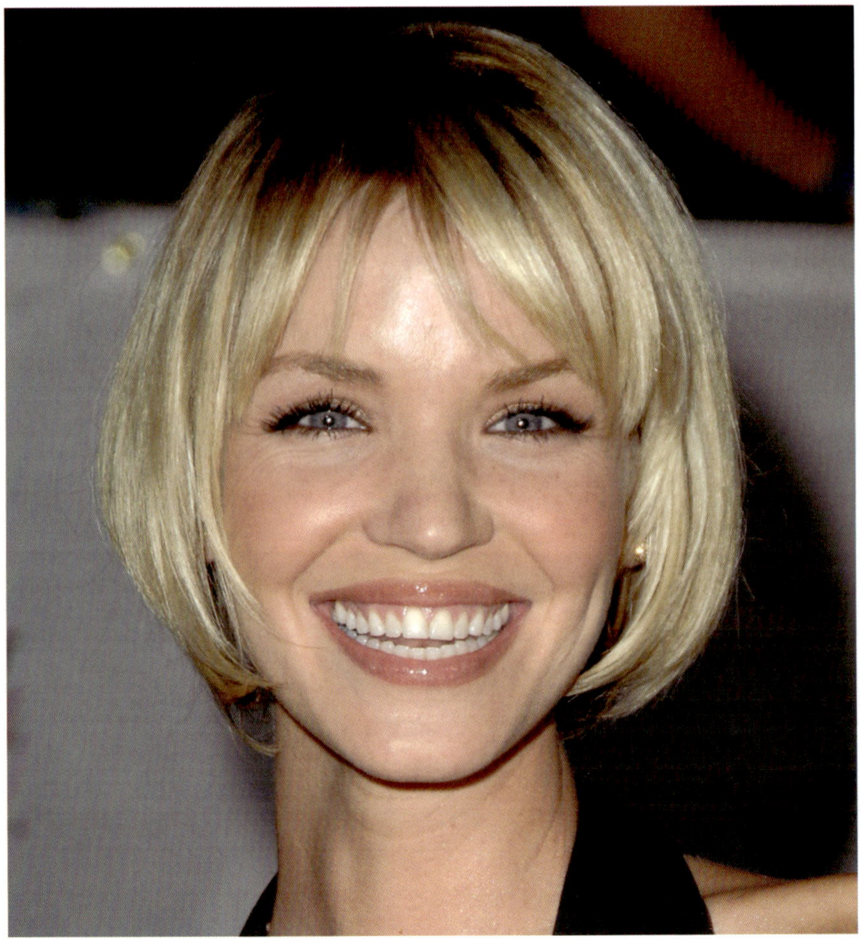

**Ashley Scott**
PHOTO: Jon Kopaloff/FilmMagic.com

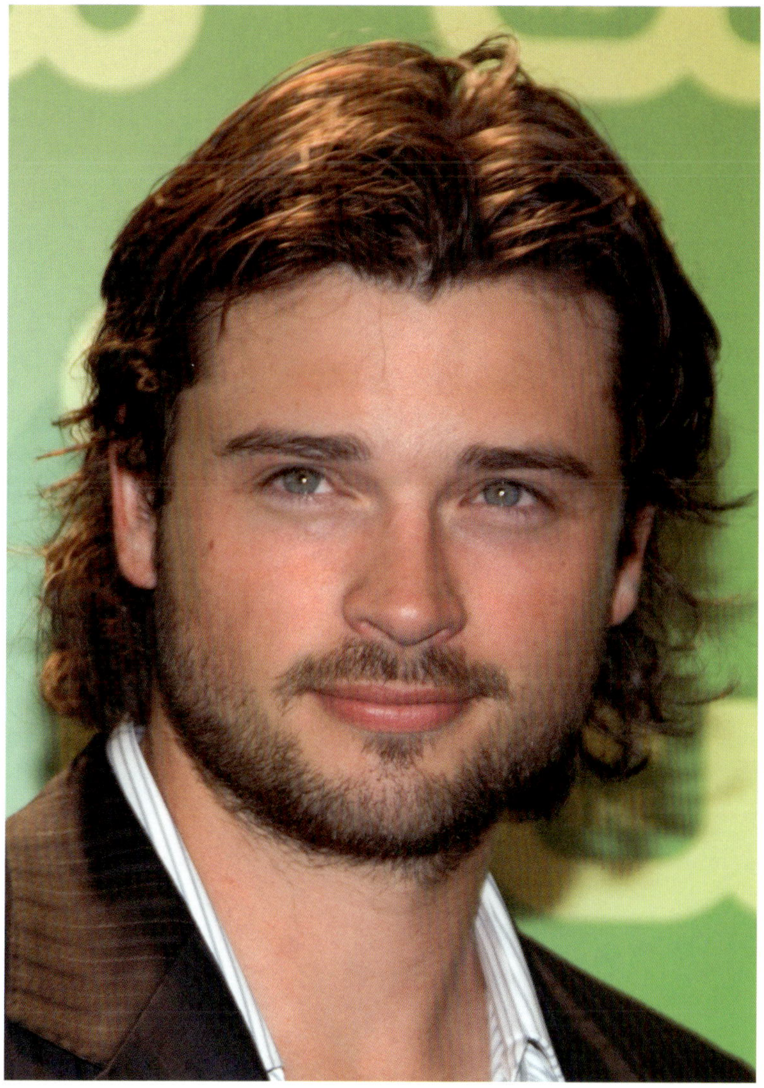

**Tom Welling**
PHOTO: Lawrence Lucier/FilmMagic.com

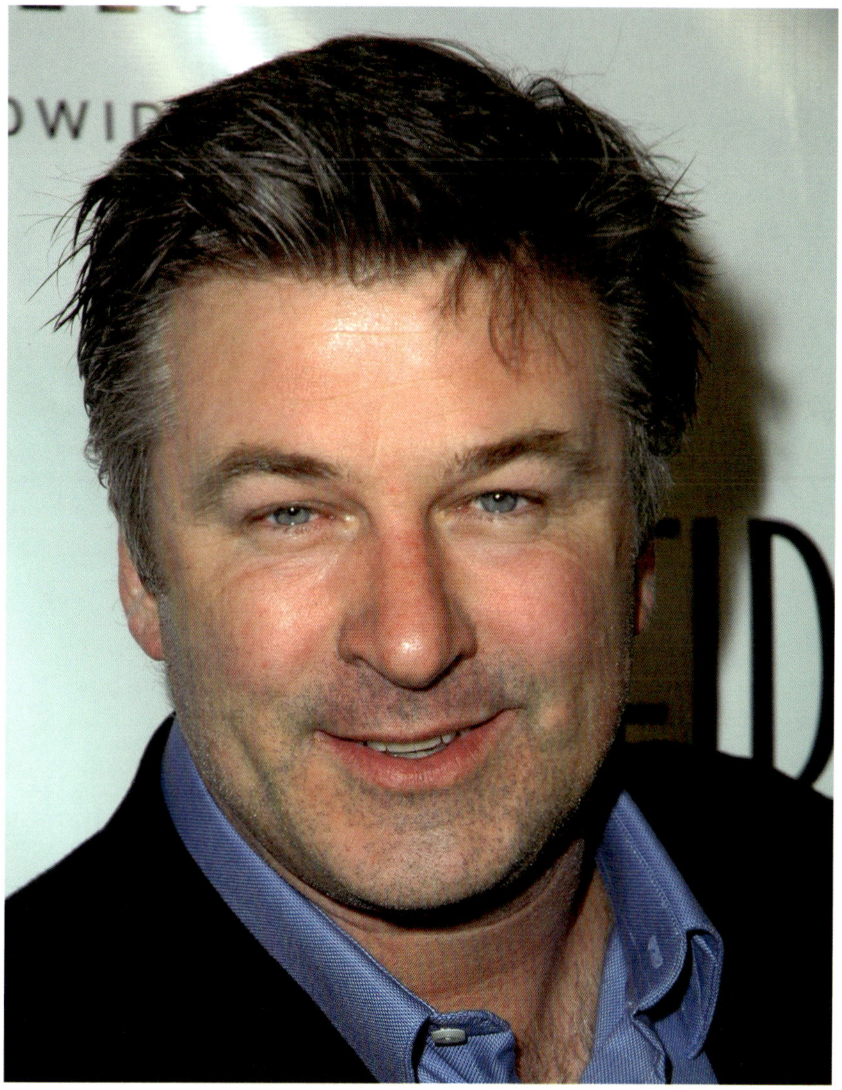

**Alec Baldwin**
PHOTO: Brandi Pettijohn/FilmMagic.com

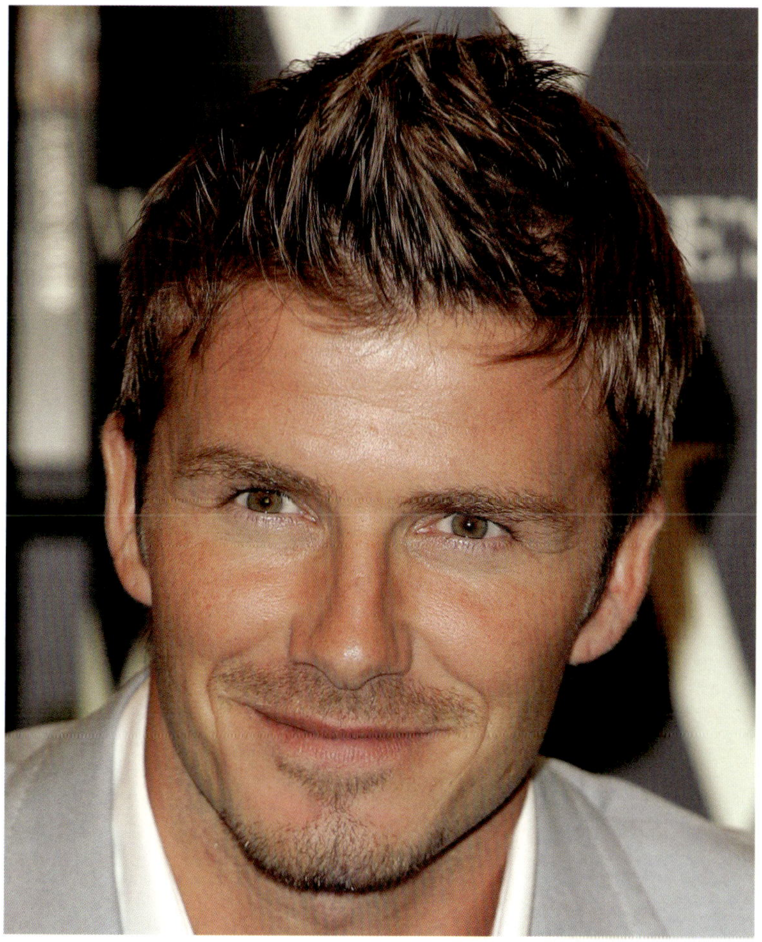

**David Beckham**
PHOTO: Fred Duval/FilmMagic.com

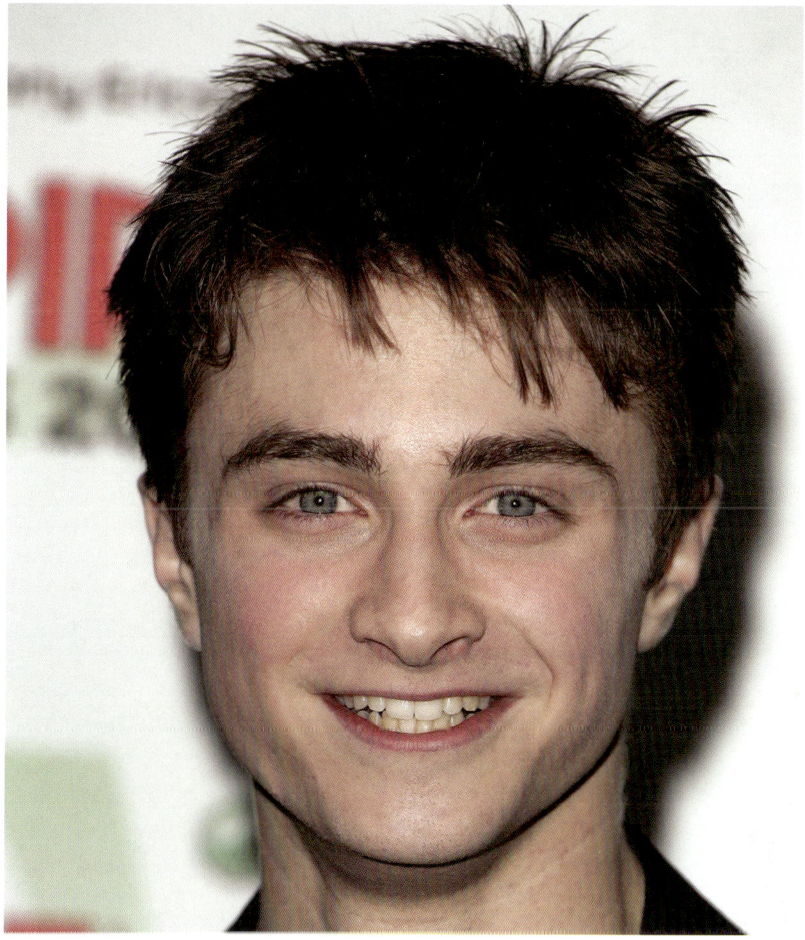

**Daniel Radcliffe**
PHOTO: Fred Duval/FilmMagic.com

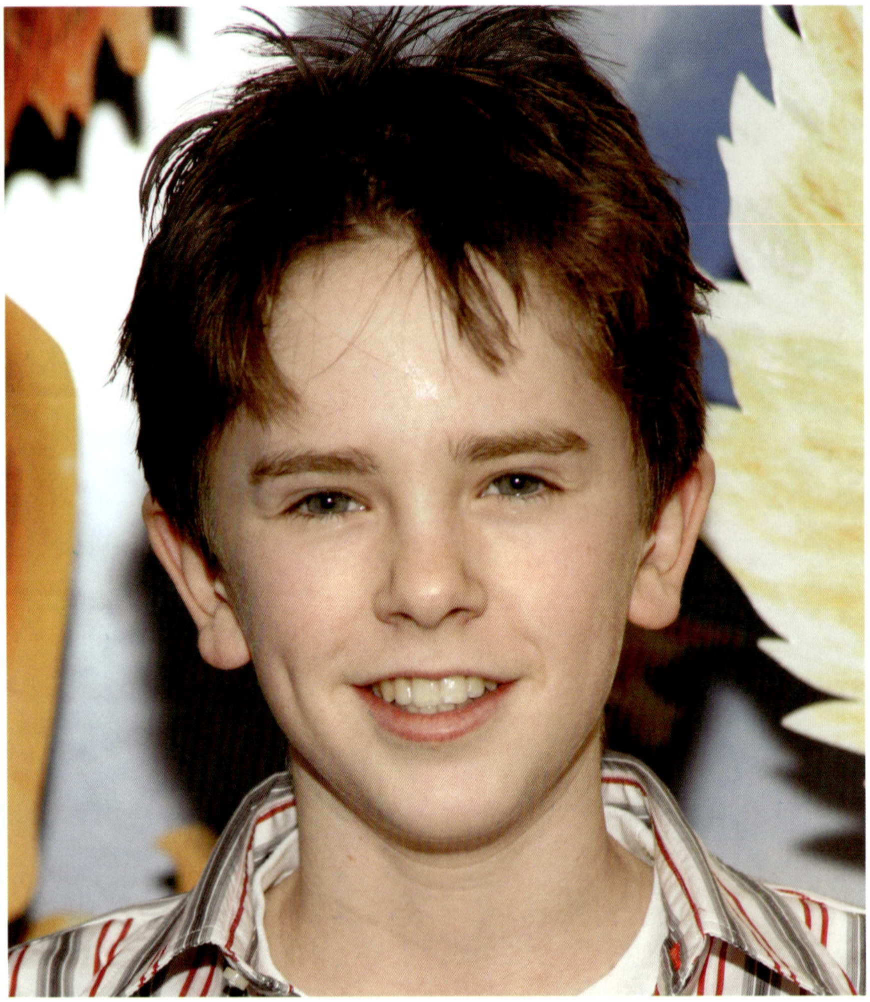

**Freddie Highmore**
PHOTO: Sylvian Gaboury/FilmMagic.com

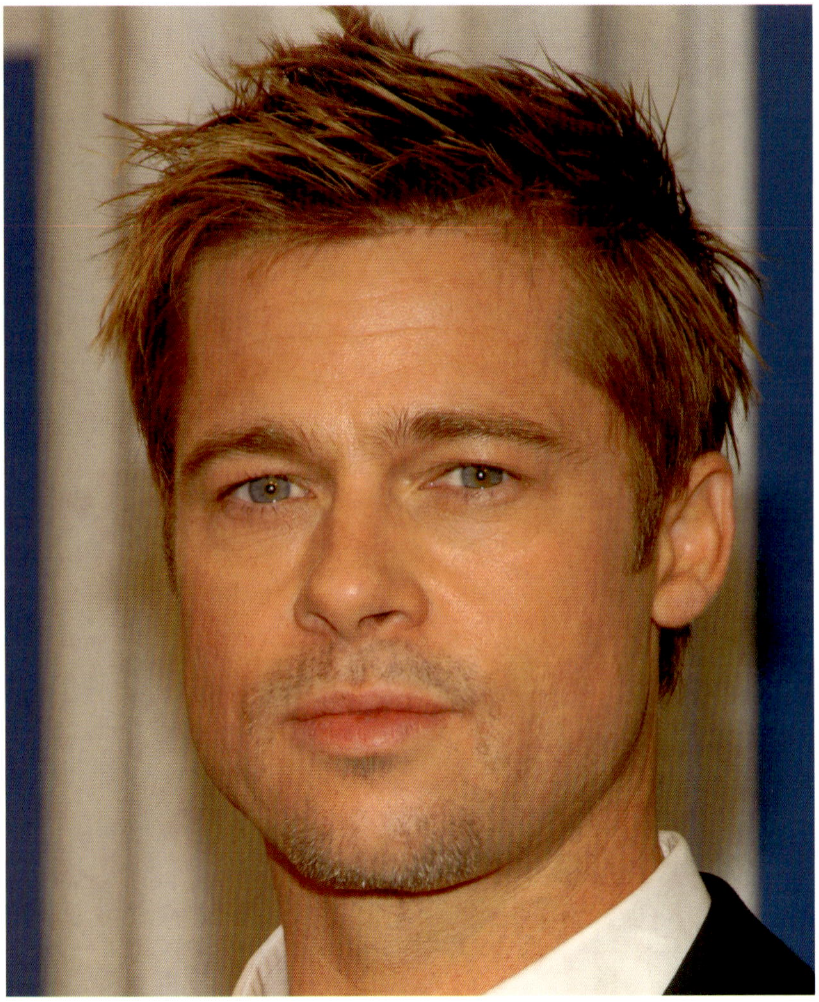

**Brad Pitt**
PHOTO: Michael Tompkins/FilmMagic.com

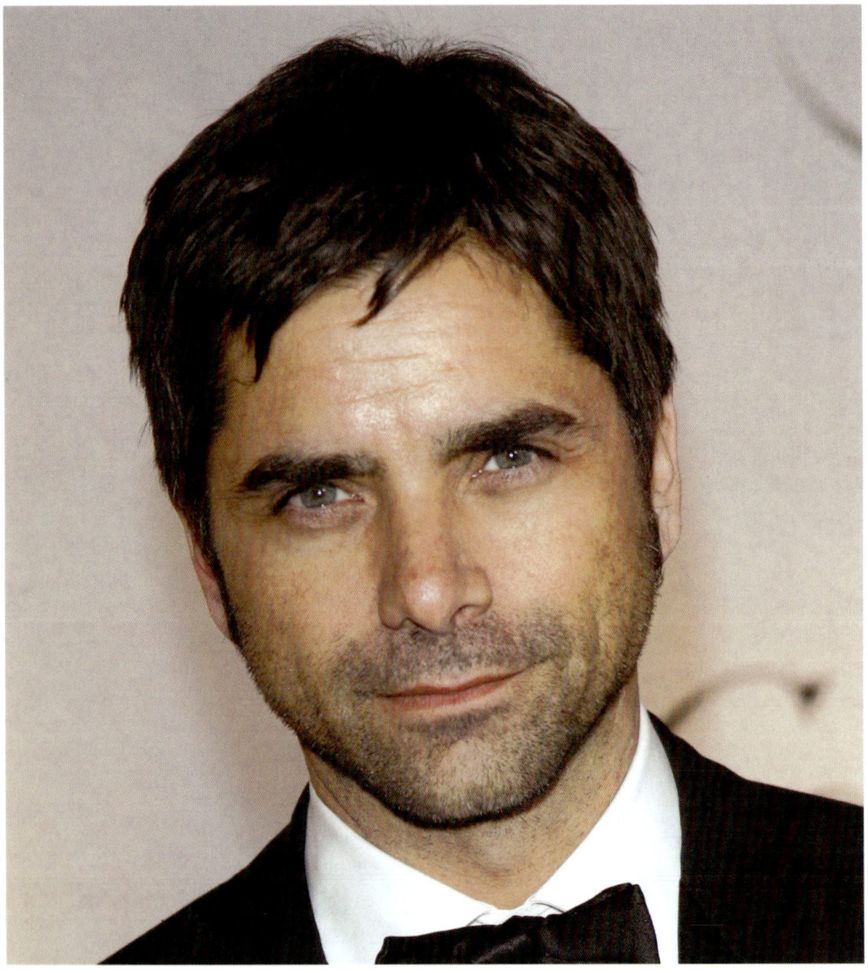

**John Stamos**
PHOTO: Michael Tran/FilmMagic.com

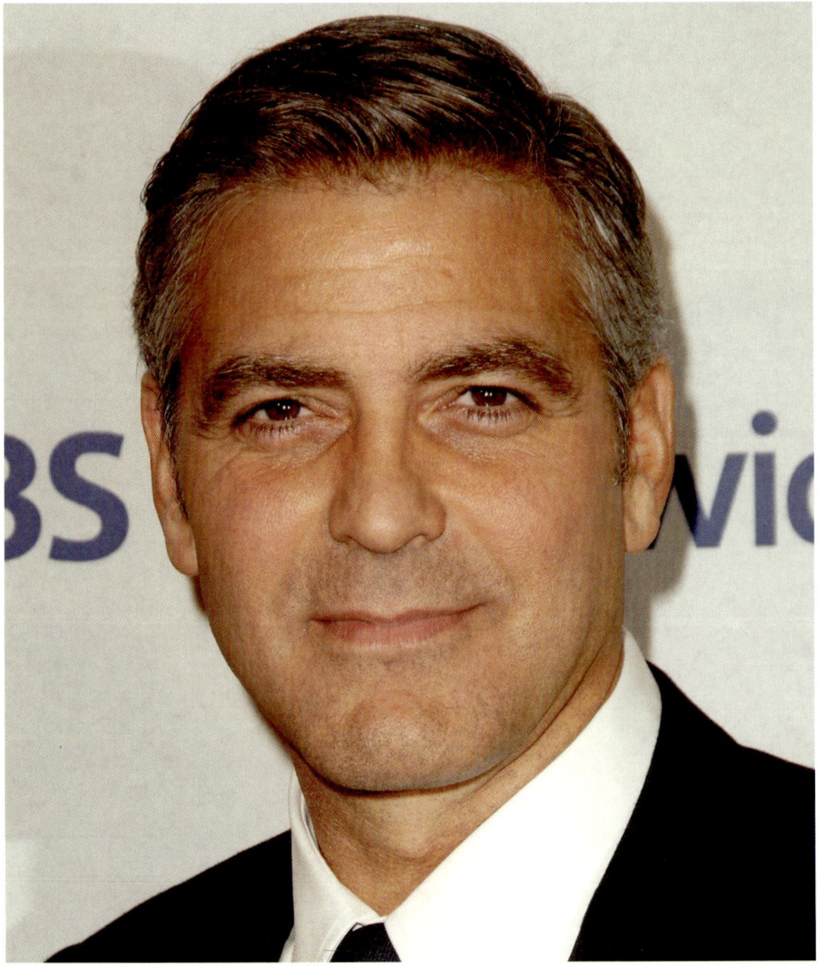


**George Clooney**
PHOTO: Jon Kopaloff/FilmMagic.com

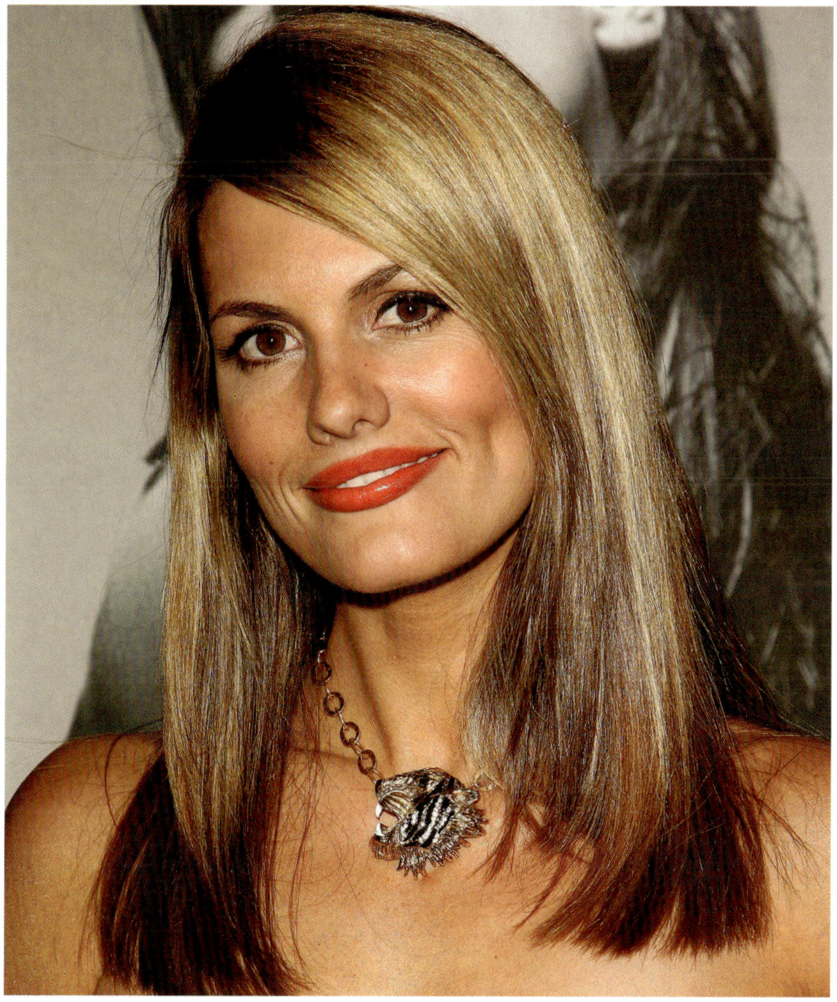

**Courtney Hansen**
PHOTO: Jason Merritt/FilmMagic.com

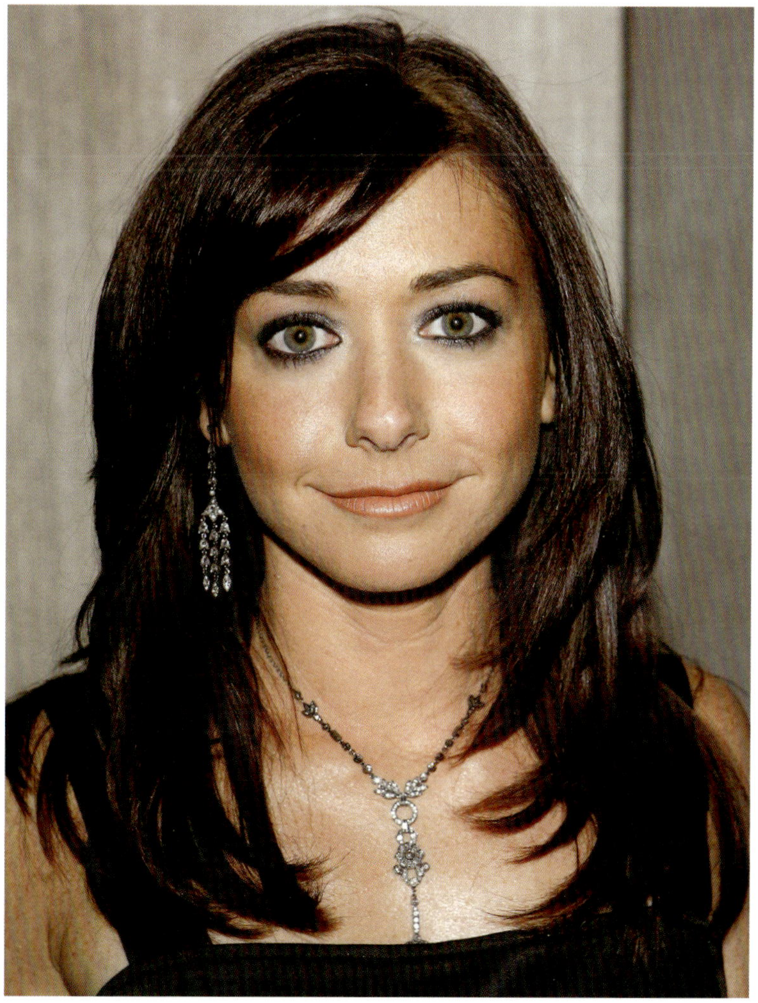

**Alyson Hannigan**
PHOTO: Michael Tran/FilmMagic.com

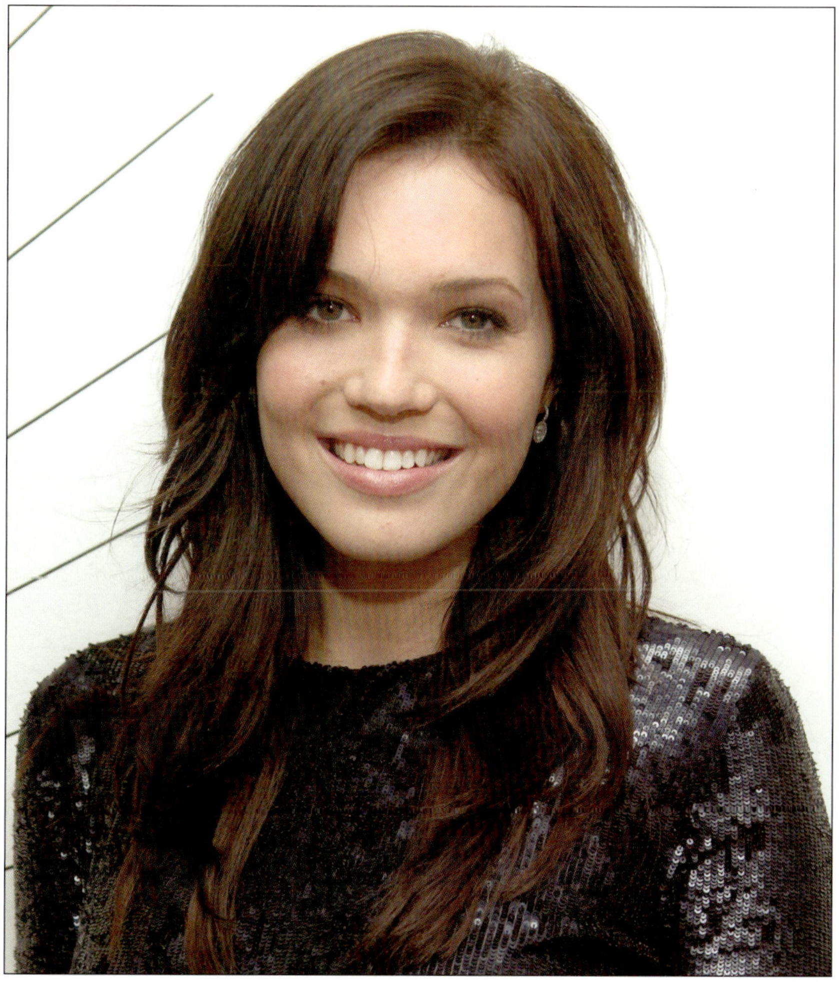

**Mandy Moore**
PHOTO: Michael Loccisano/FilmMagic.com

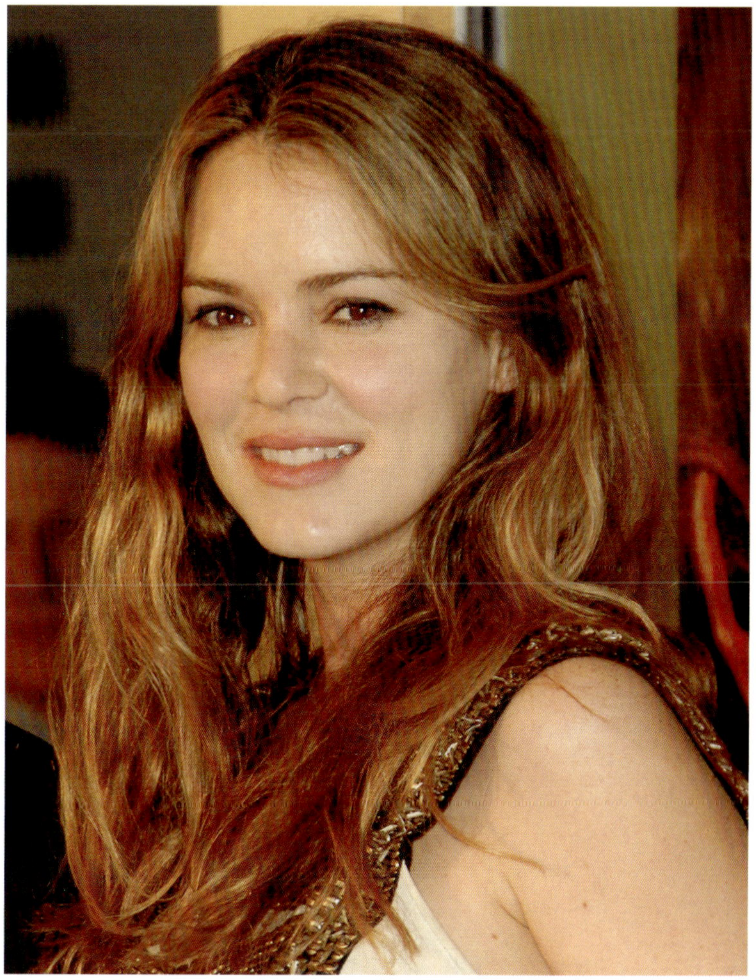

**Jacinda Barrette**
PHOTO: Jon Kopaloff/FilmMagic.com

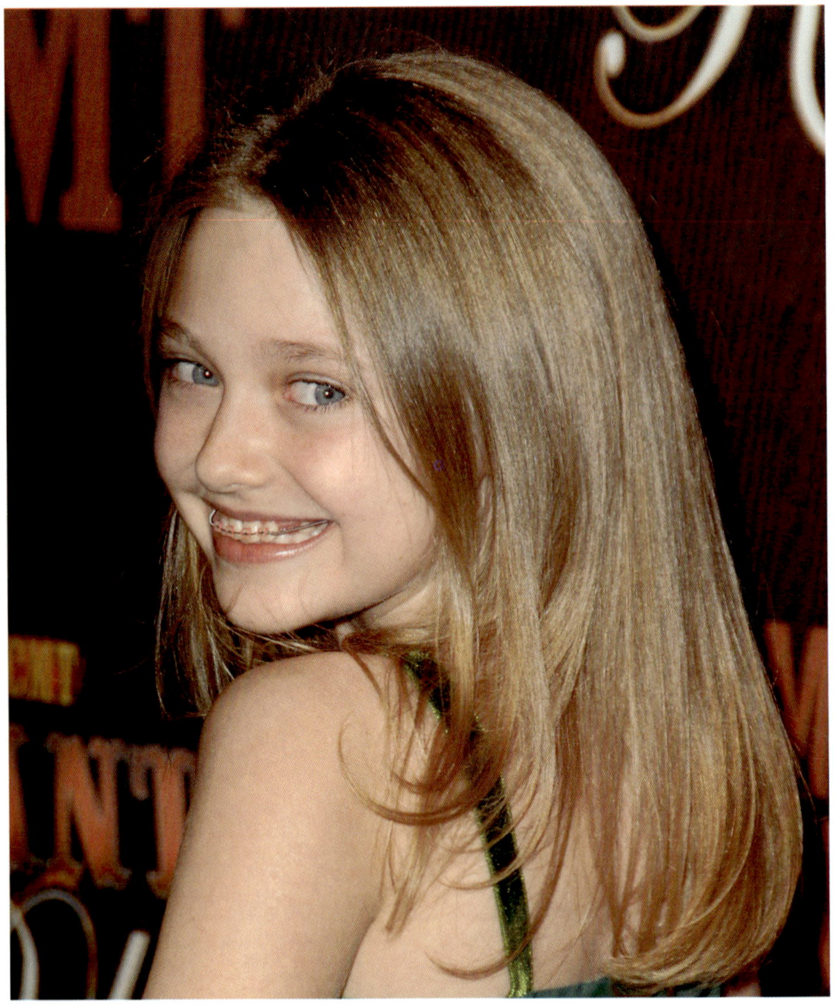

**Dakota Fanning**
PHOTO: Jon Kopaloff/FilmMagic.com

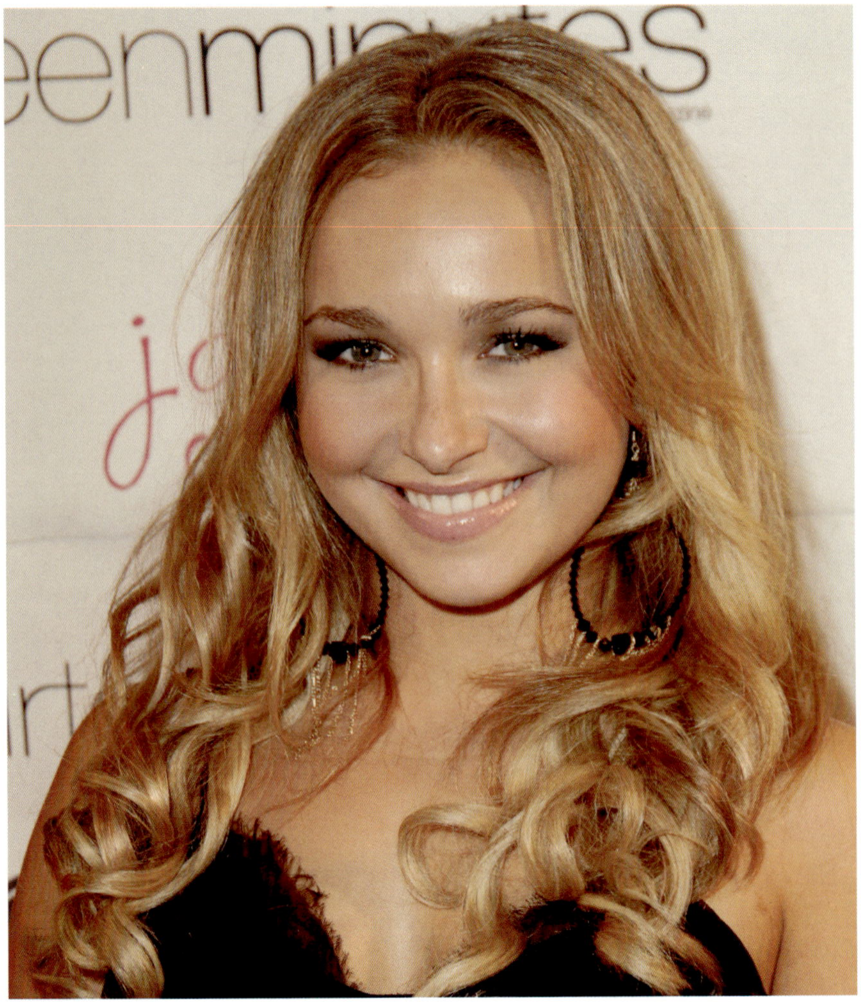

**Hayden Panettiere**
PHOTO: Jon Kopaloff/FilmMagic.com

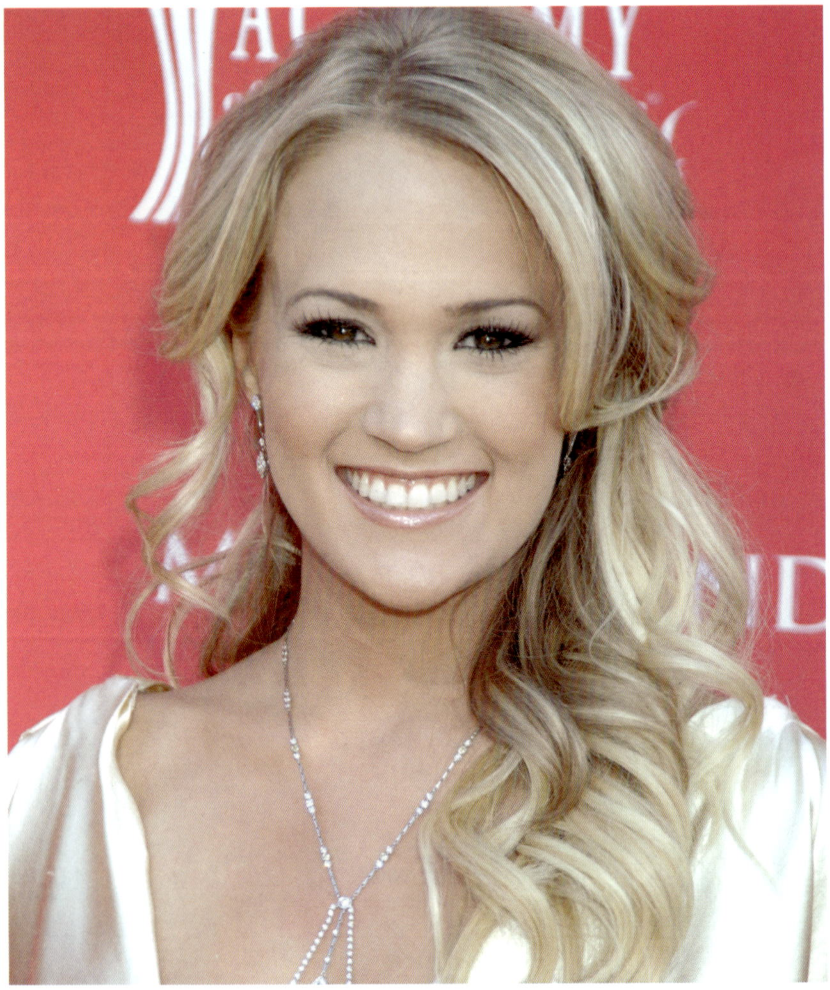

**Carrie Underwood**
PHOTO: Jeff Kravitz/FilmMagic.com

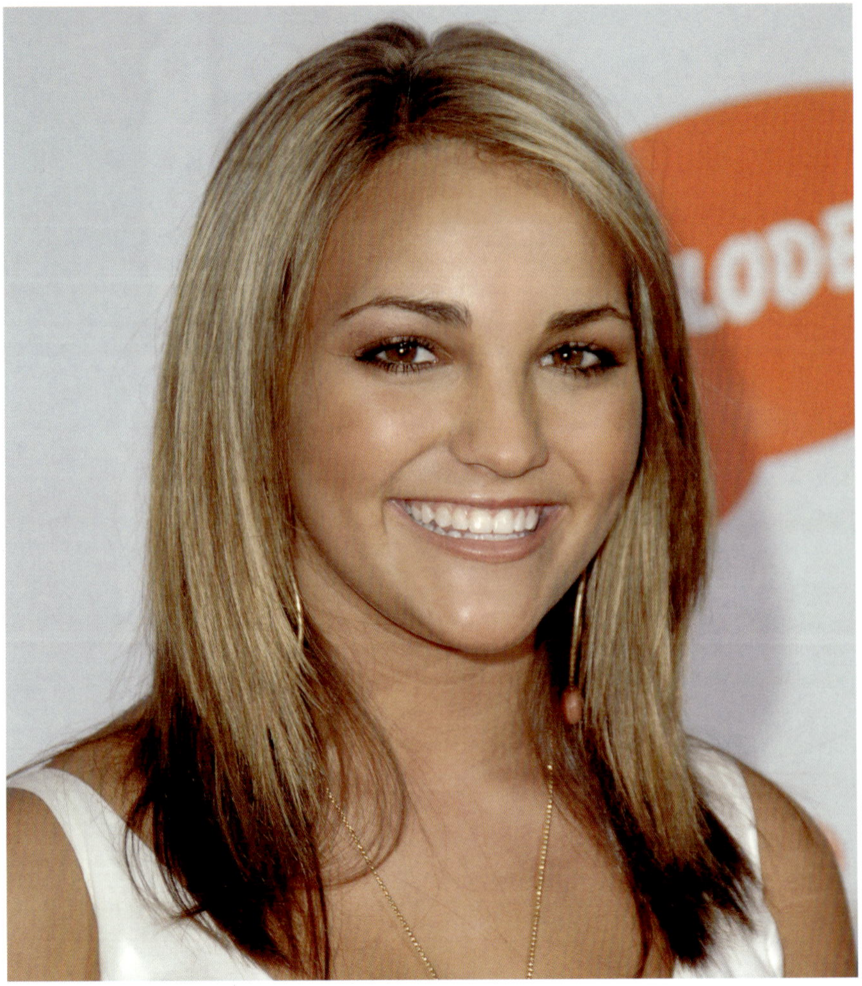

**Jamie Lynn Spears**
PHOTO: John Kopaloff/FilmMagic.com

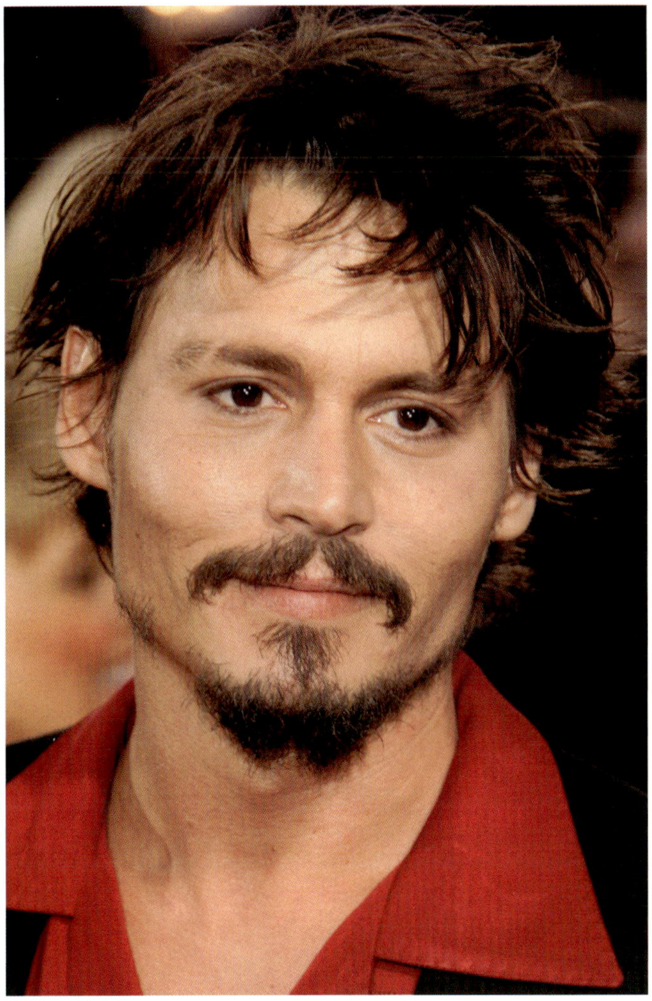

**Johnny Depp**
PHOTO: Tyler Michaels/FilmMagic.com

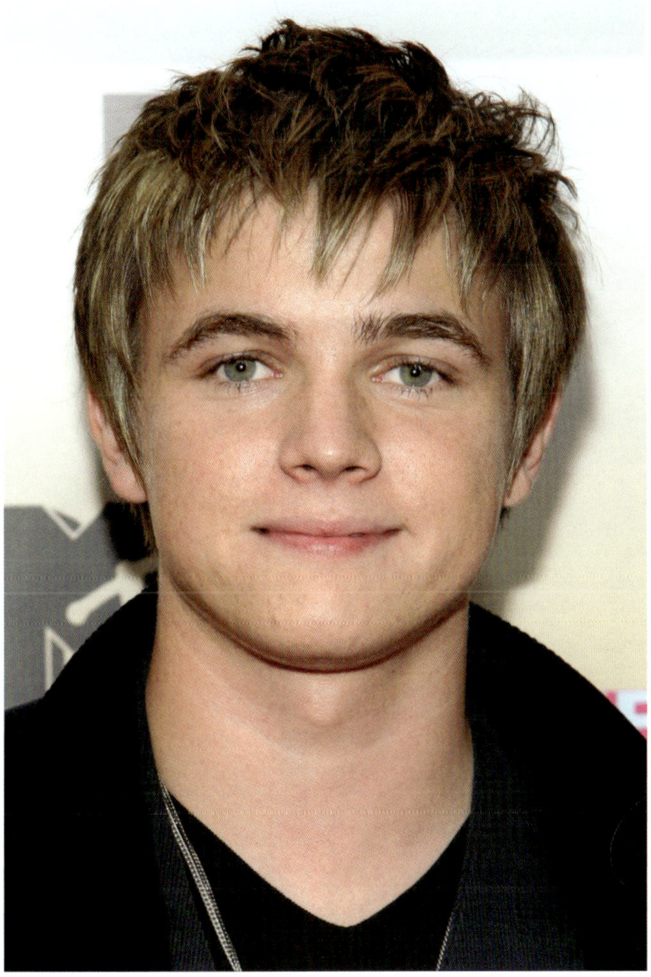

**Jesse McCartney**
PHOTO: Mark Von Holden/FilmMagic.com

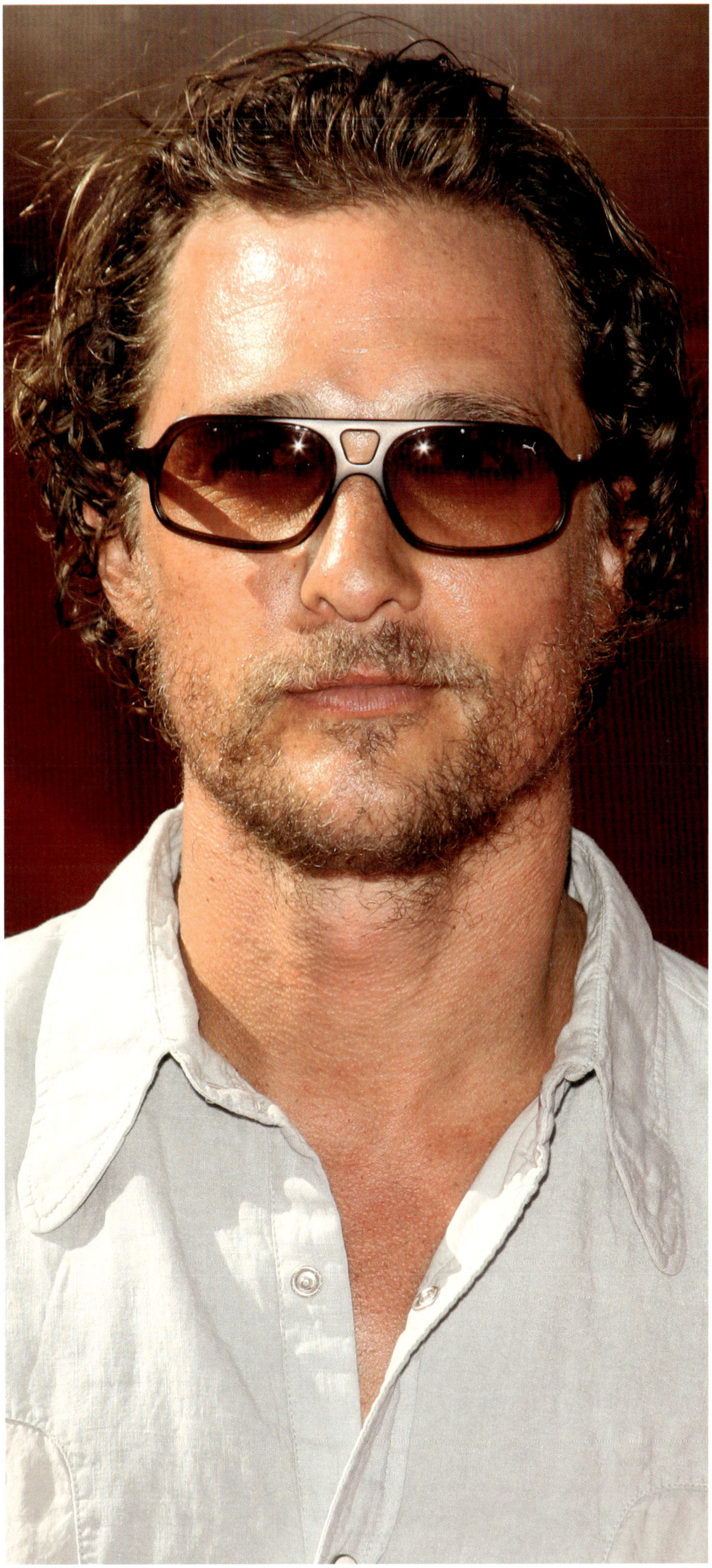

**Matthew McConaughey**
PHOTO: Jason Merritt/FilmMagic.com

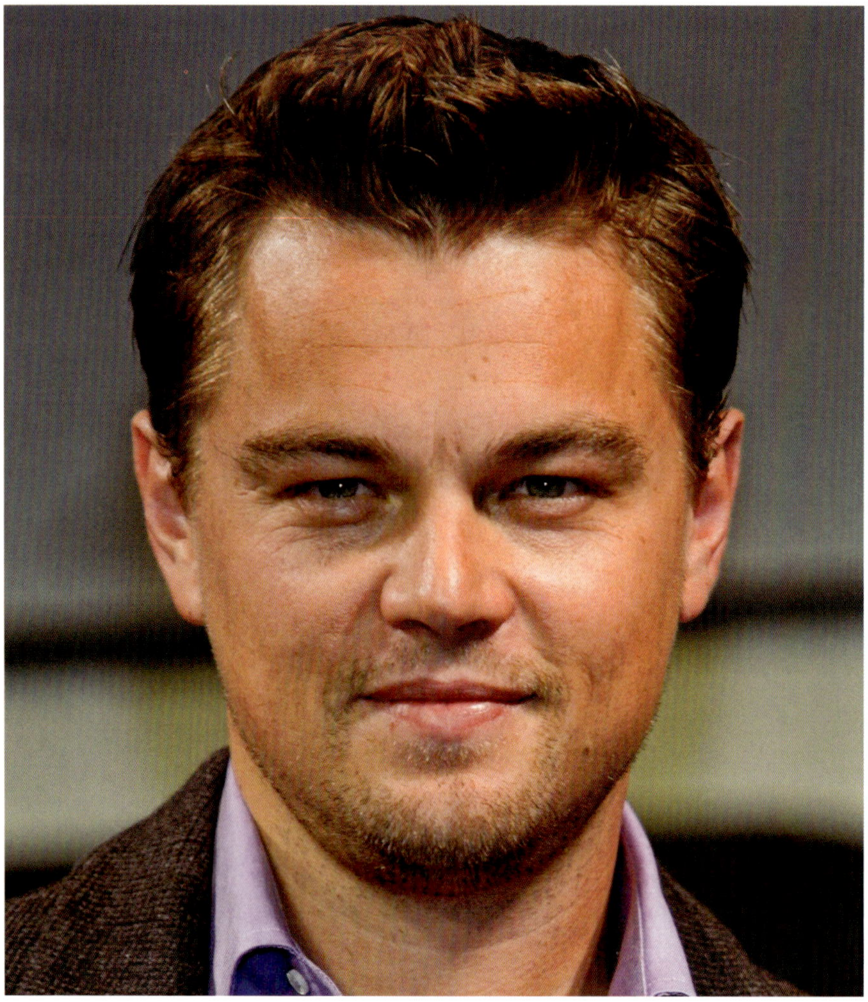

**Leonardo DiCaprio**
PHOTO: JIL Studio/FilmMagic.com

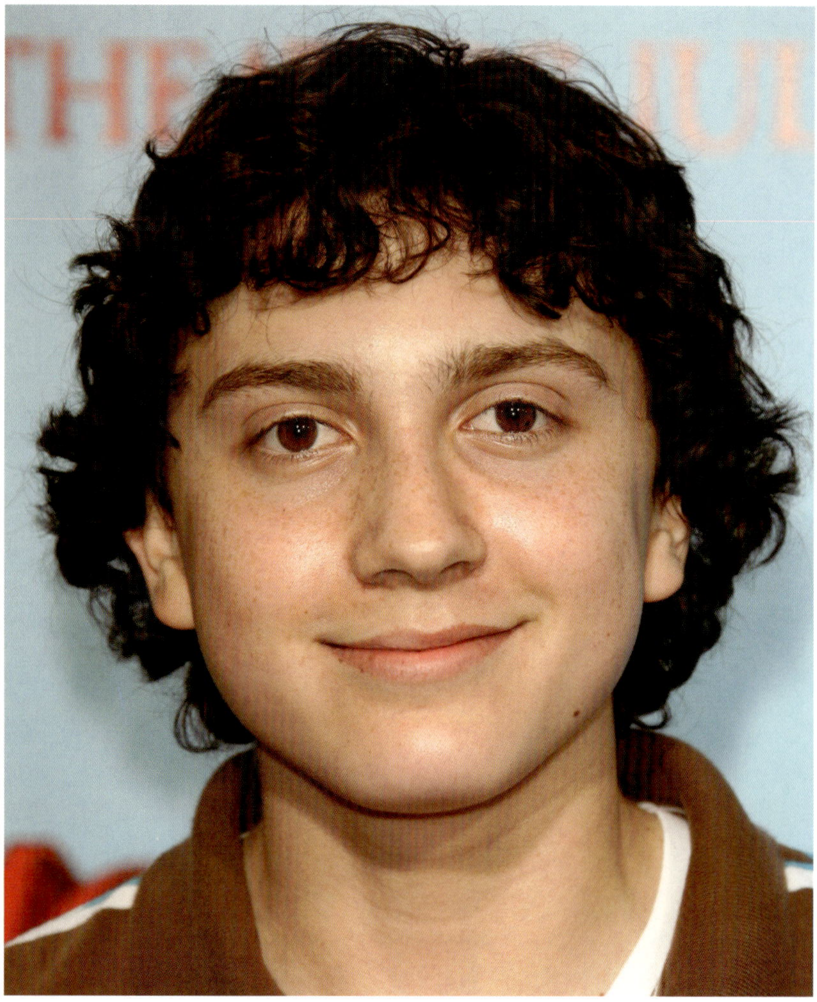

**Daryl Sabara**
PHOTO: Mirek Towski/FilmMagic.com

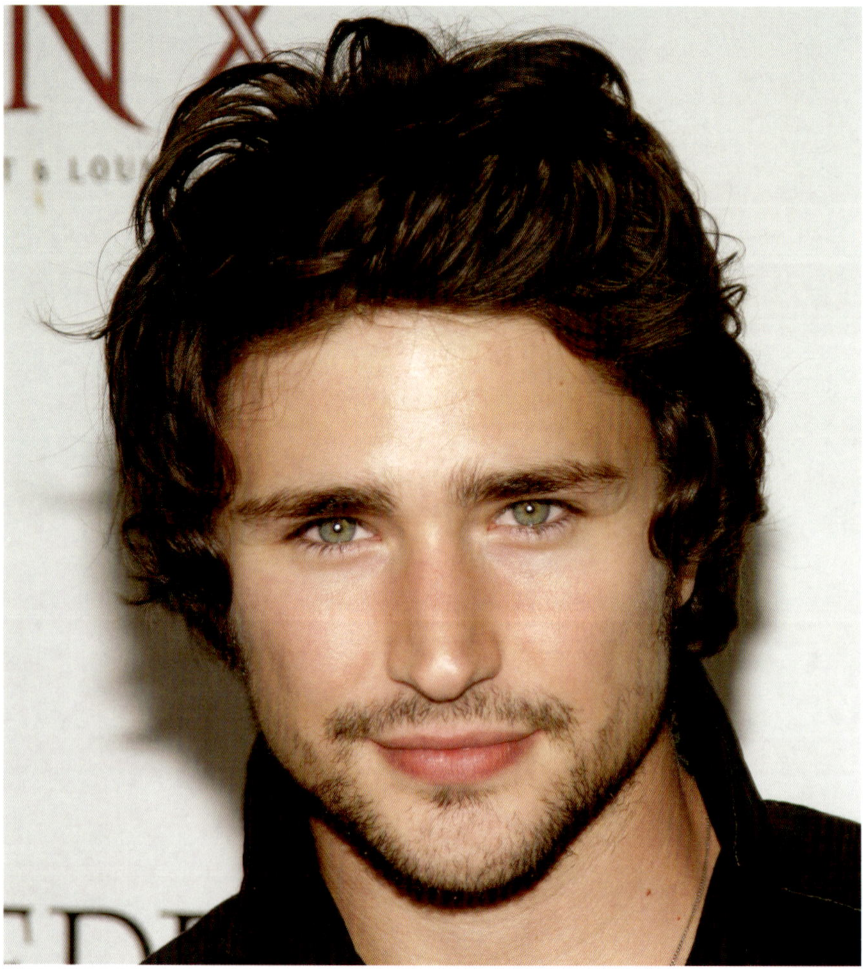

**Matt Dallas**
PHOTO: Michael Tran/FilmMagic.com

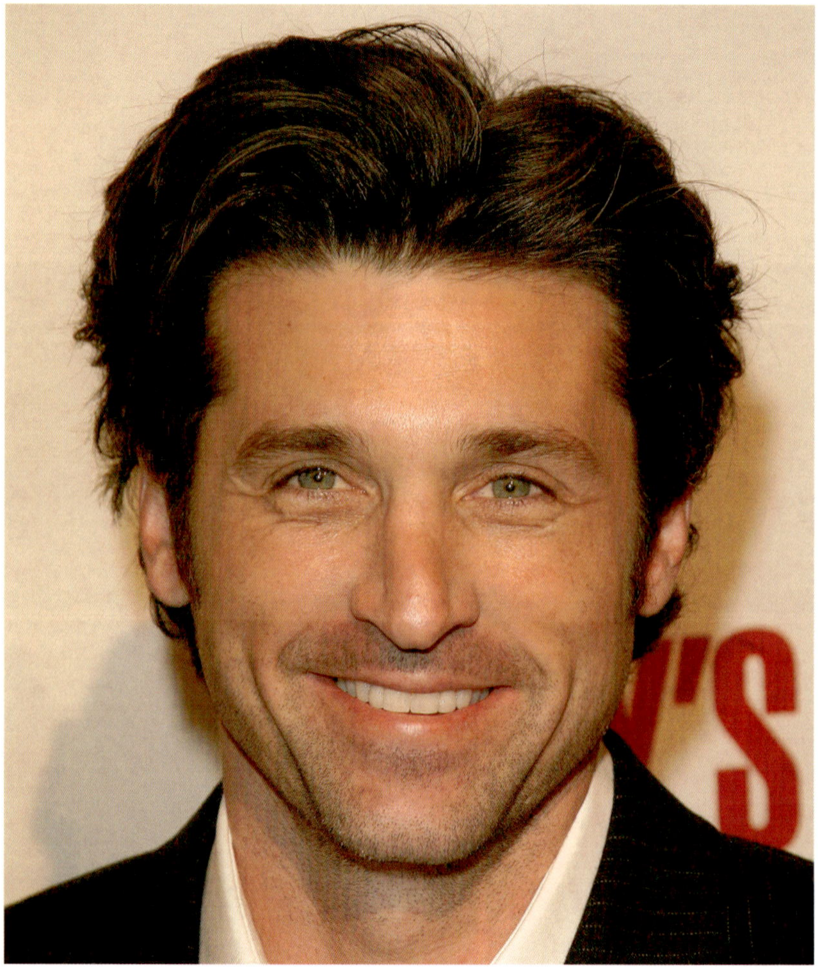

**Patrick Dempsey**
PHOTO: Jason Merritt/FilmMagic.com

**Jeri Ryan**
PHOTO: Jon Kopaloff/FilmMagic.com

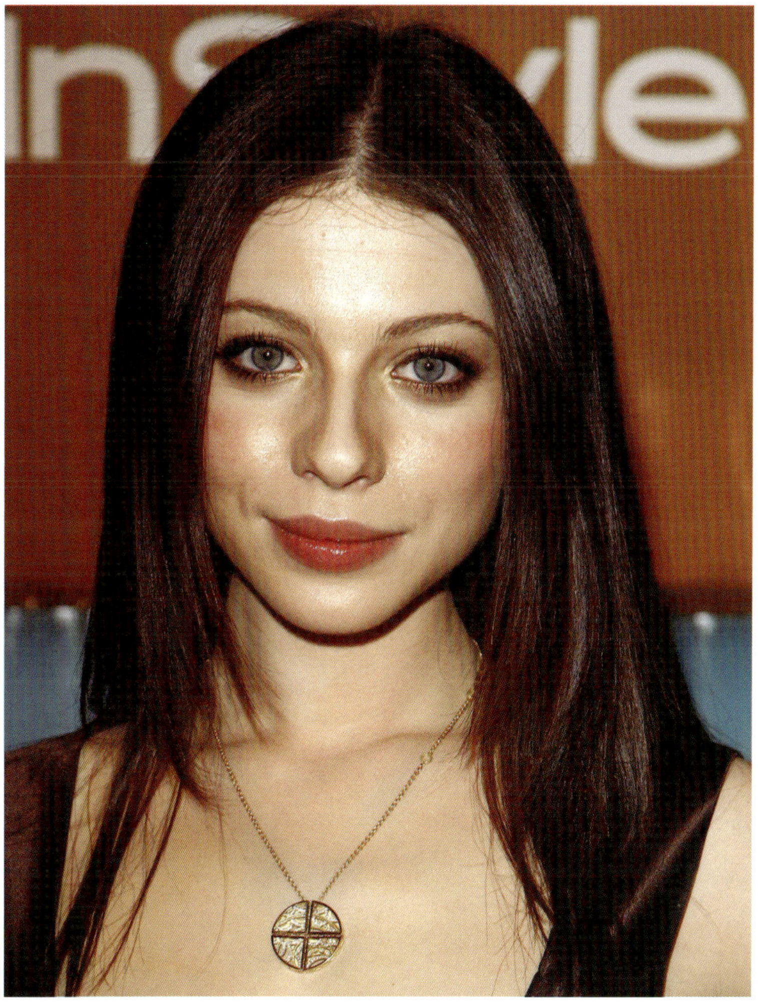

**Michelle Trachtenberg**
PHOTO: Chris Polk/FilmMagic.com

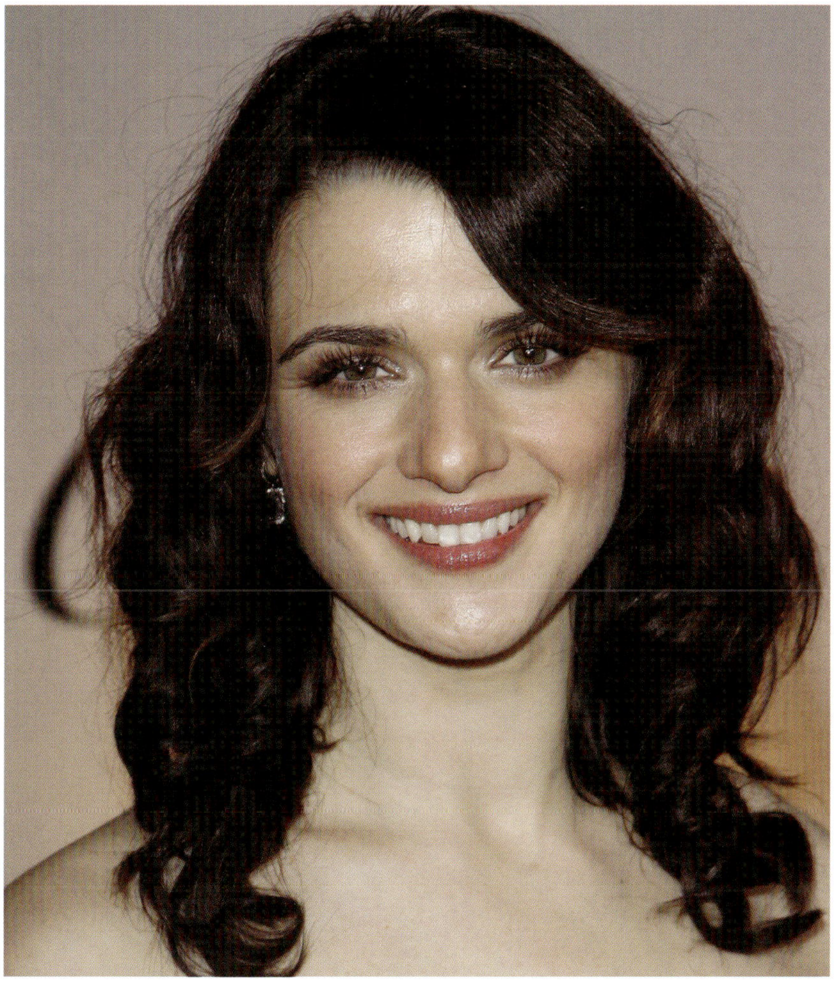

**Rachel Weisz**
PHOTO: Michael Tran/FilmMagic.com

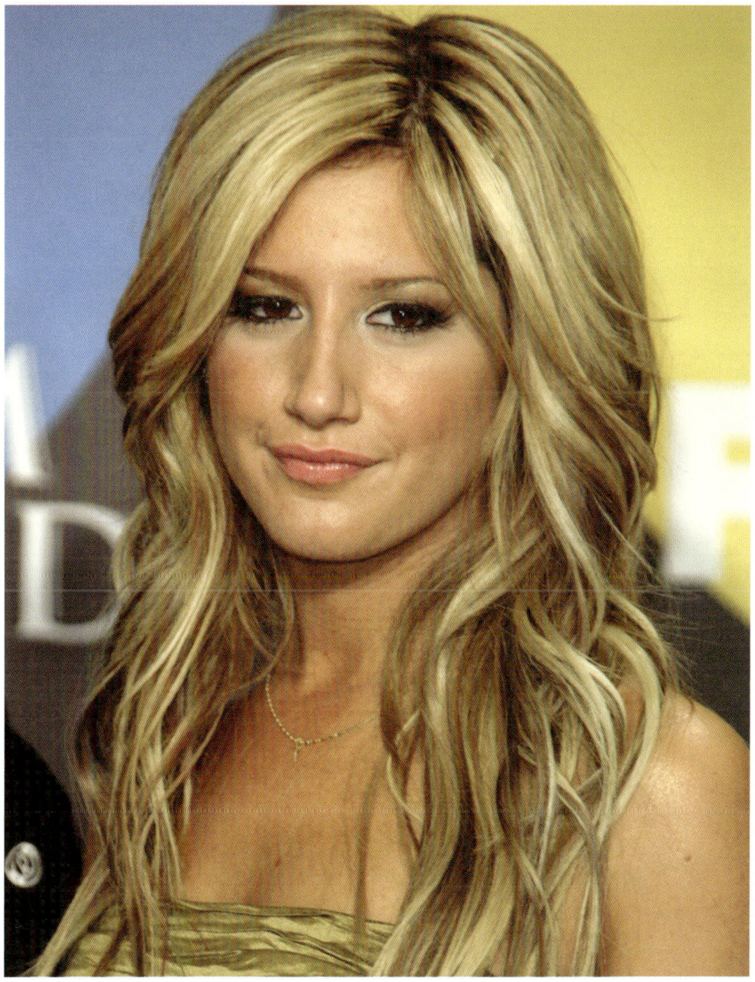

**Ashley Tisdale**
PHOTO: Todd Williamson/FilmMagic.com

**Goldwell**
HAIR: Trend Zoom 06 Team

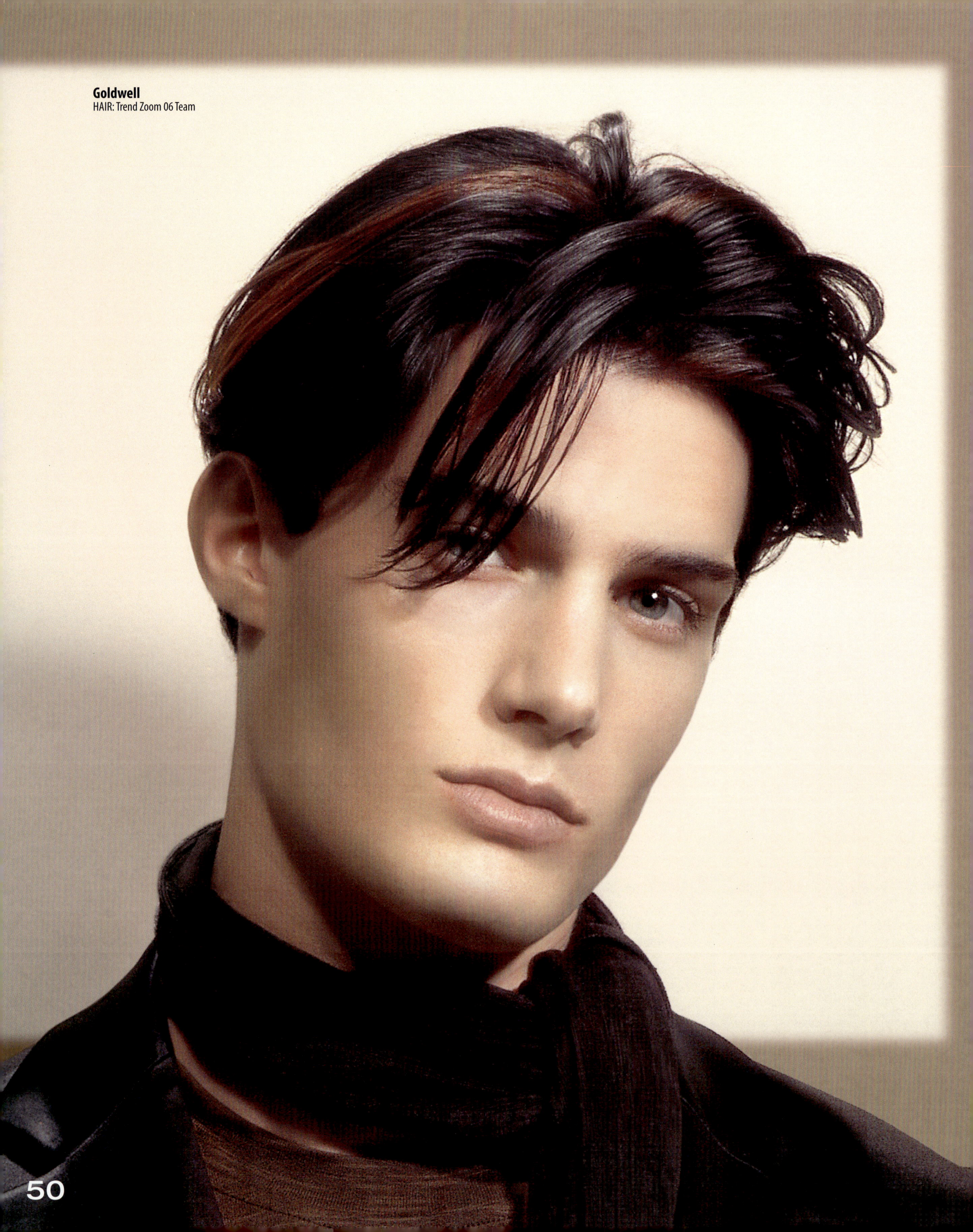

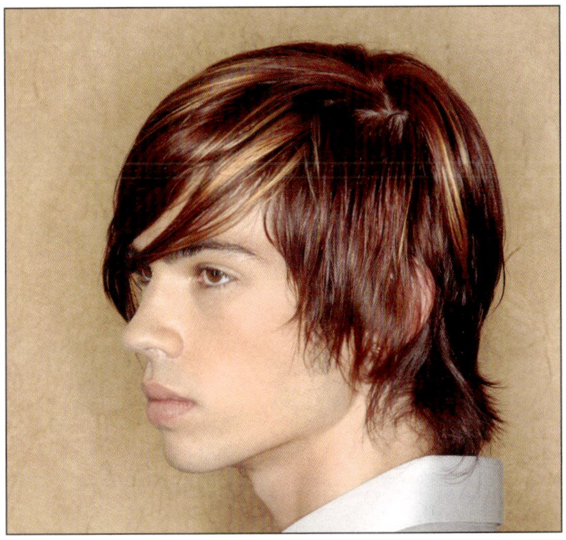

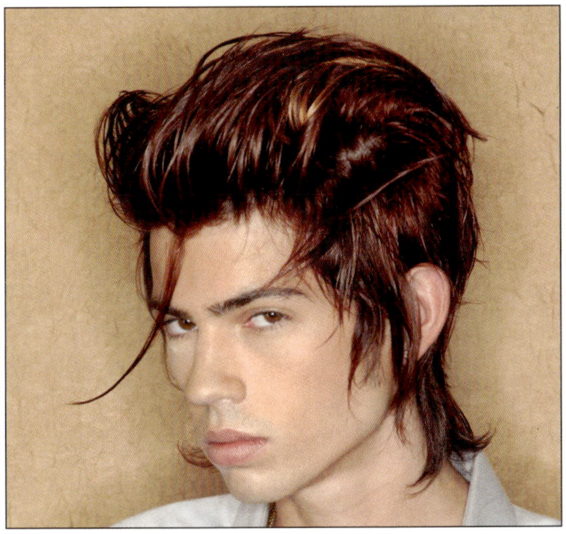

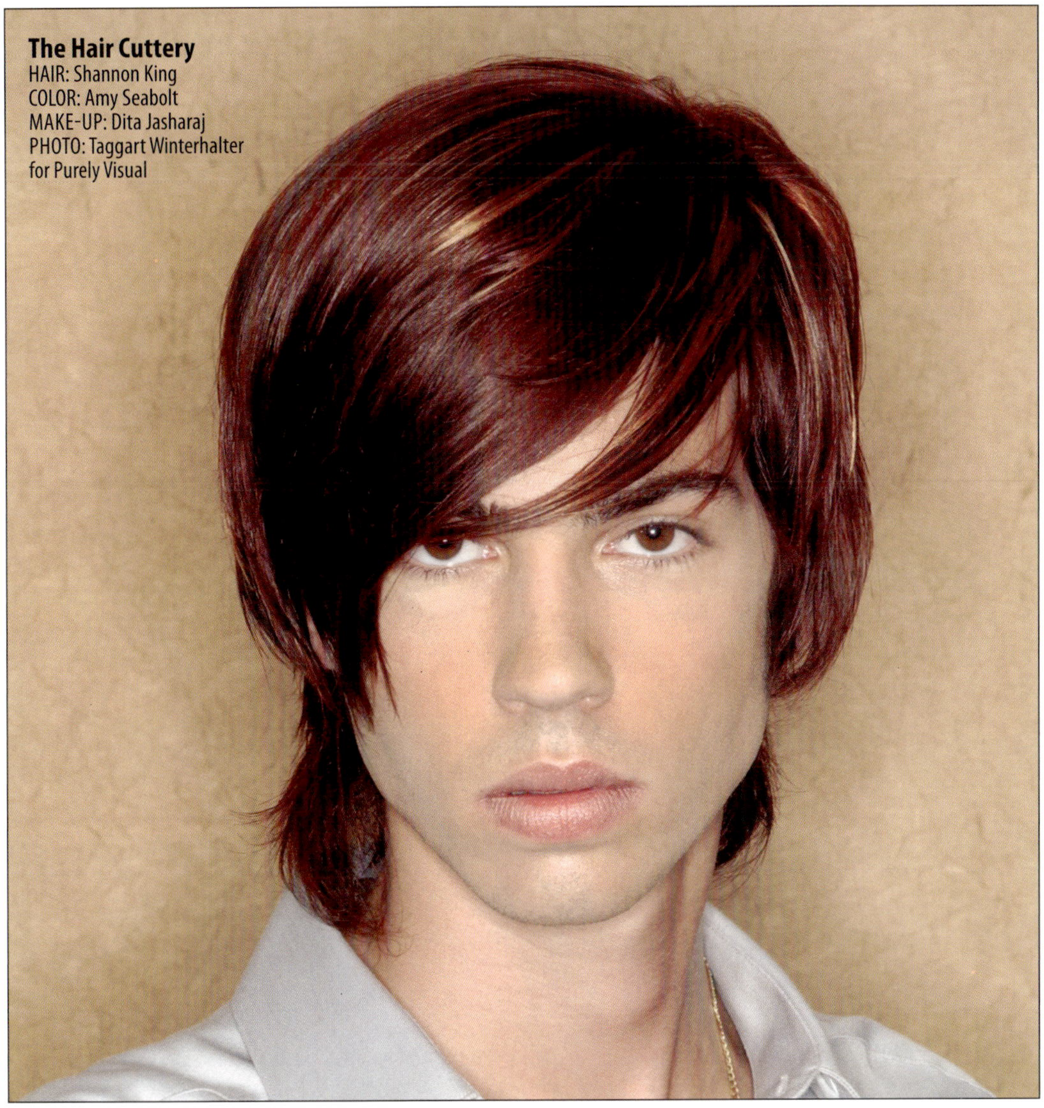

**The Hair Cuttery**
HAIR: Shannon King
COLOR: Amy Seabolt
MAKE-UP: Dita Jasharaj
PHOTO: Taggart Winterhalter for Purely Visual

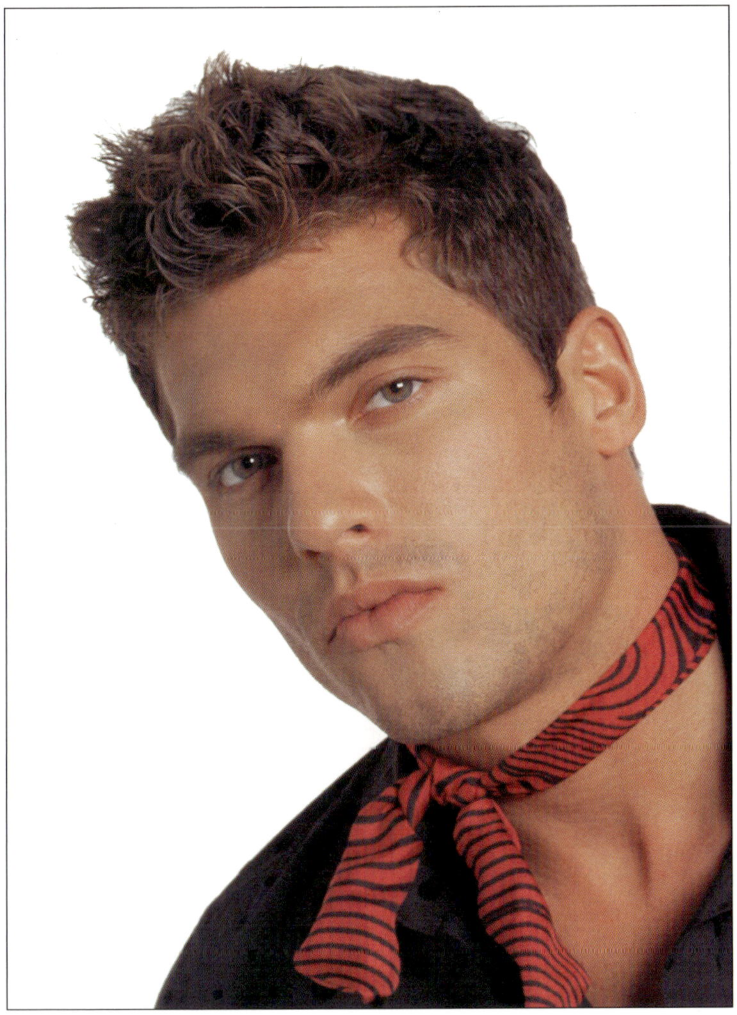

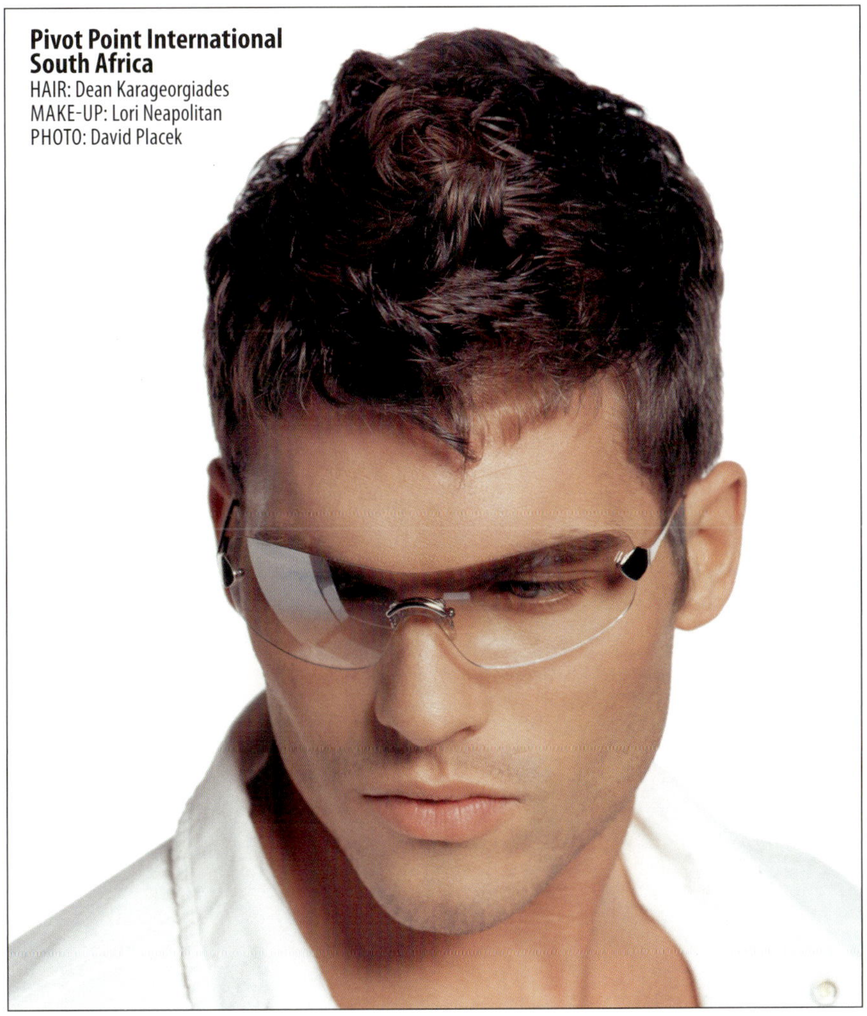

**Pivot Point International South Africa**
HAIR: Dean Karageorgiades
MAKE-UP: Lori Neapolitan
PHOTO: David Placek

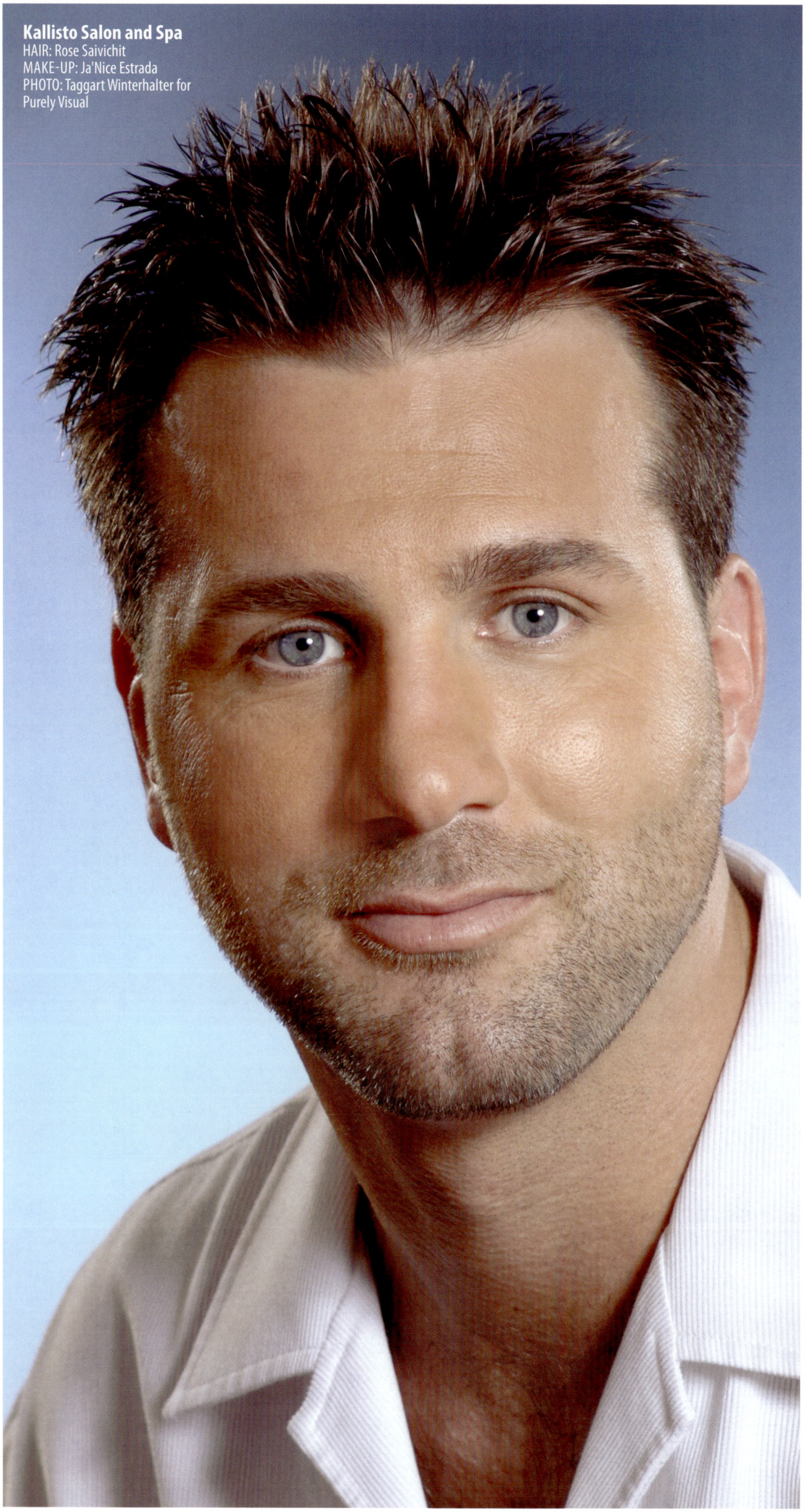

**Kallisto Salon and Spa**
HAIR: Rose Saivichit
MAKE-UP: Ja'Nice Estrada
PHOTO: Taggart Winterhalter for Purely Visual

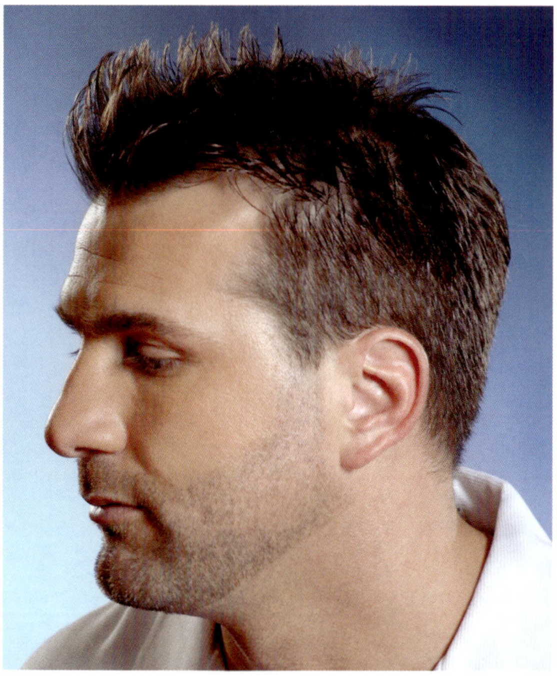

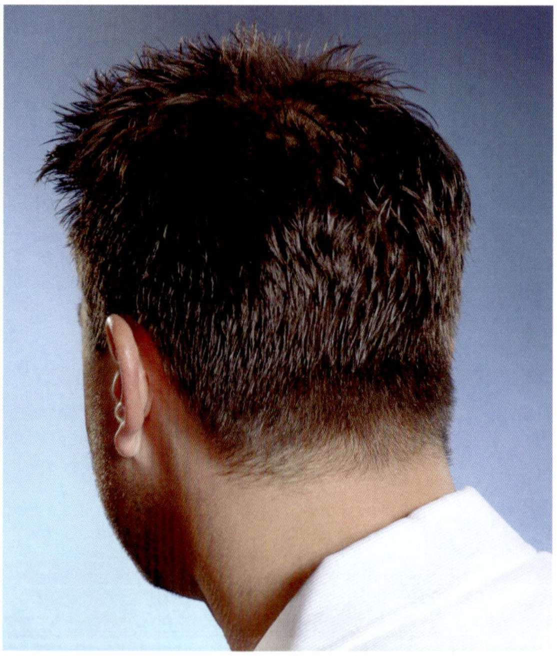

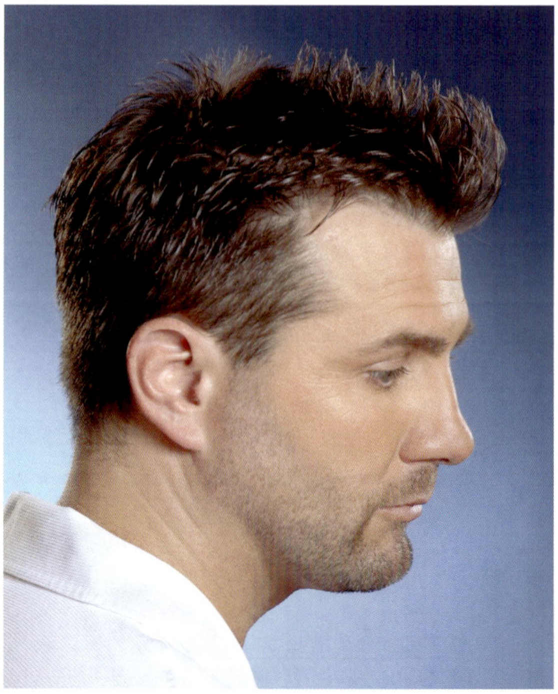

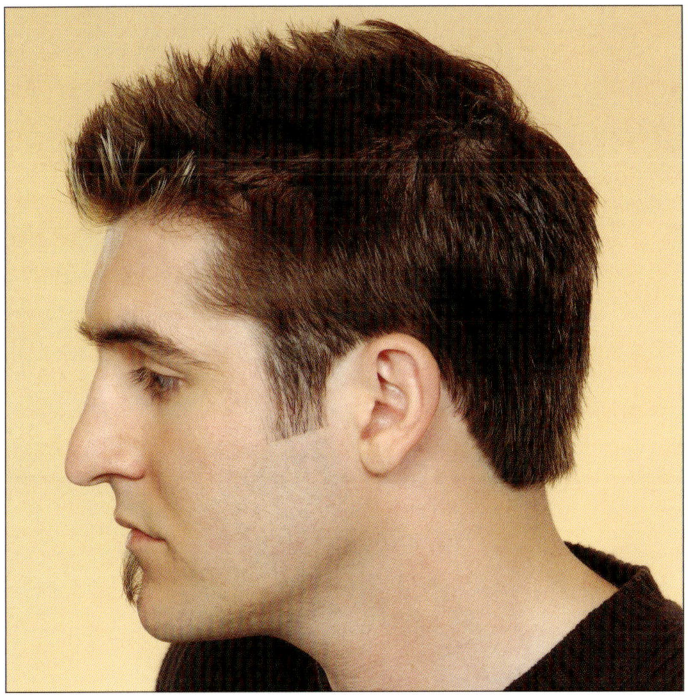

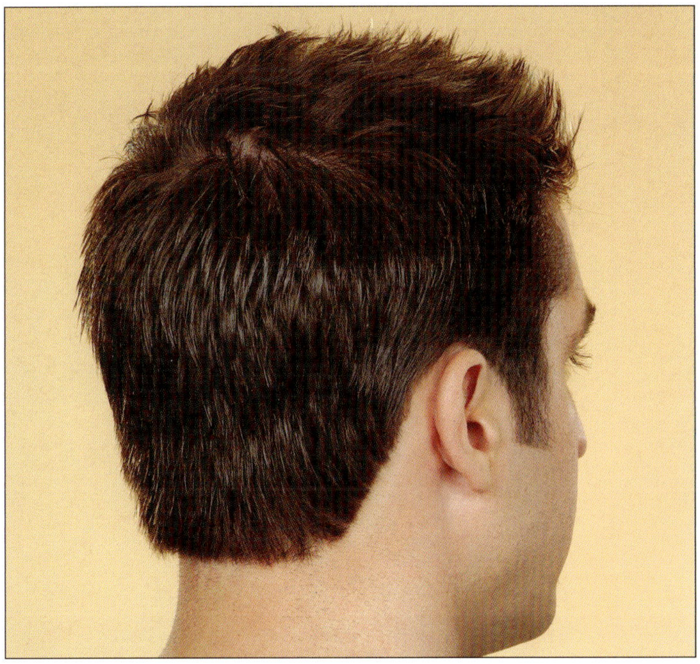

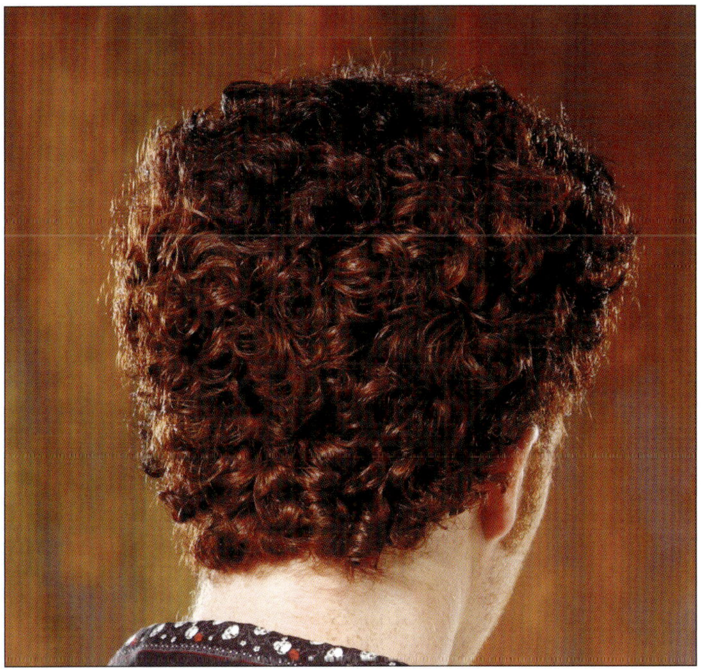

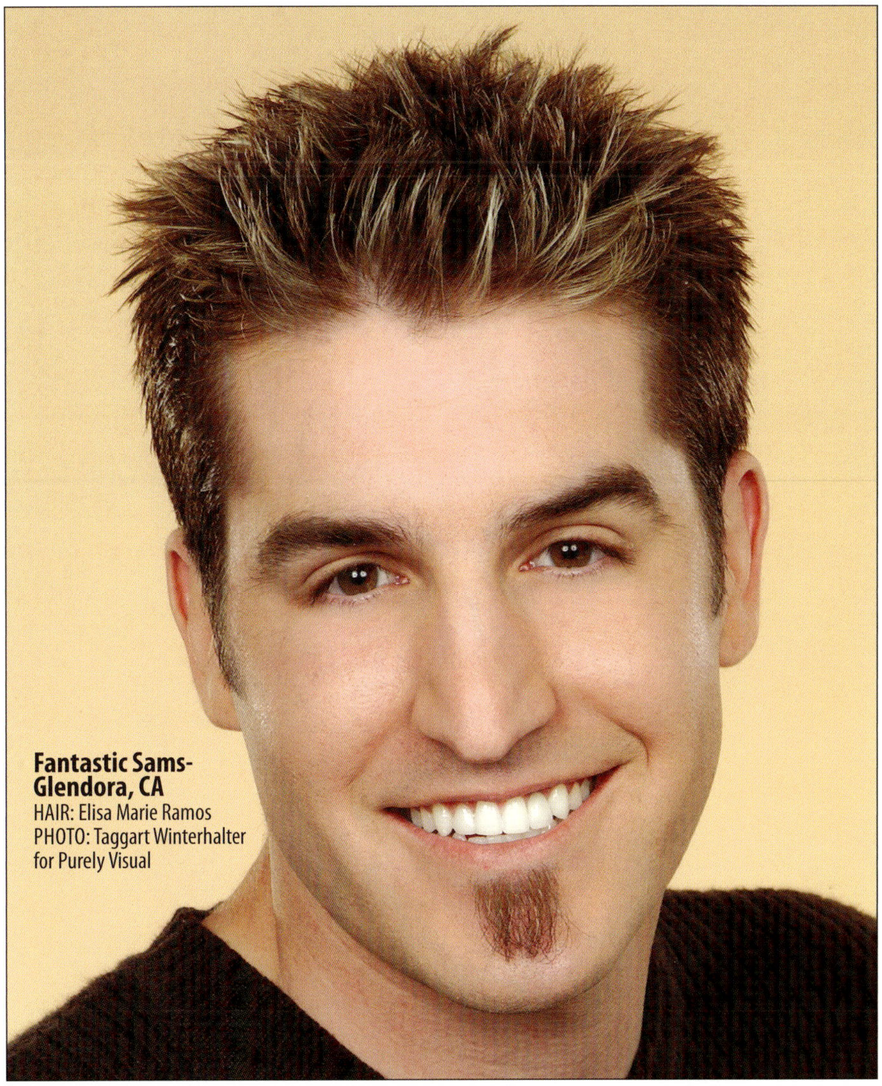

**Fantastic Sams-Glendora, CA**
HAIR: Elisa Marie Ramos
PHOTO: Taggart Winterhalter for Purely Visual

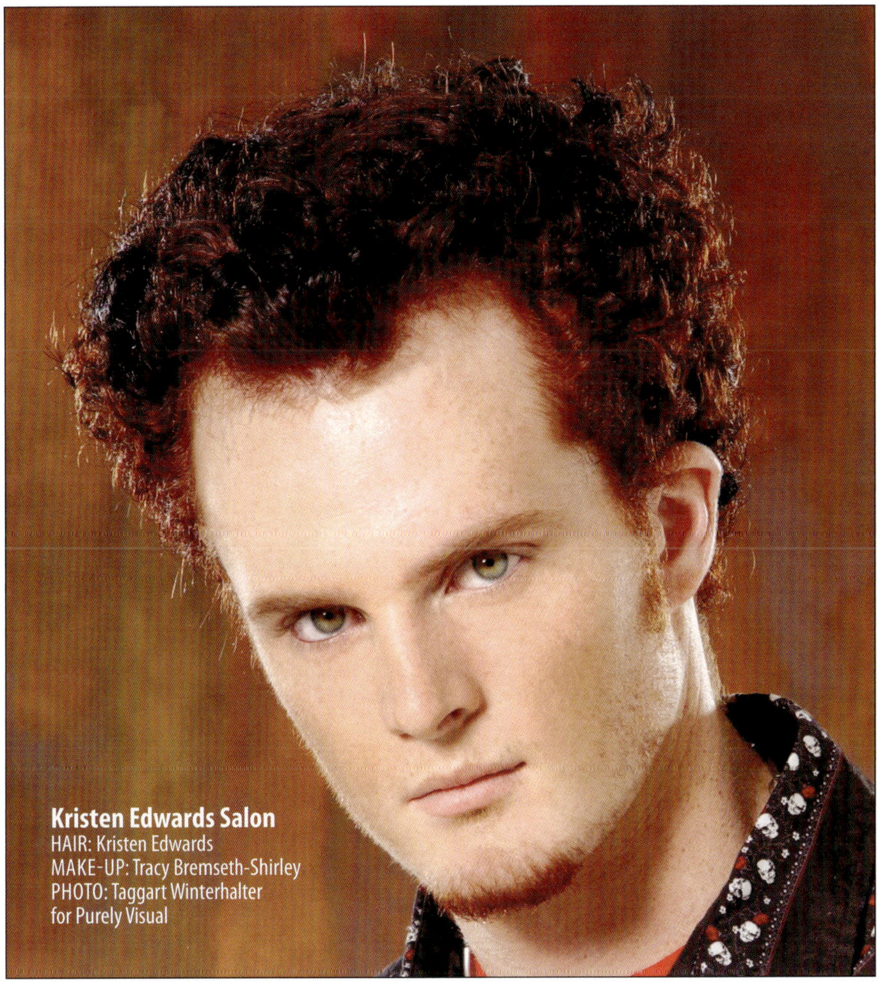

**Kristen Edwards Salon**
HAIR: Kristen Edwards
MAKE-UP: Tracy Bremseth-Shirley
PHOTO: Taggart Winterhalter for Purely Visual

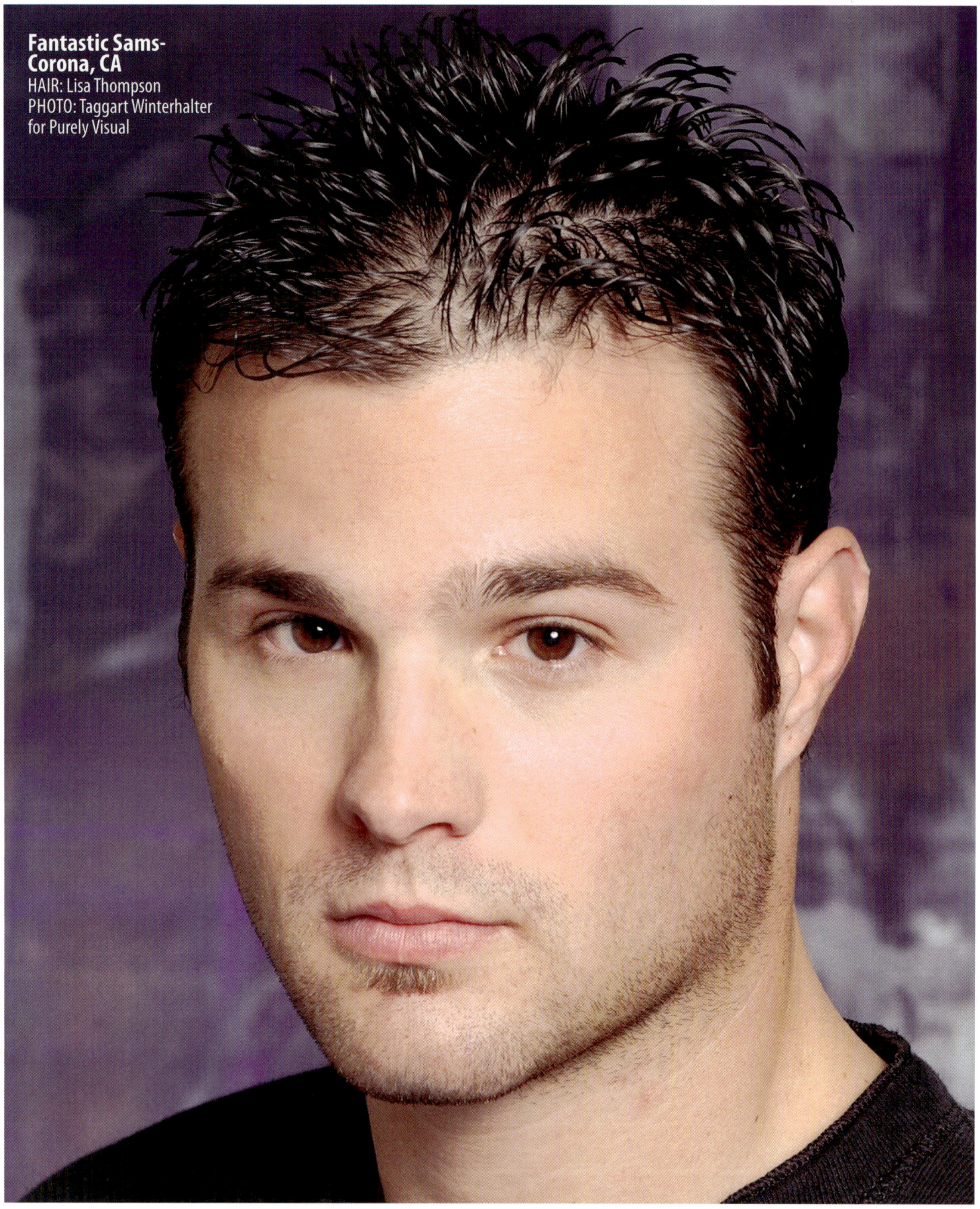

**Fantastic Sams-
Corona, CA**
HAIR: Lisa Thompson
PHOTO: Taggart Winterhalter
for Purely Visual

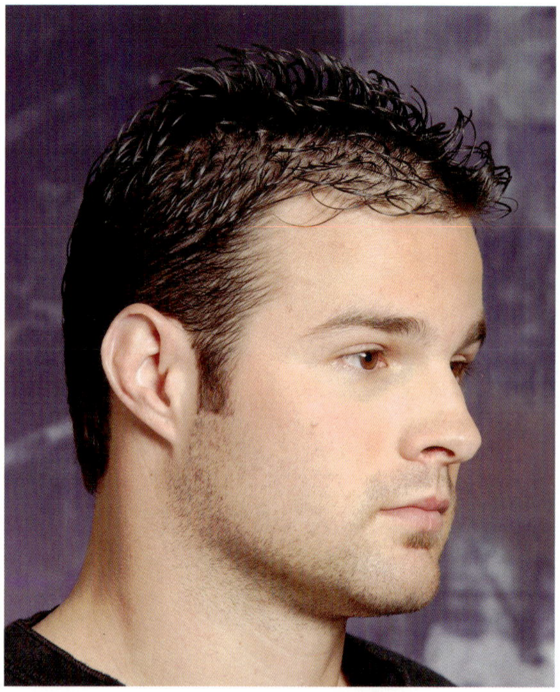

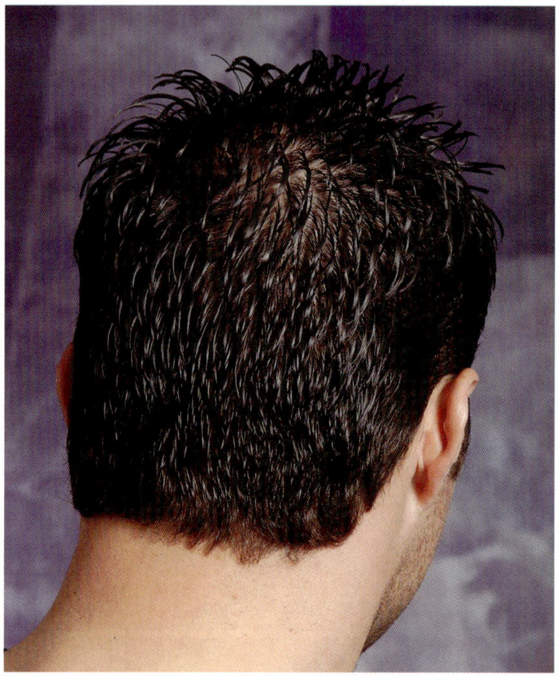

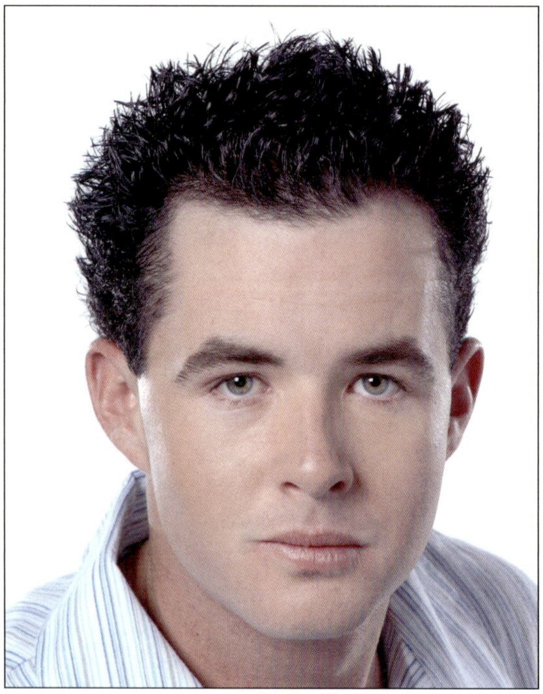

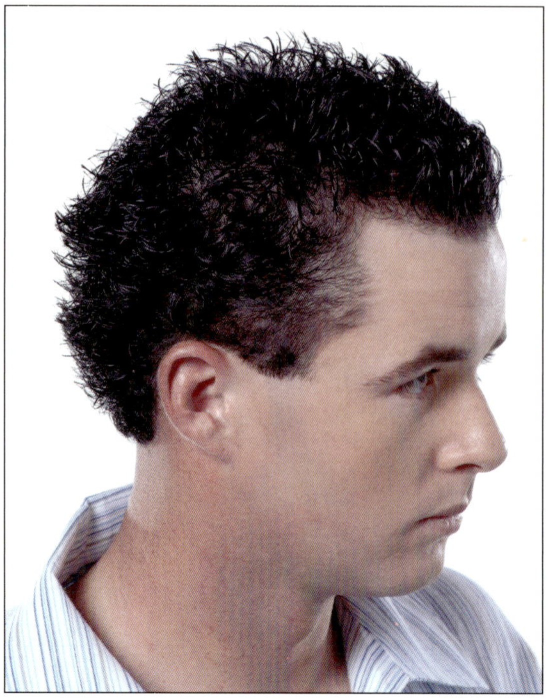

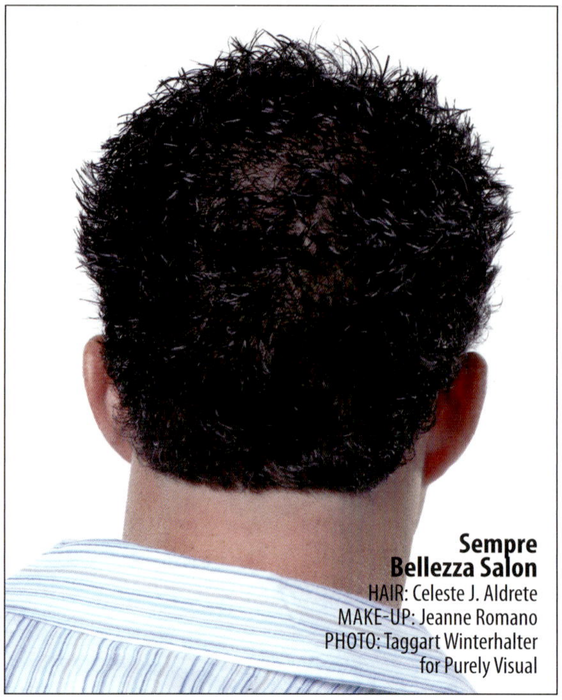

**Sempre
Bellezza Salon**
HAIR: Celeste J. Aldrete
MAKE-UP: Jeanne Romano
PHOTO: Taggart Winterhalter
for Purely Visual

**Goldwell**
HAIR: Trend Zoom 06 Team

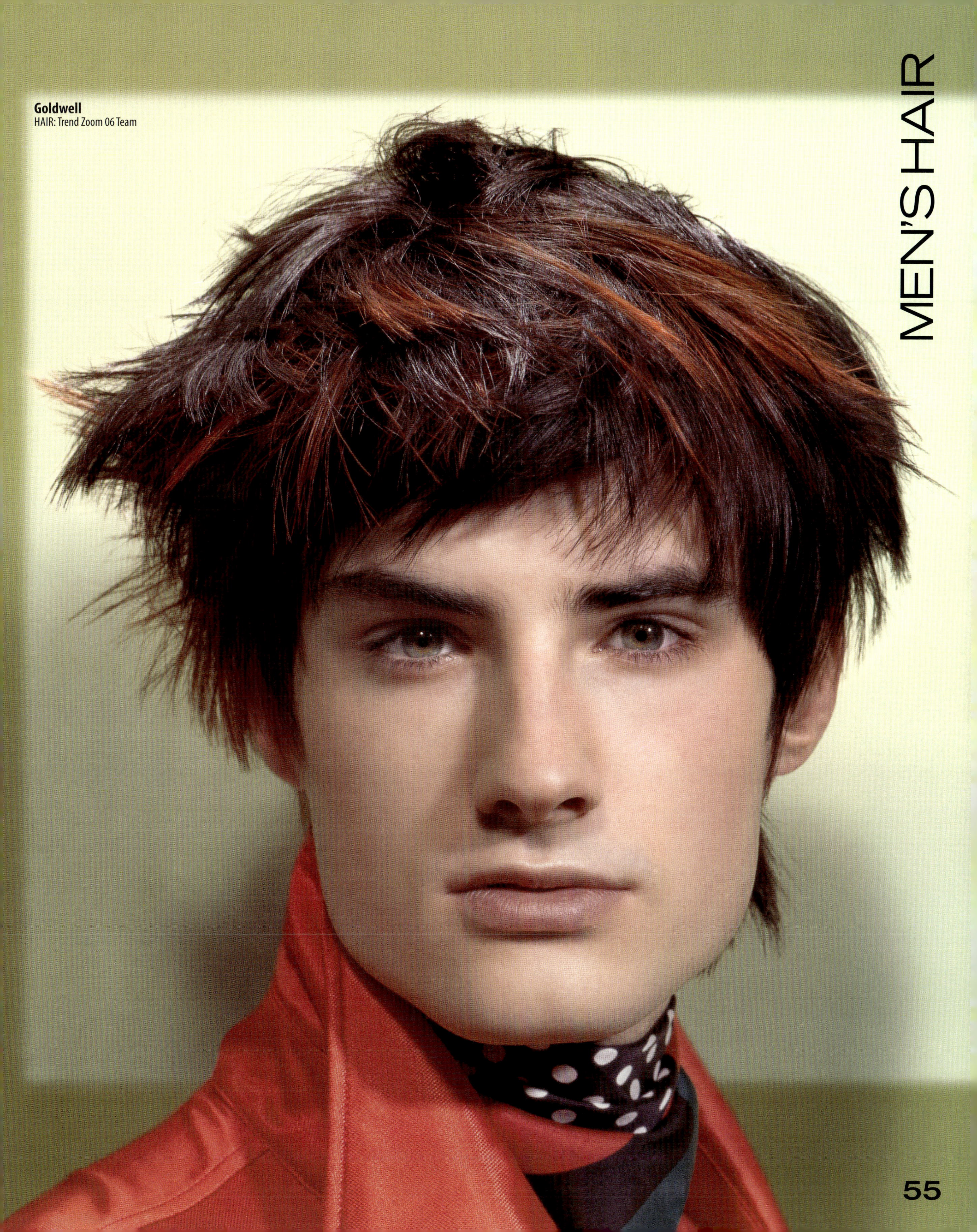

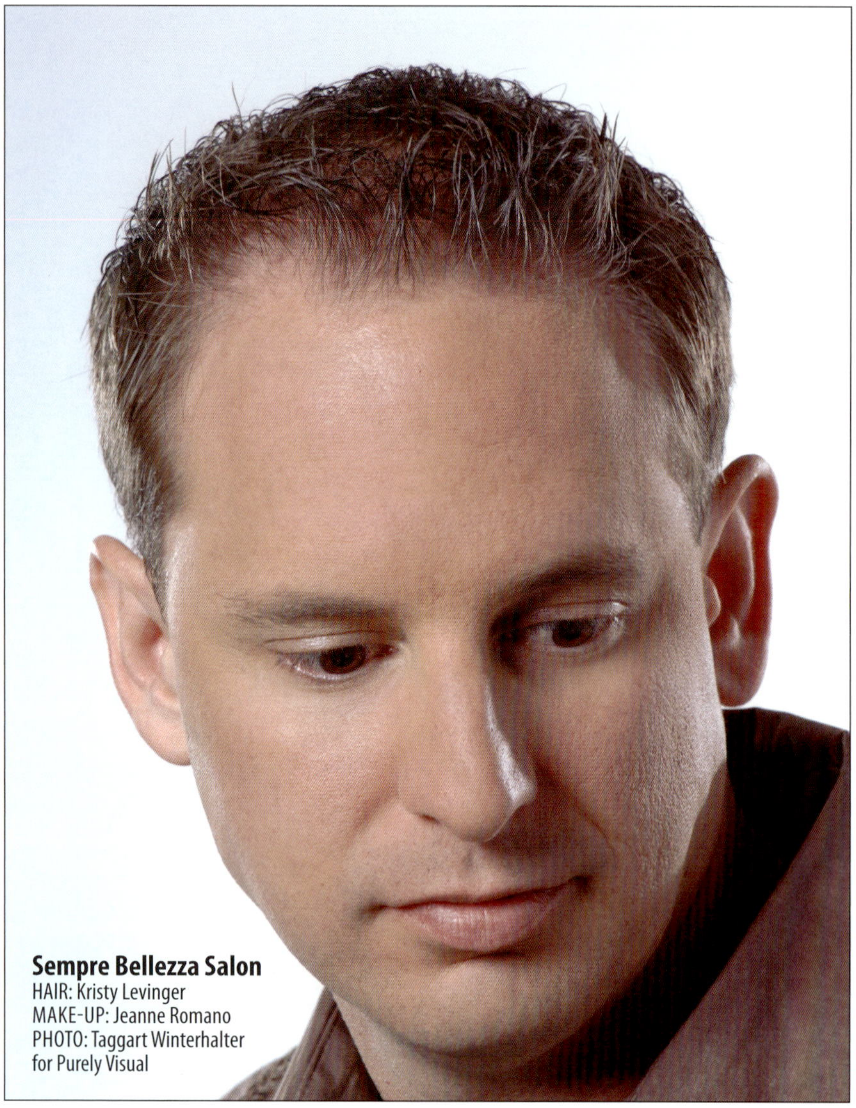

**Sempre Bellezza Salon**
HAIR: Kristy Levinger
MAKE-UP: Jeanne Romano
PHOTO: Taggart Winterhalter for Purely Visual

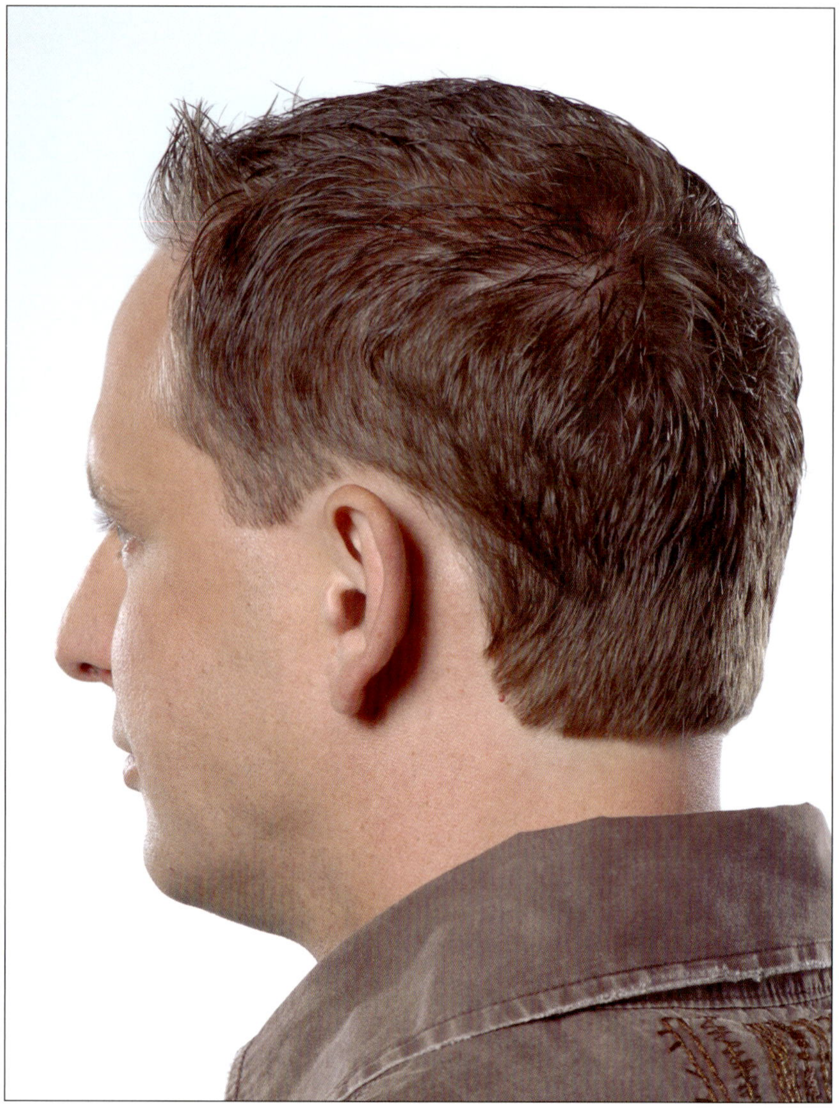

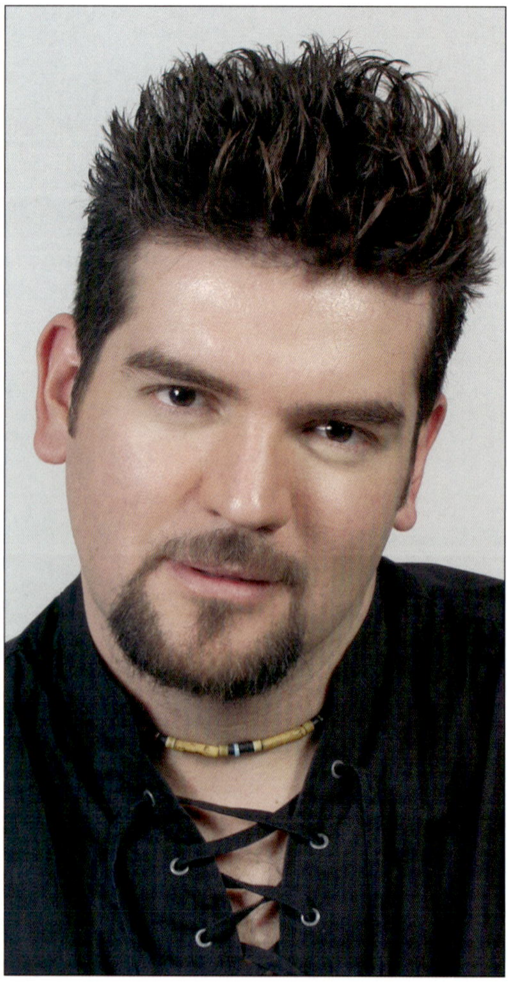

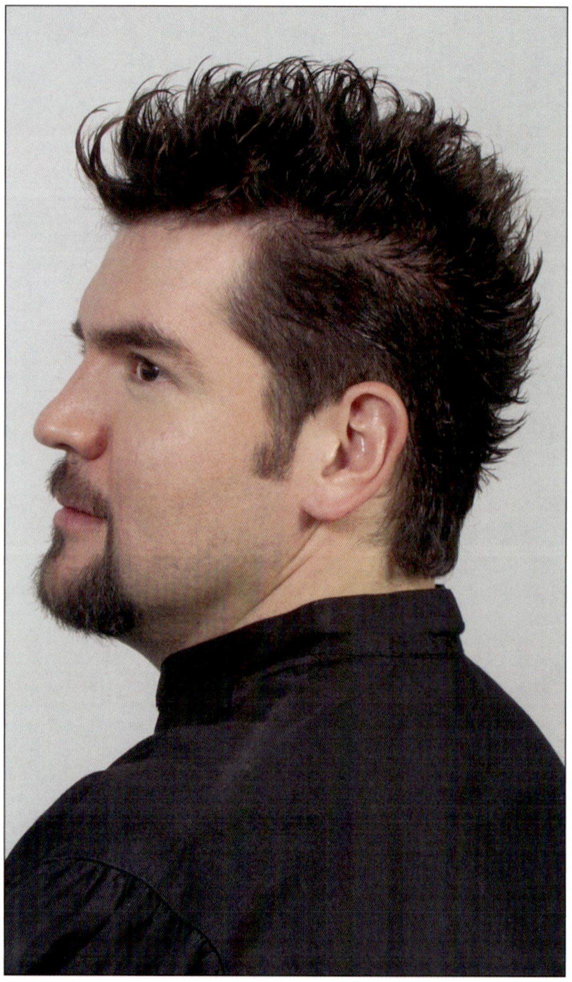

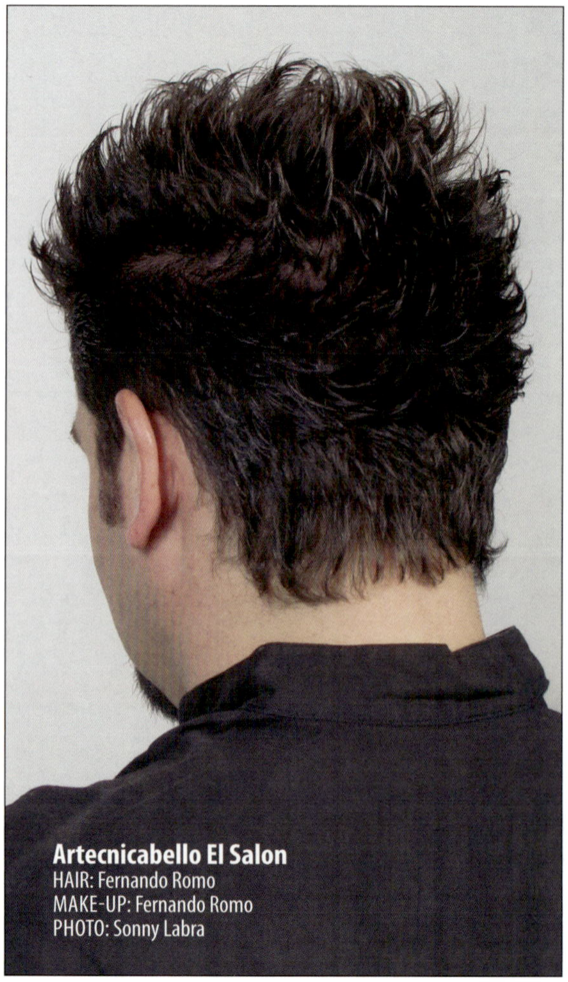

**Artecnicabello El Salon**
HAIR: Fernando Romo
MAKE-UP: Fernando Romo
PHOTO: Sonny Labra

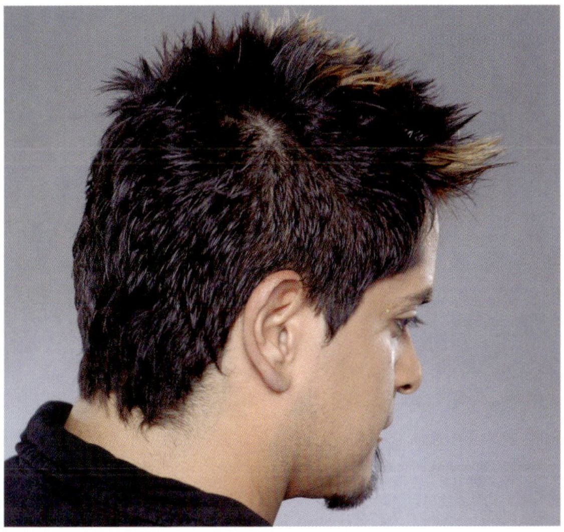

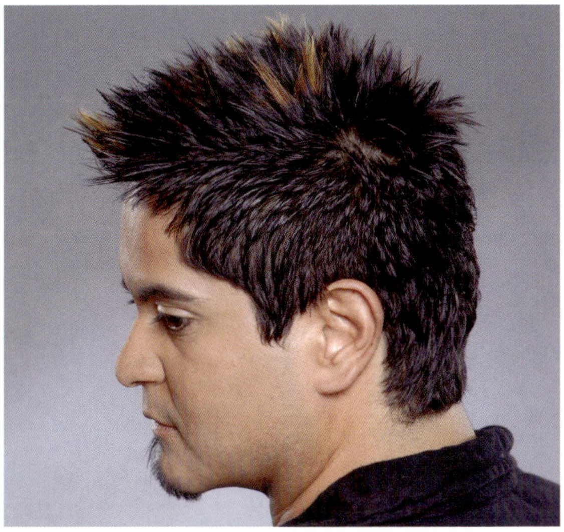

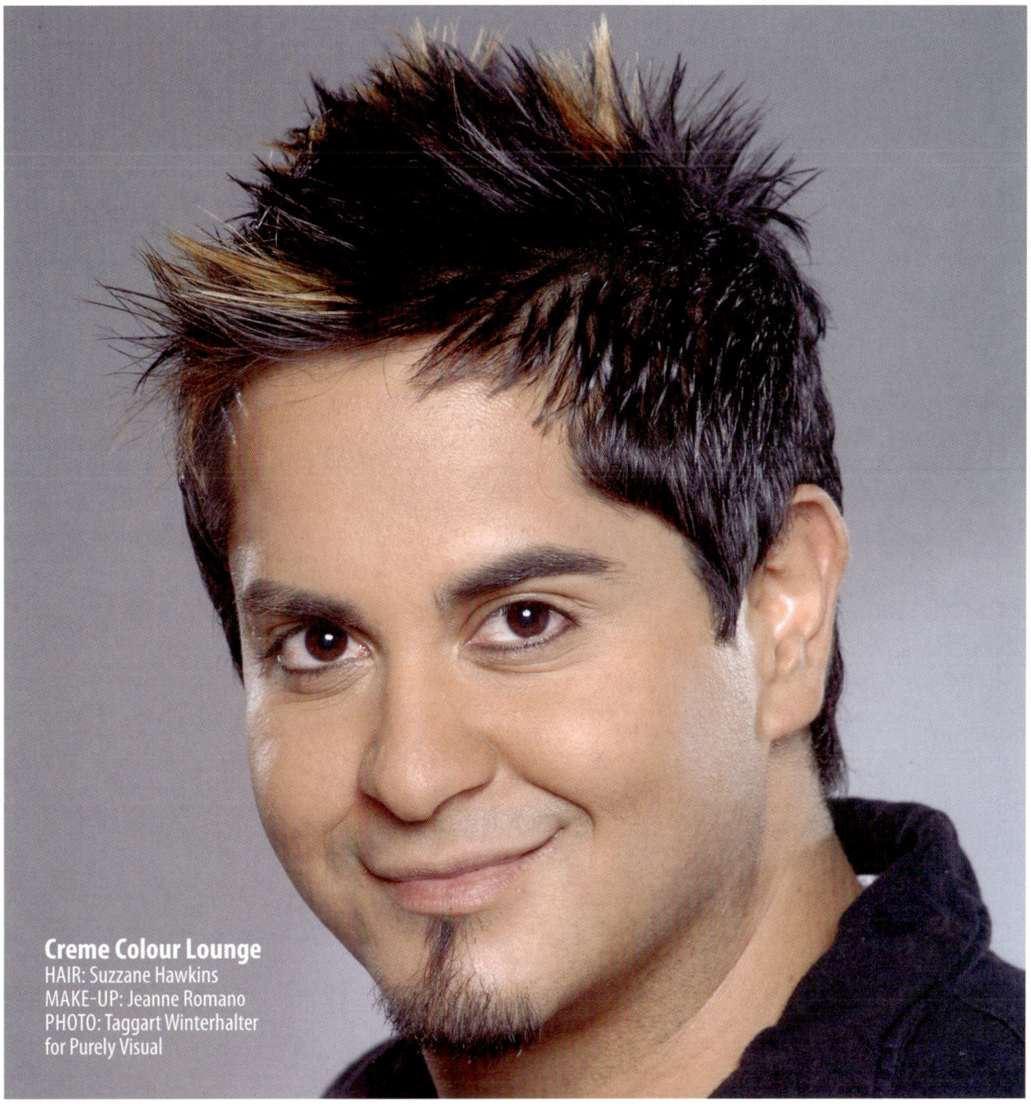

**Creme Colour Lounge**
HAIR: Suzzane Hawkins
MAKE-UP: Jeanne Romano
PHOTO: Taggart Winterhalter for Purely Visual

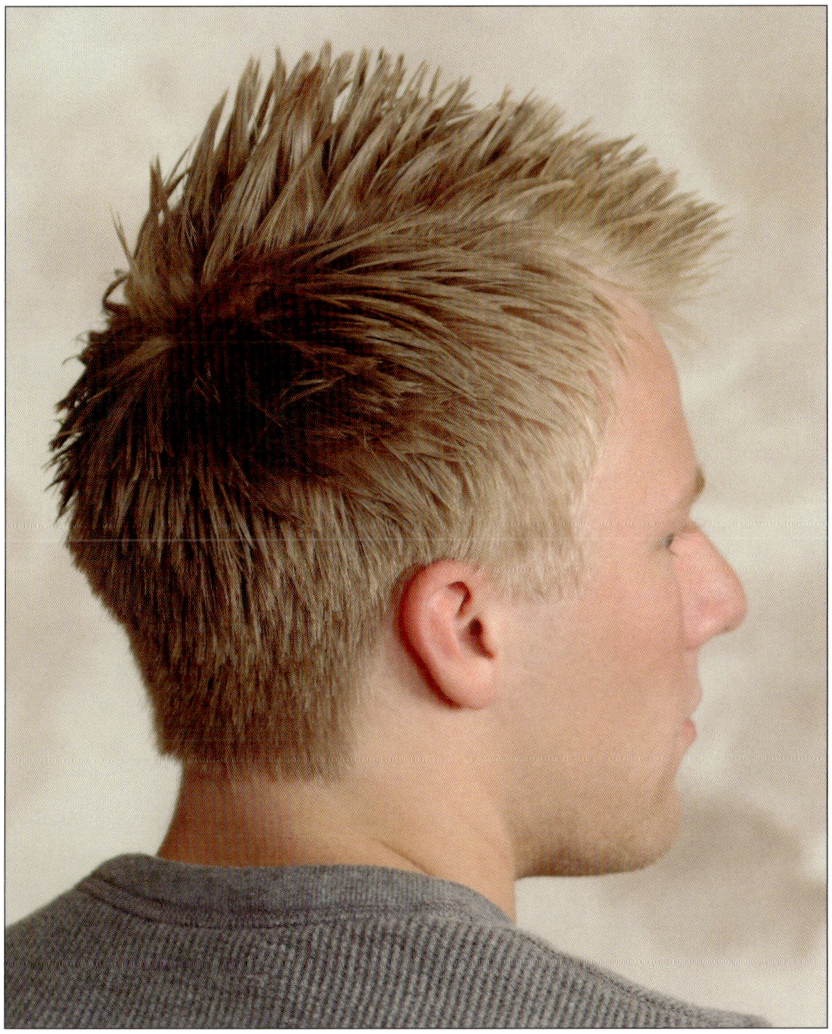

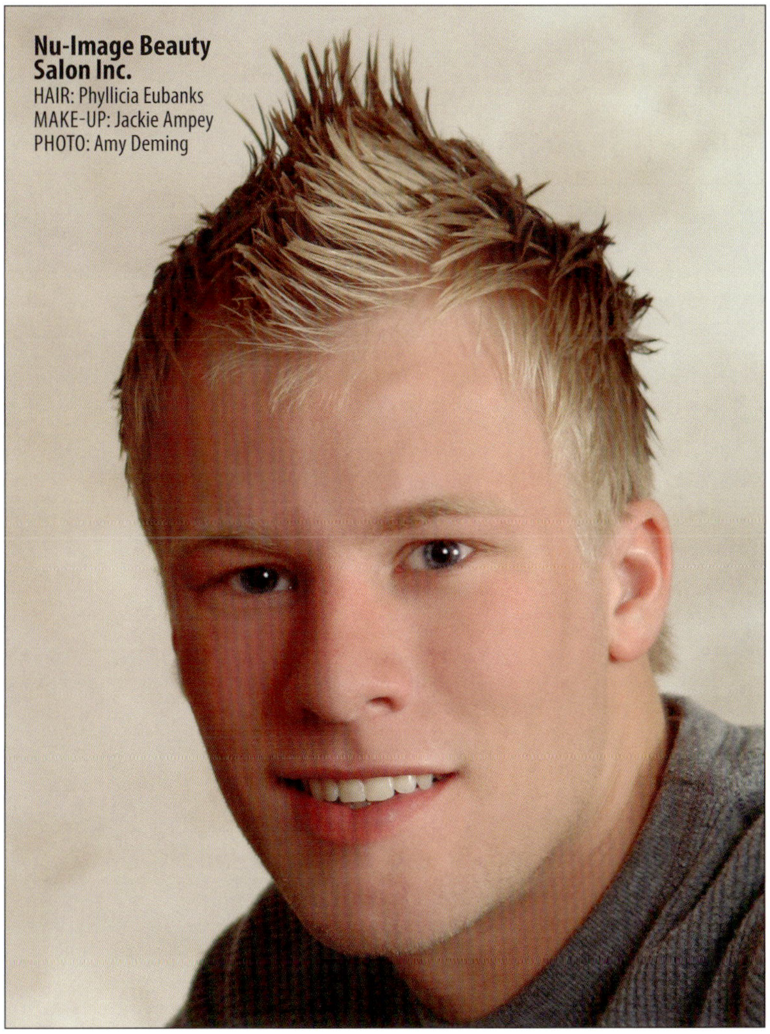

**Nu-Image Beauty Salon Inc.**
HAIR: Phyllicia Eubanks
MAKE-UP: Jackie Ampey
PHOTO: Amy Deming

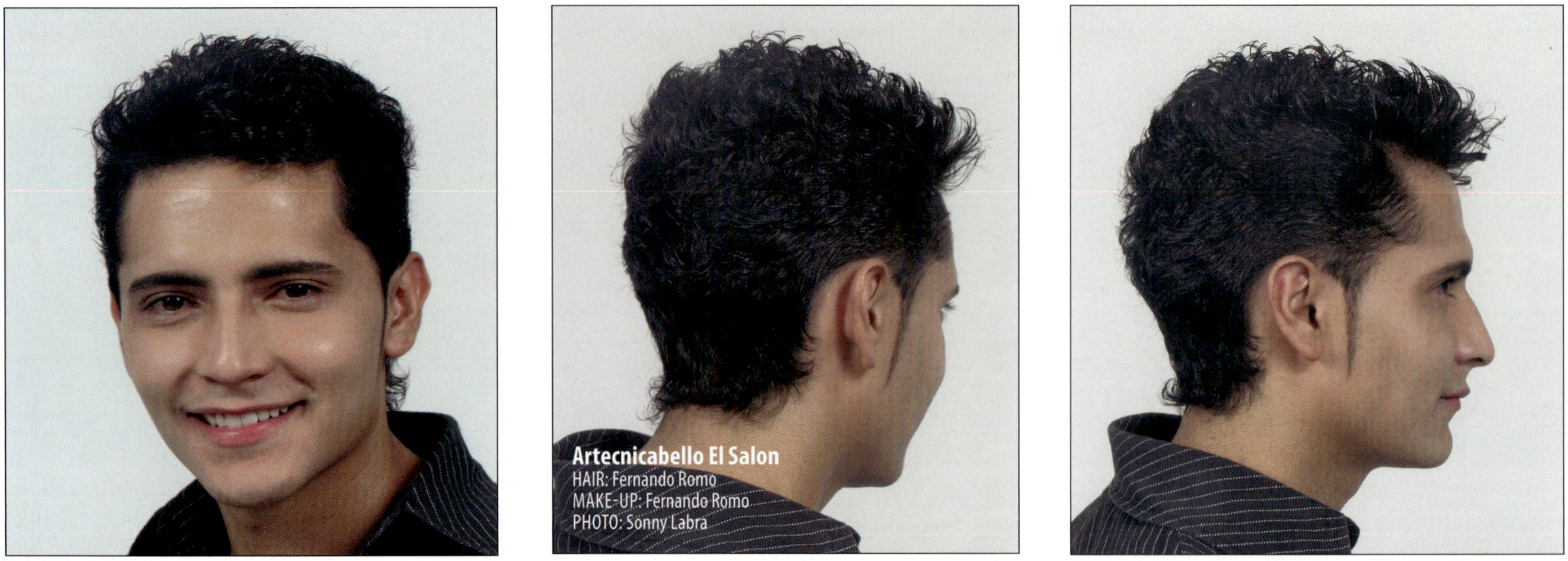

**Artecnicabello El Salon**
HAIR: Fernando Romo
MAKE-UP: Fernando Romo
PHOTO: Sonny Labra

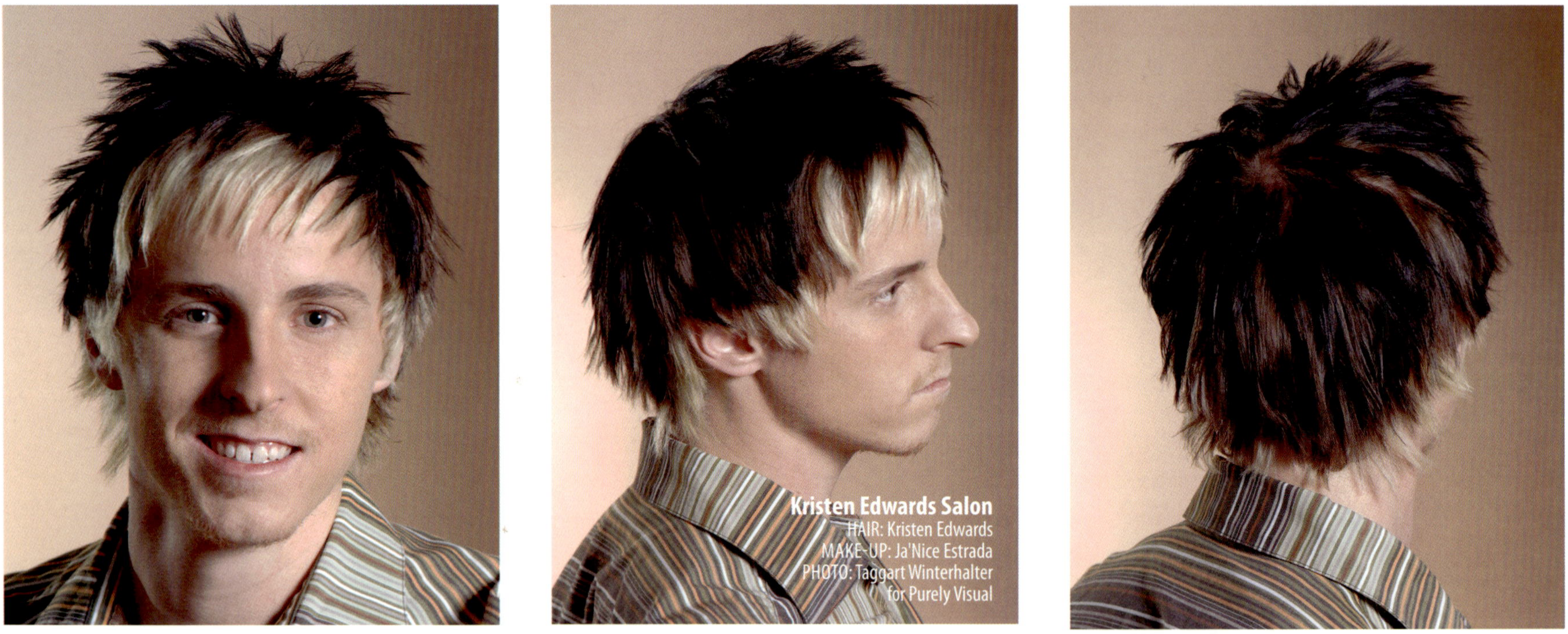

**Kristen Edwards Salon**
HAIR: Kristen Edwards
MAKE-UP: Ja'Nice Estrada
PHOTO: Taggart Winterhalter for Purely Visual

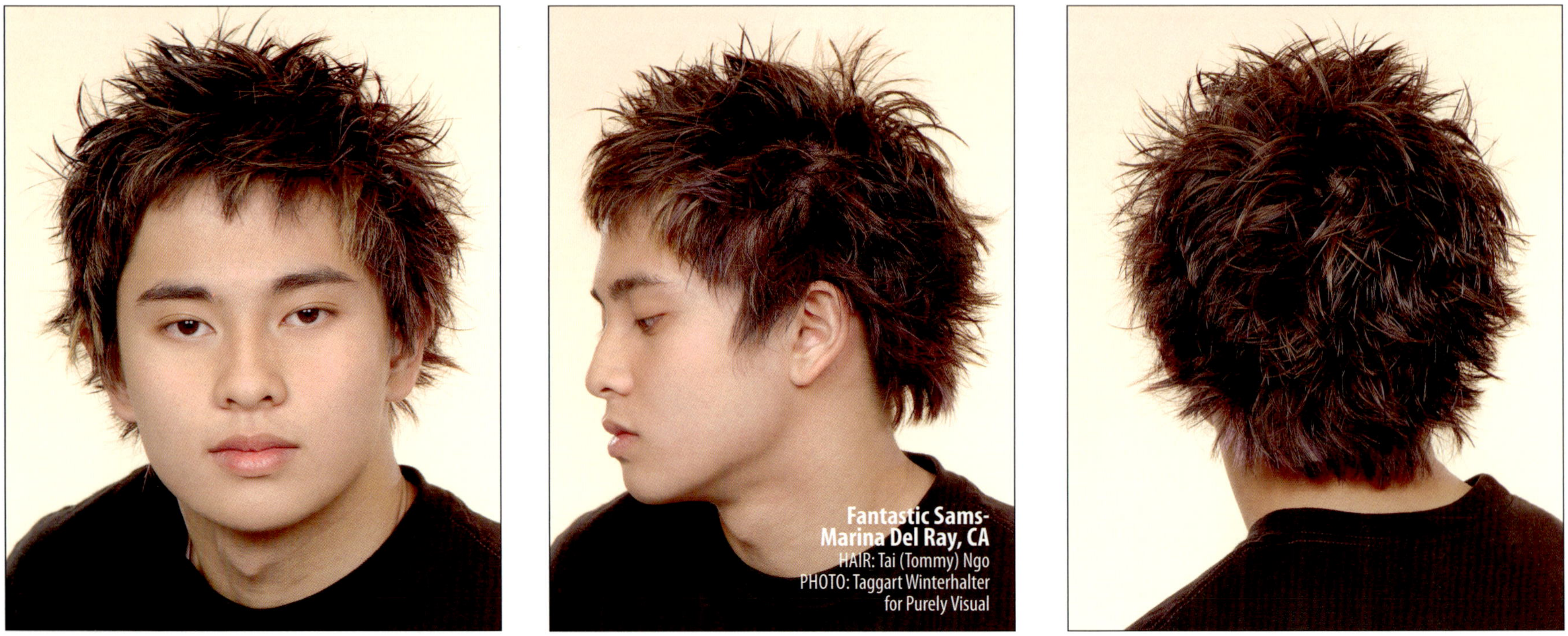

**Fantastic Sams-Marina Del Ray, CA**
HAIR: Tai (Tommy) Ngo
PHOTO: Taggart Winterhalter for Purely Visual

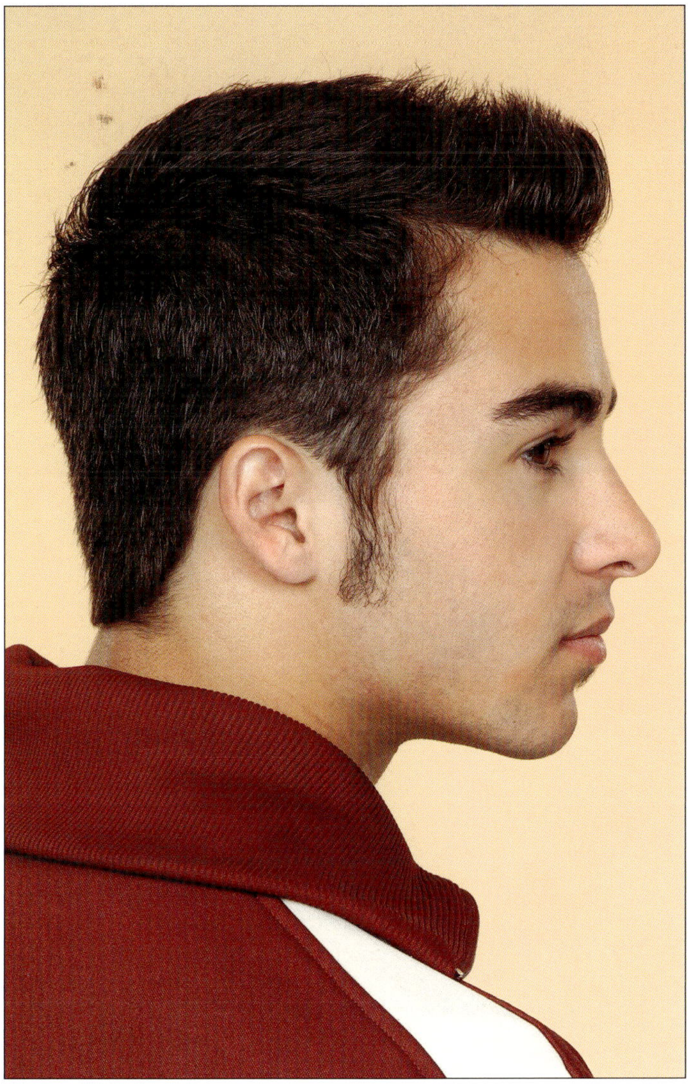

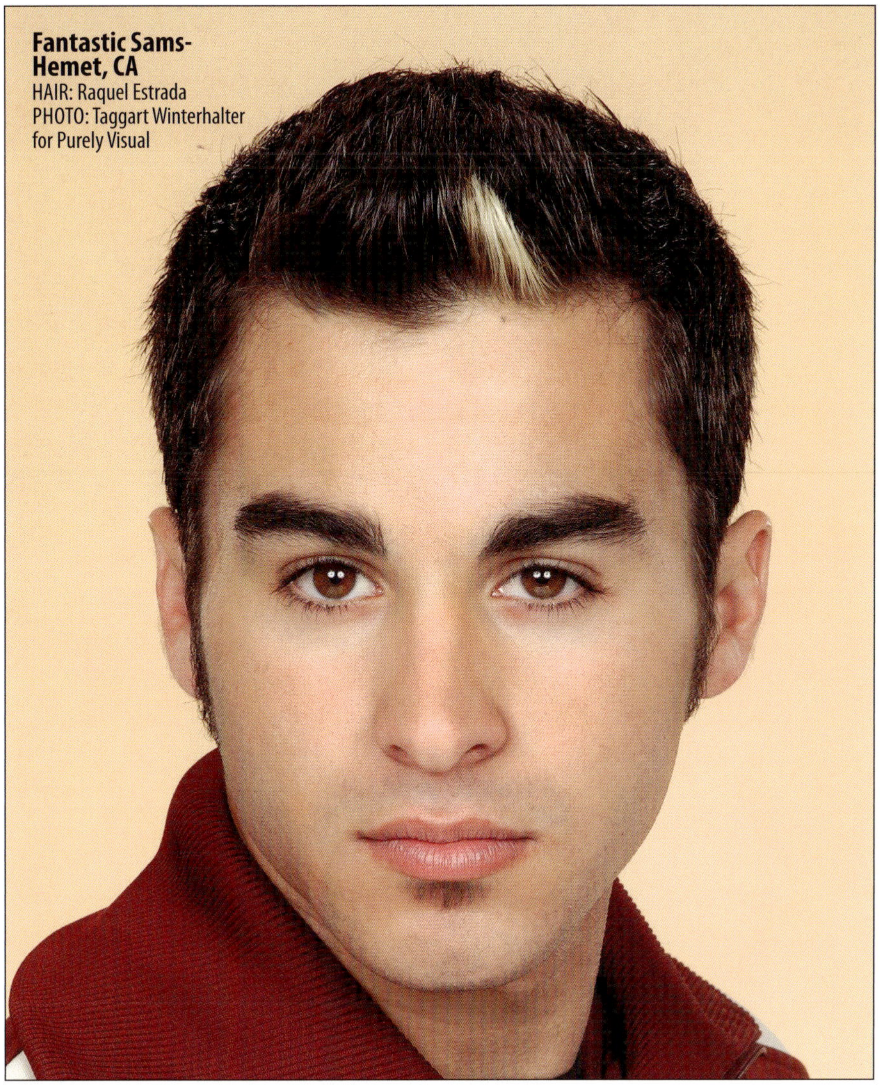

**Fantastic Sams-**
**Hemet, CA**
HAIR: Raquel Estrada
PHOTO: Taggart Winterhalter for Purely Visual

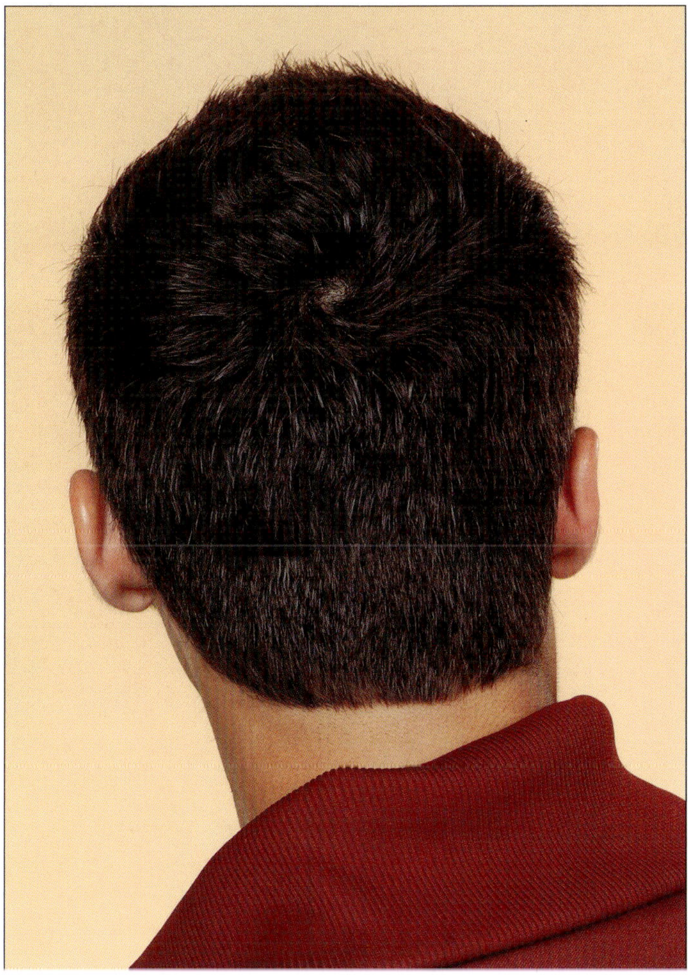

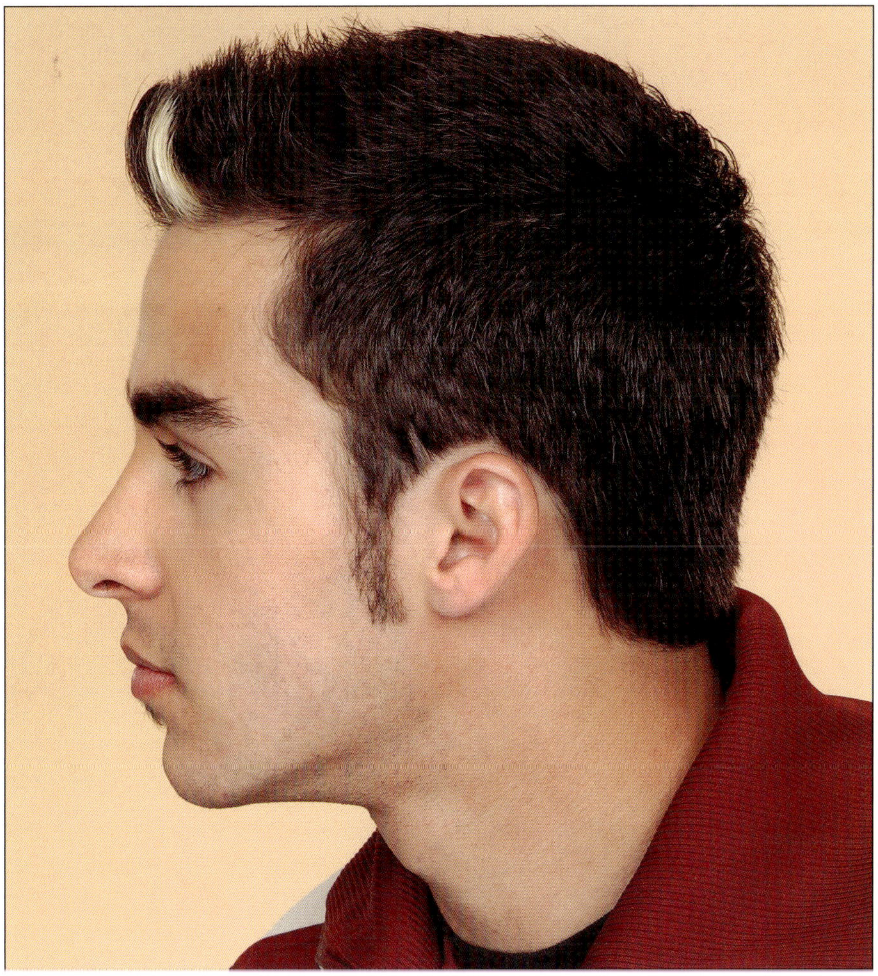

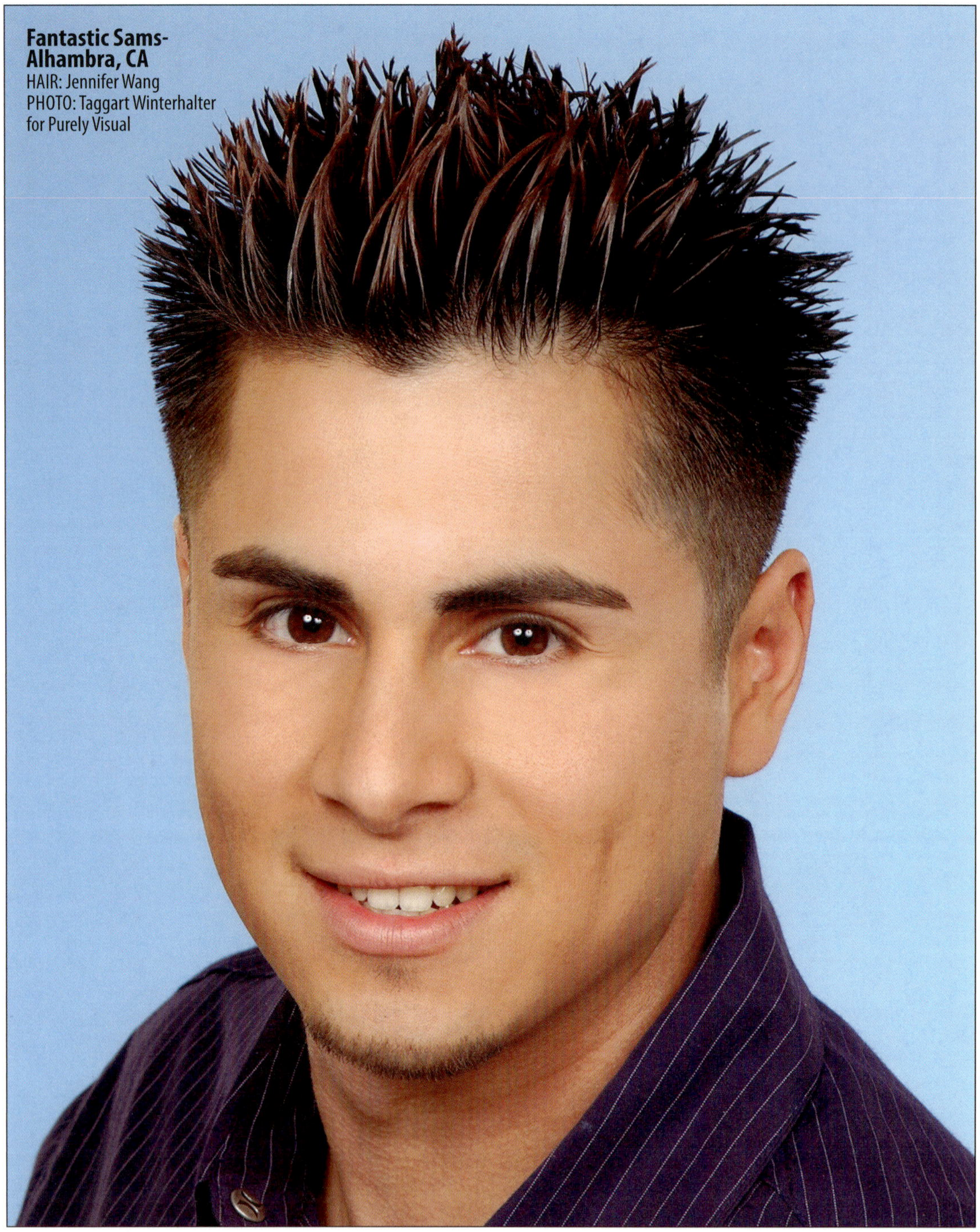

**Fantastic Sams-**
**Alhambra, CA**
HAIR: Jennifer Wang
PHOTO: Taggart Winterhalter
for Purely Visual

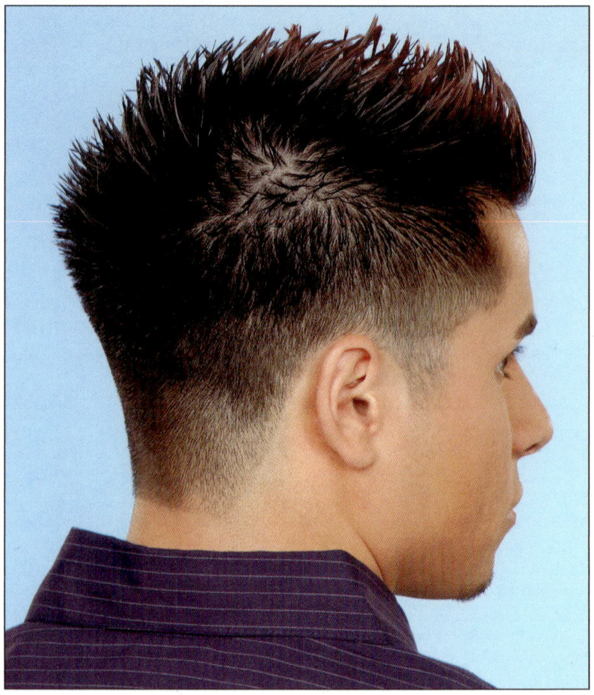

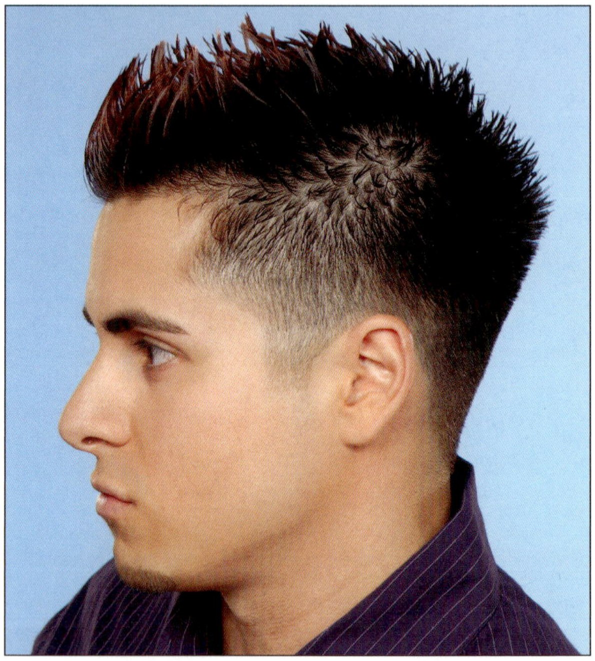

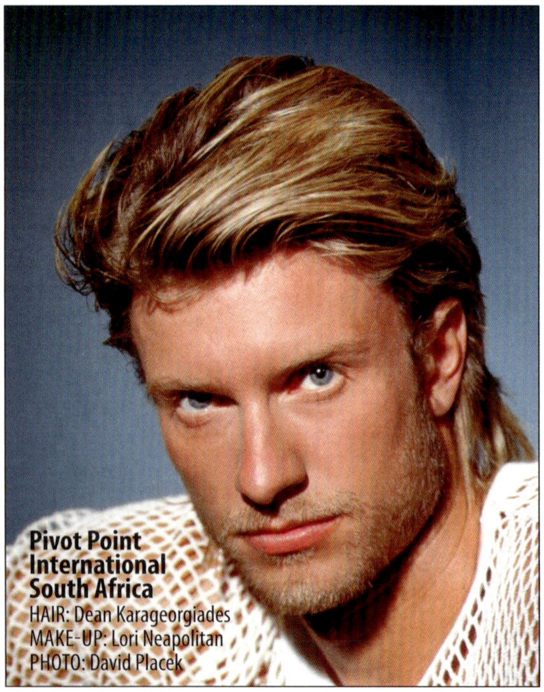

**Pivot Point**
**International**
**South Africa**
HAIR: Dean Karageorgiades
MAKE-UP: Lori Neapolitan
PHOTO: David Placek

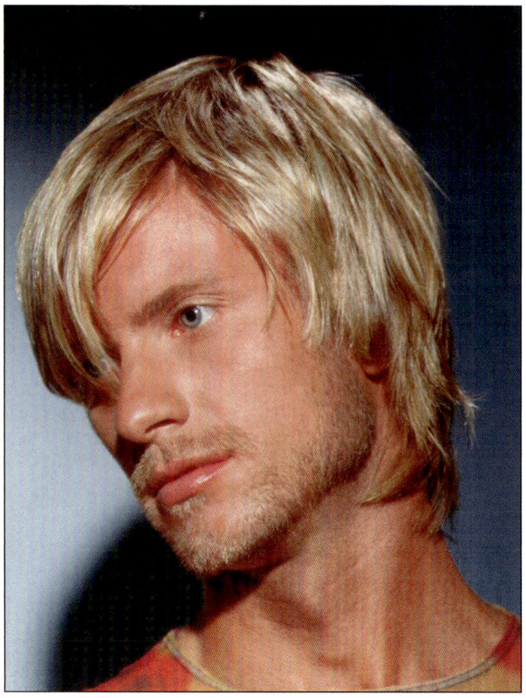

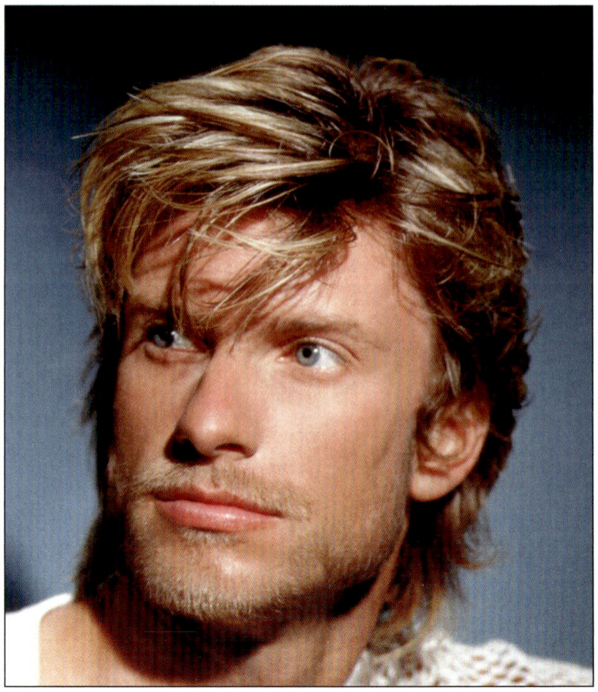

**Coiffure Hair Sun, Switzerland**
HAIR: Hair Sun-Team
MAKE-UP: Hair Sun-Team
PHOTO: Raphael Bonjouor

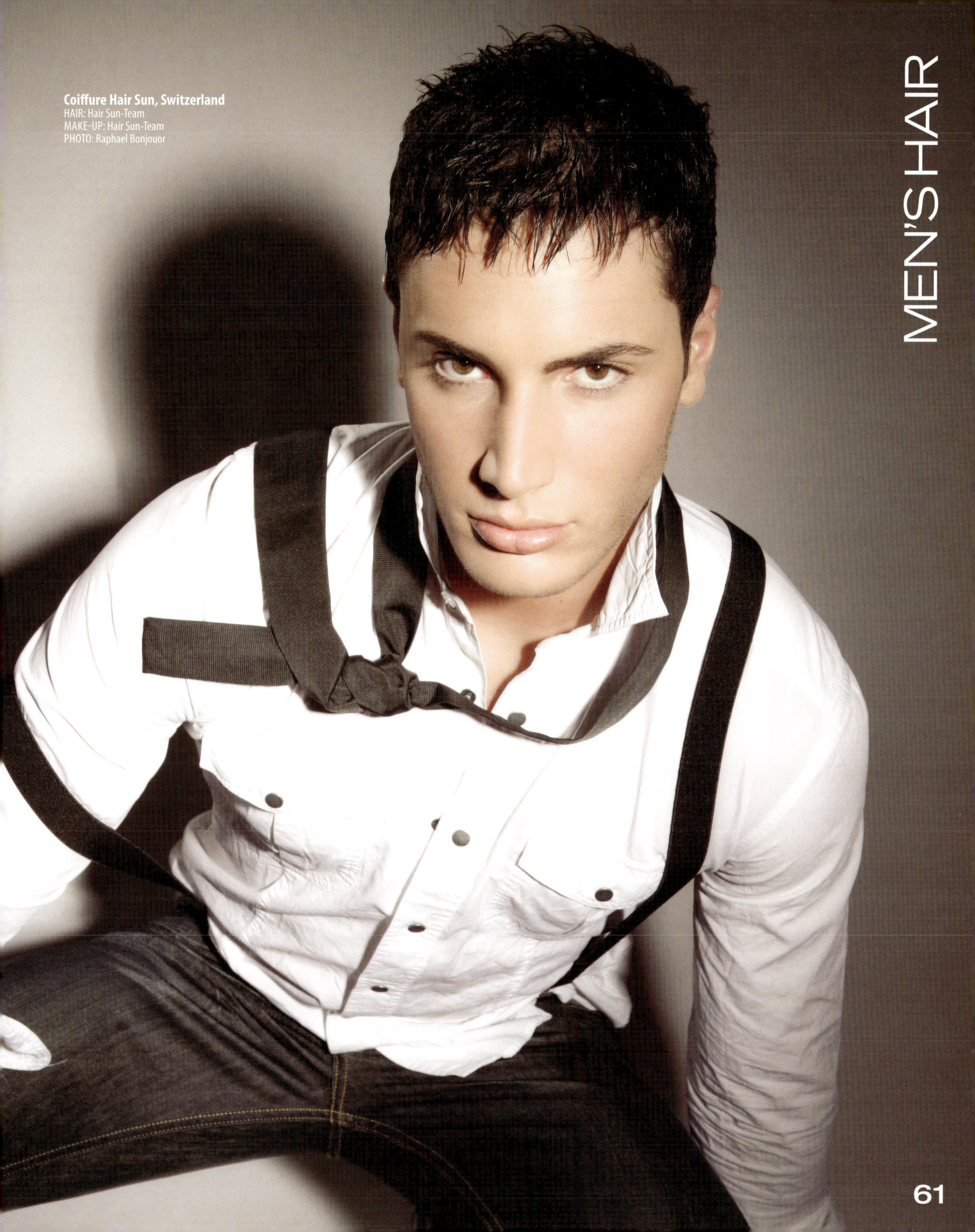

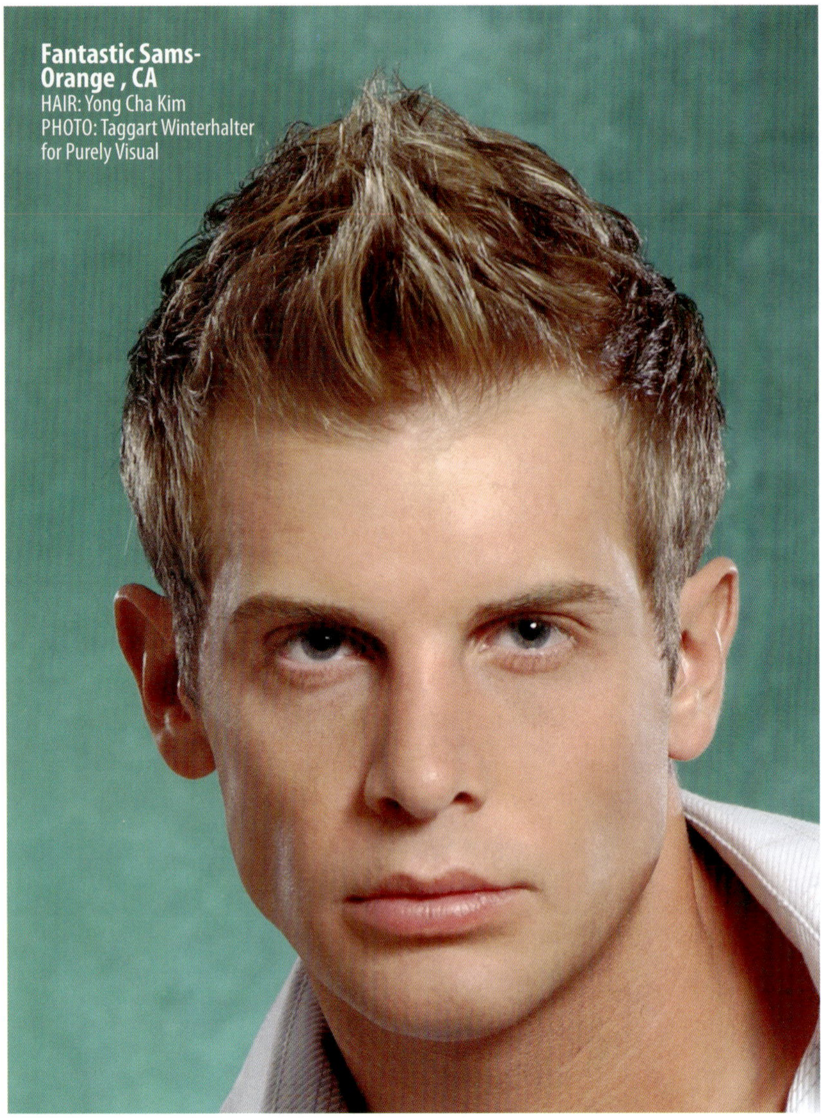

Fantastic Sams-
Orange , CA
HAIR: Yong Cha Kim
PHOTO: Taggart Winterhalter
for Purely Visual

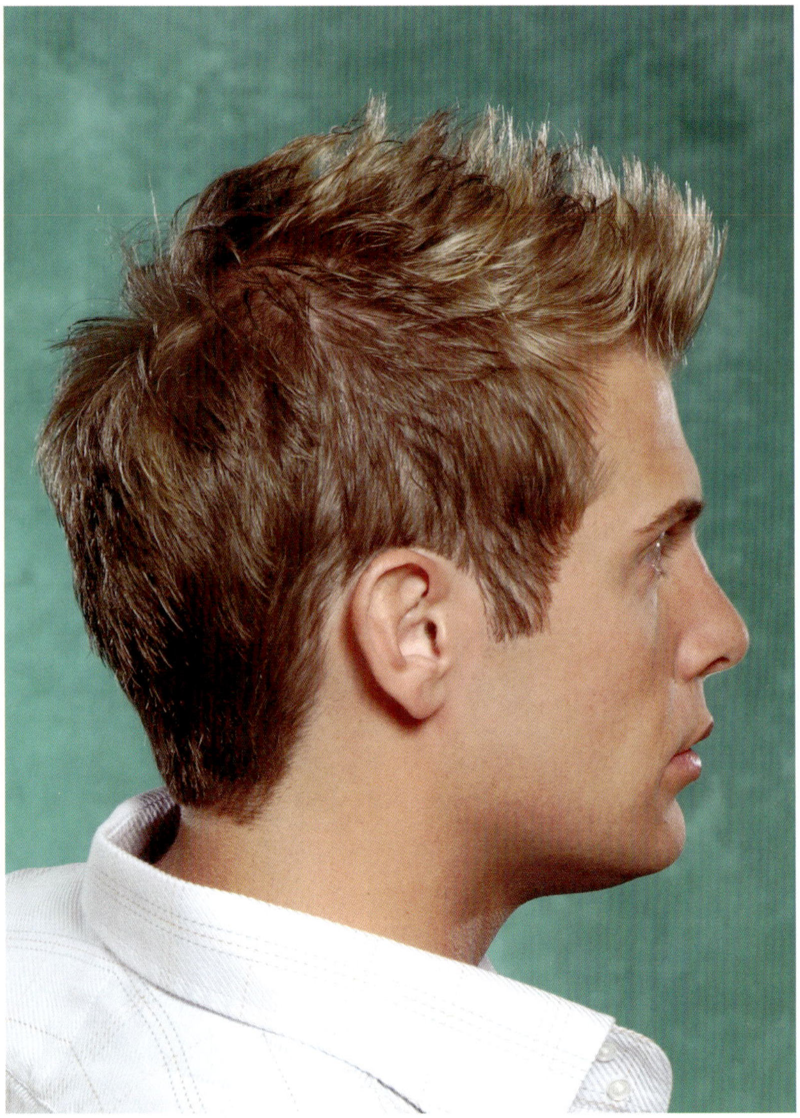

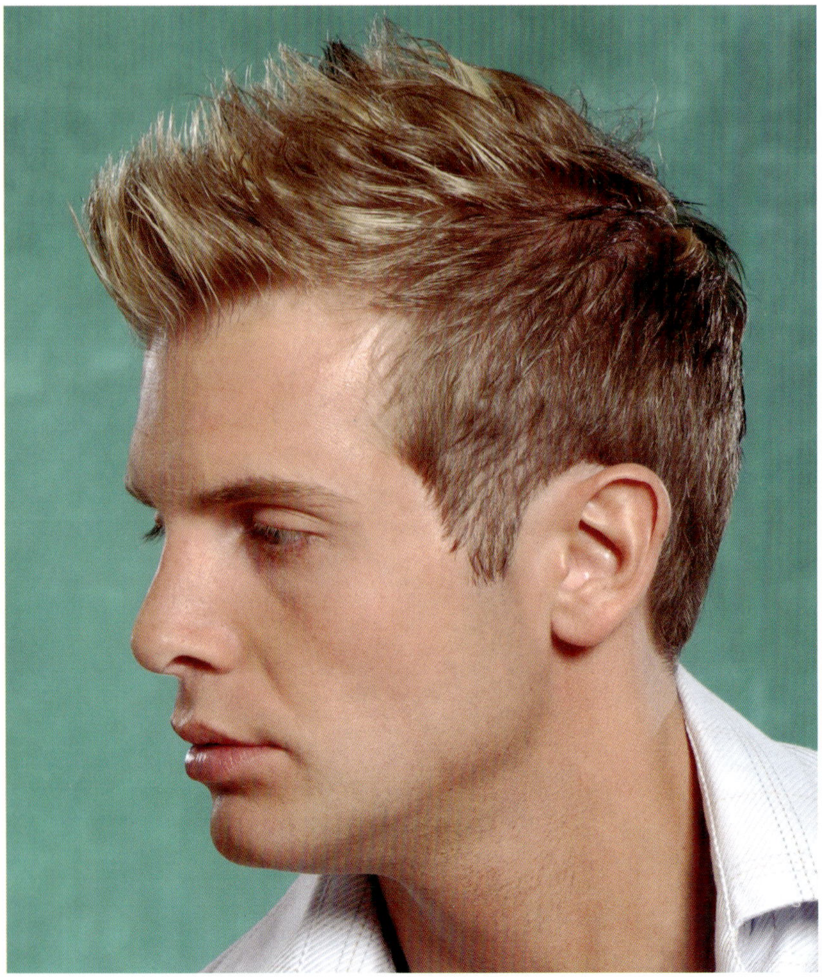

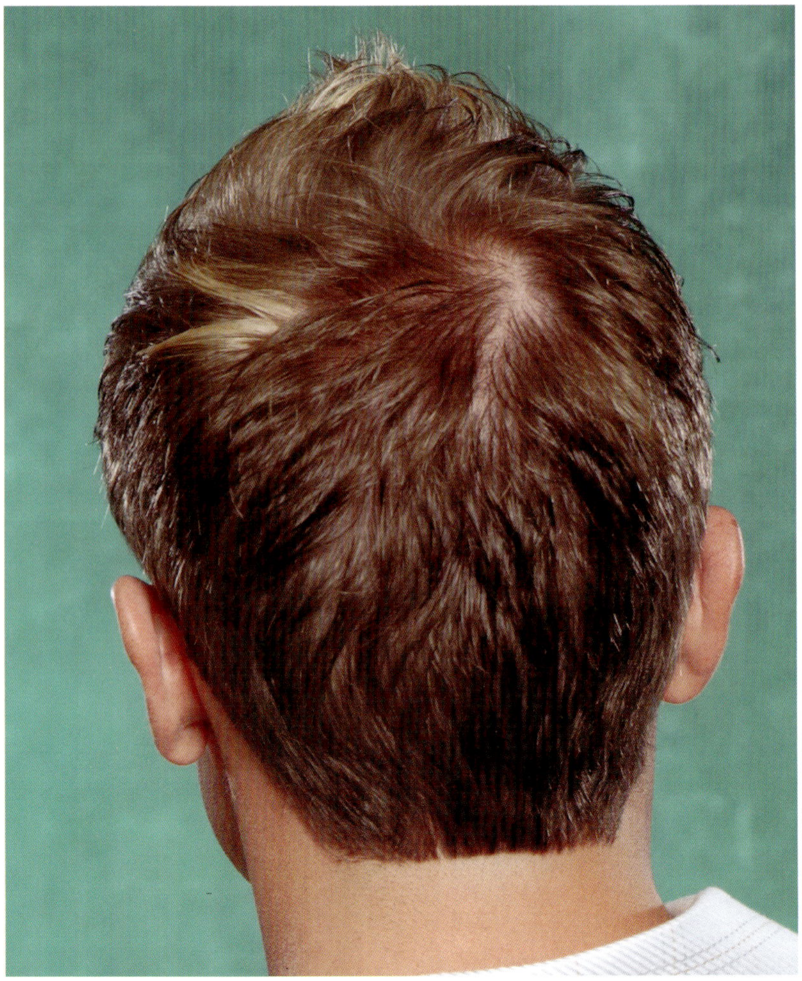

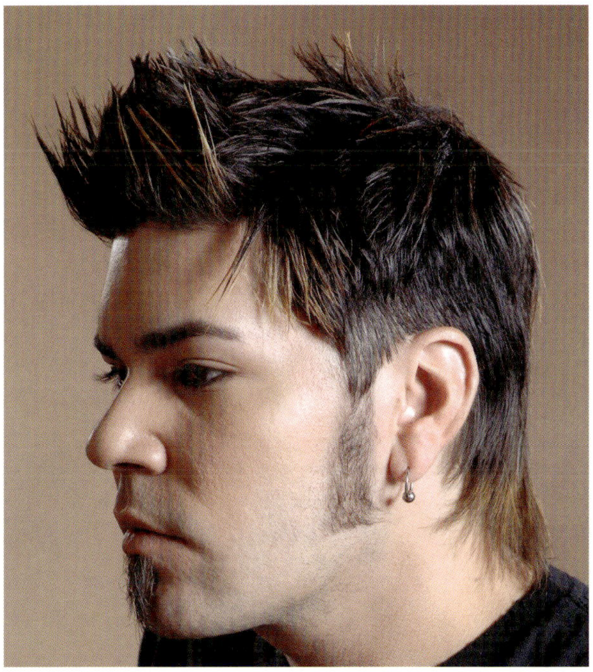

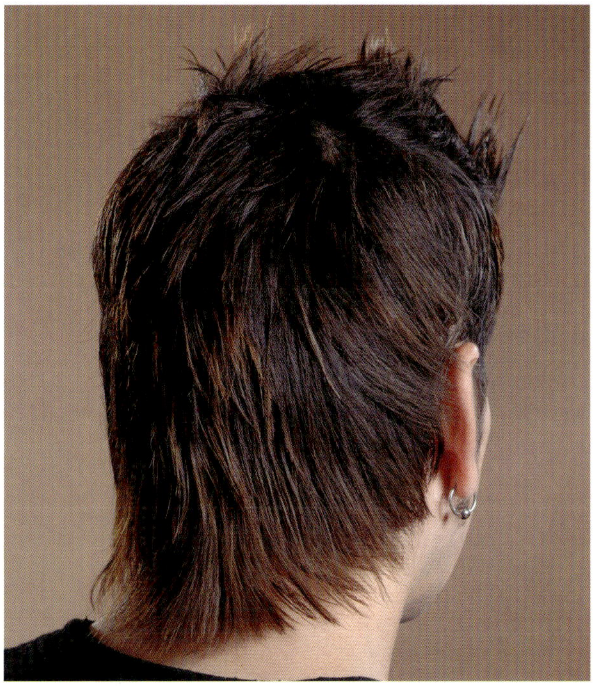

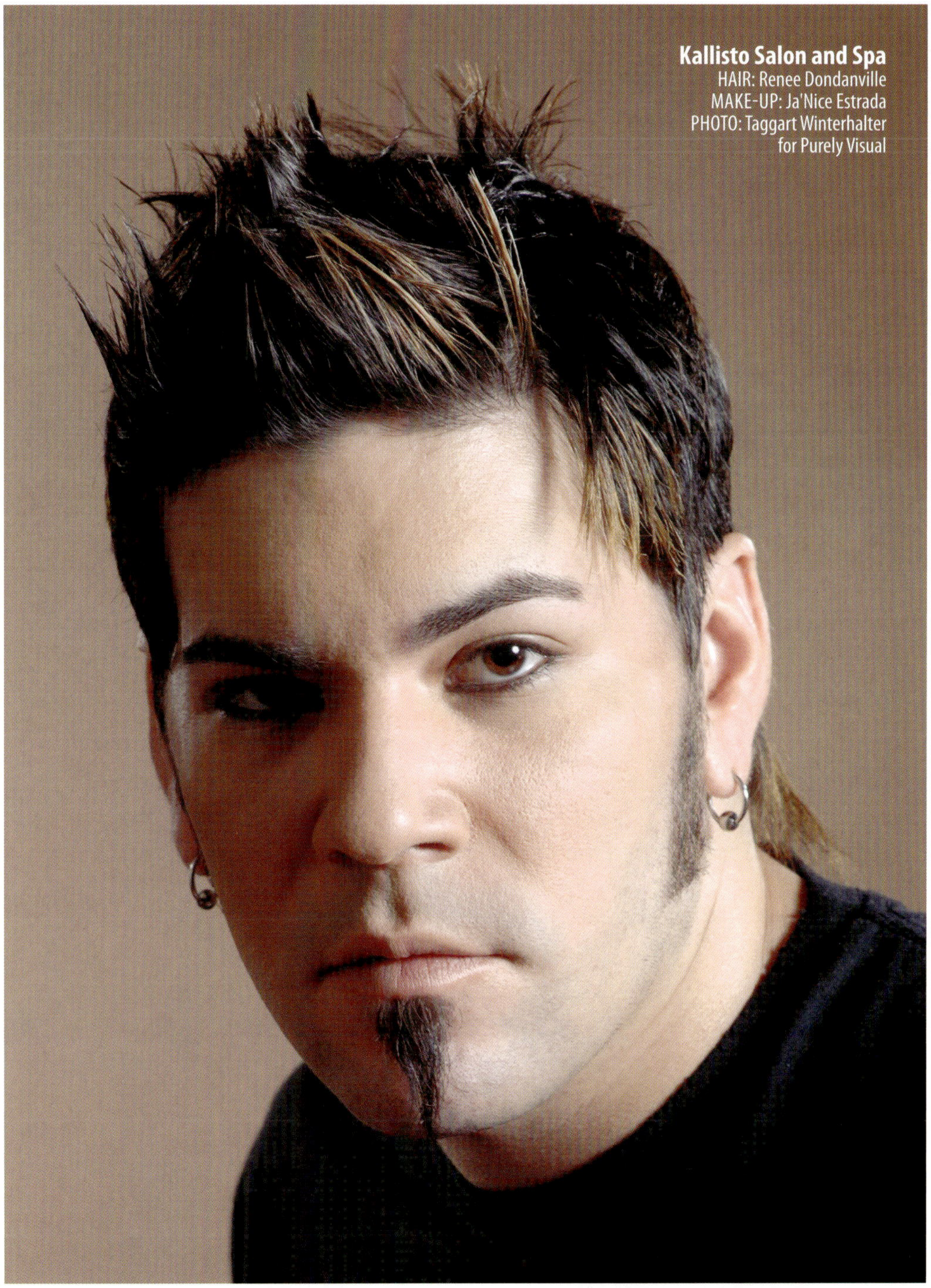

**Kallisto Salon and Spa**
HAIR: Renee Dondanville
MAKE-UP: Ja'Nice Estrada
PHOTO: Taggart Winterhalter for Purely Visual

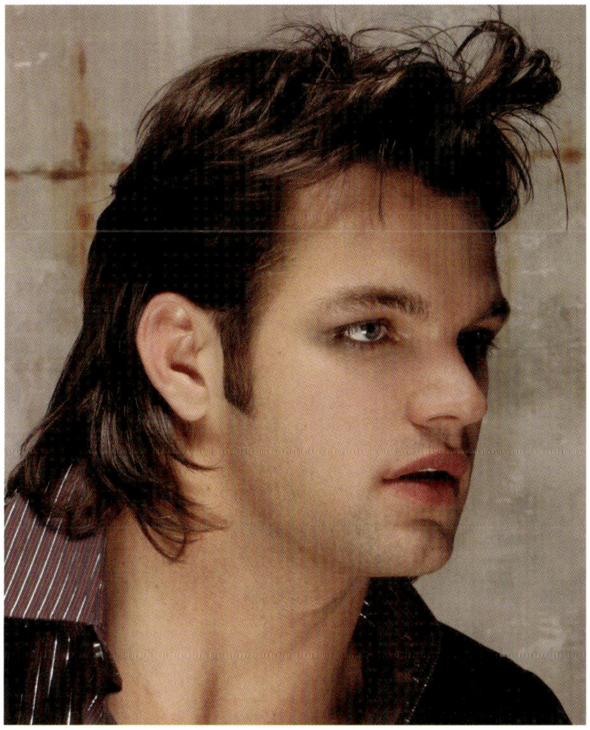

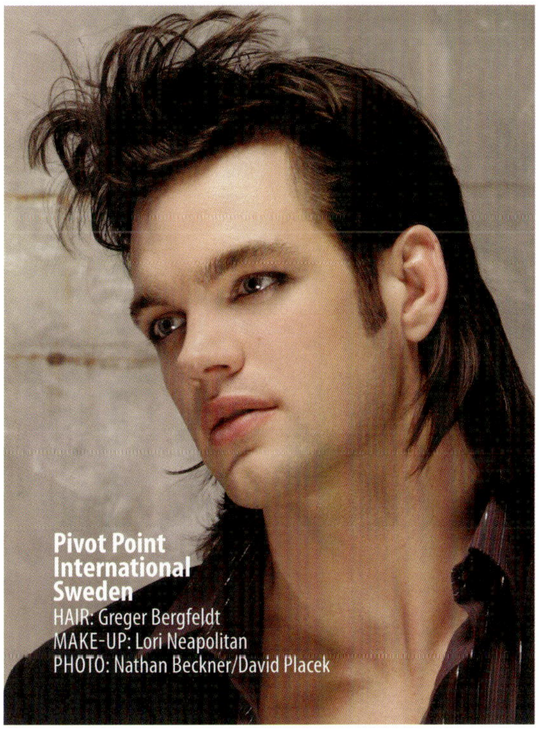

**Pivot Point International Sweden**
HAIR: Greger Bergfeldt
MAKE-UP: Lori Neapolitan
PHOTO: Nathan Beckner/David Placek

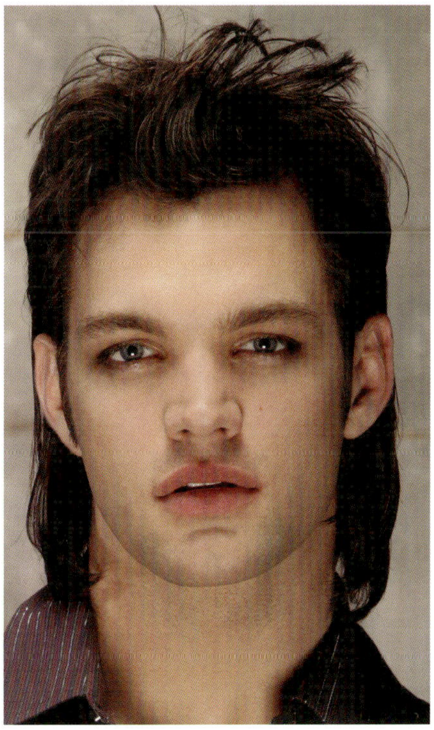

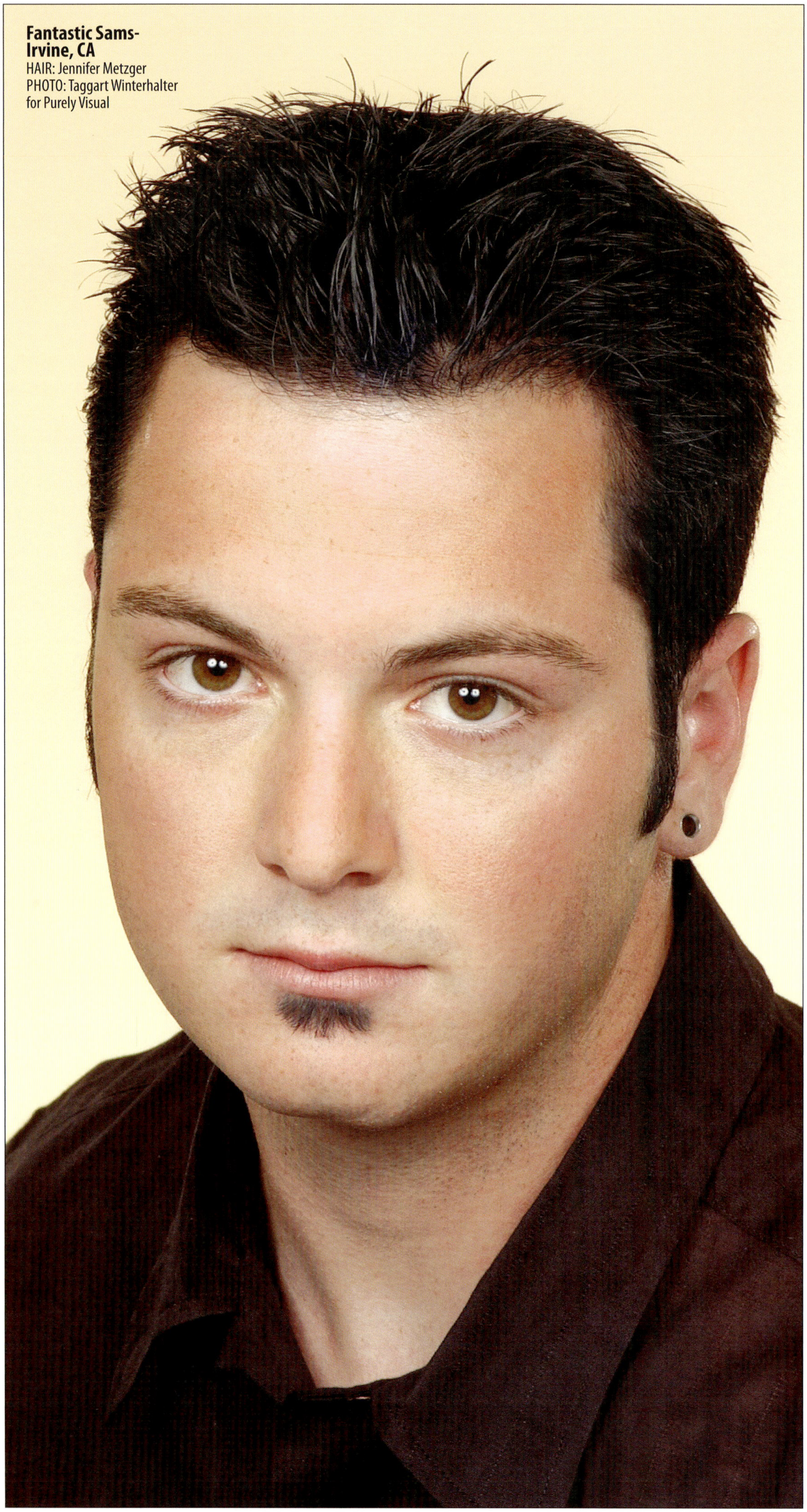

**Fantastic Sams-
Irvine, CA**
HAIR: Jennifer Metzger
PHOTO: Taggart Winterhalter
for Purely Visual

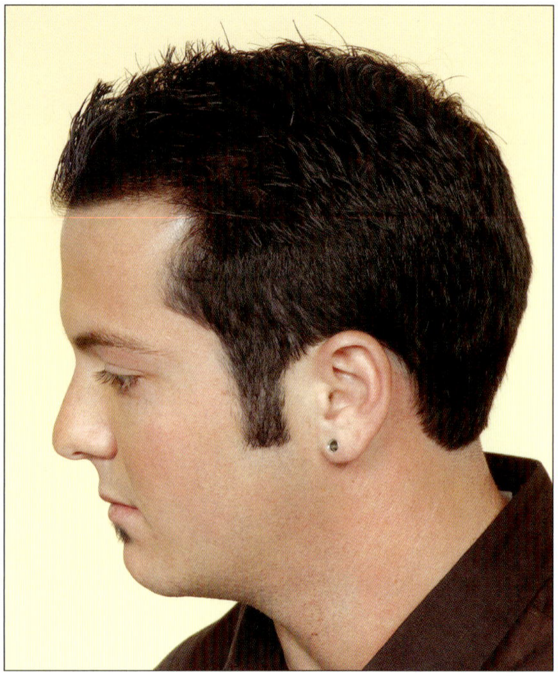

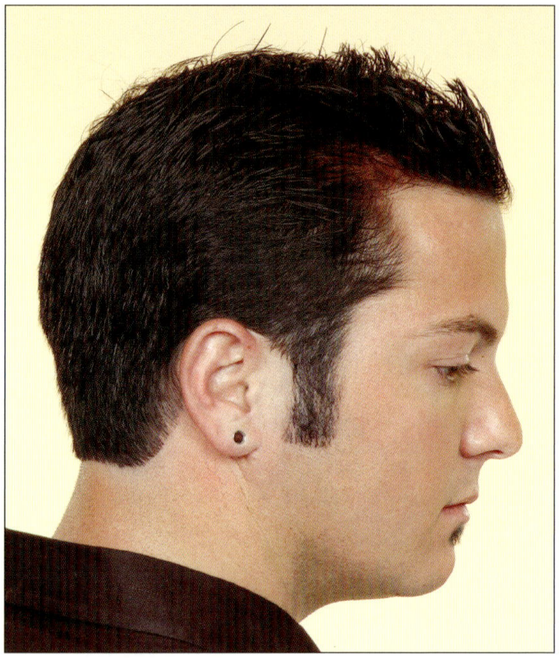

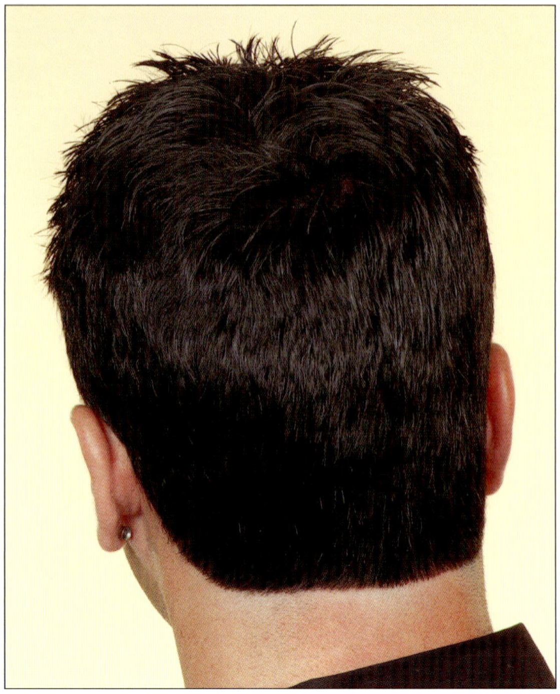

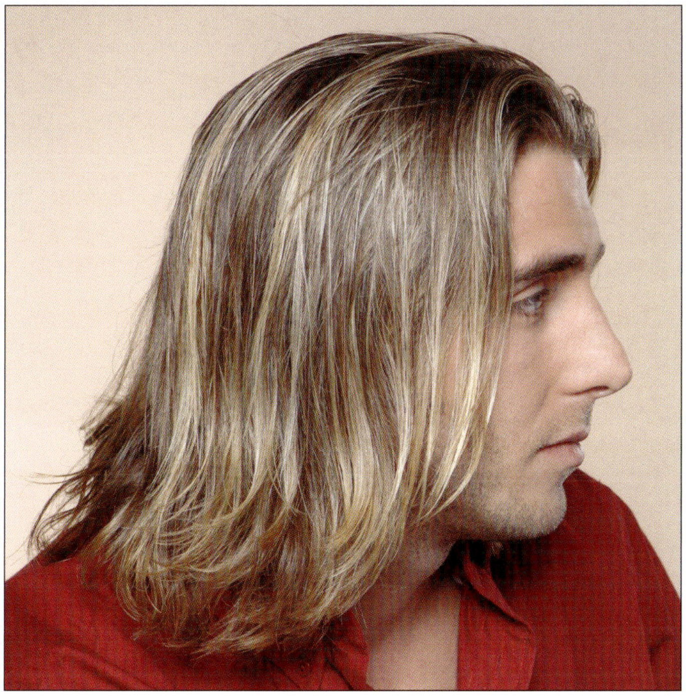

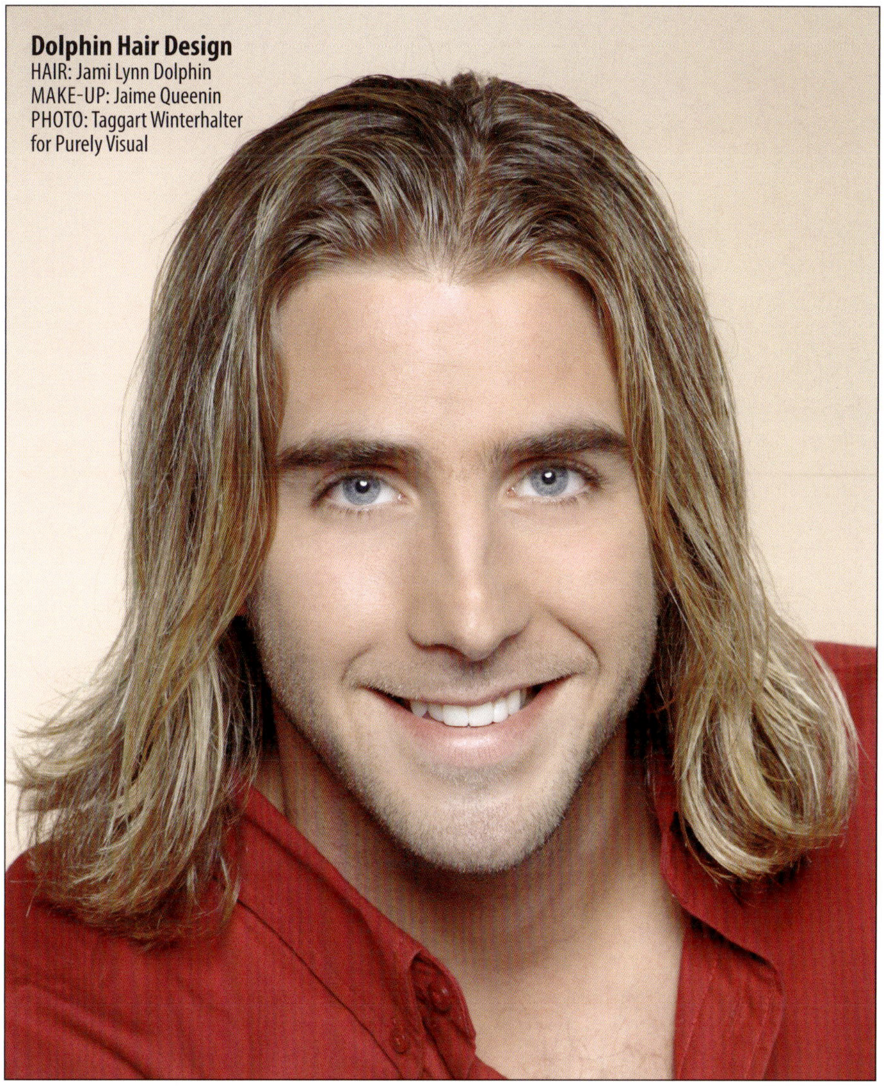

**Dolphin Hair Design**
HAIR: Jami Lynn Dolphin
MAKE-UP: Jaime Queenin
PHOTO: Taggart Winterhalter for Purely Visual

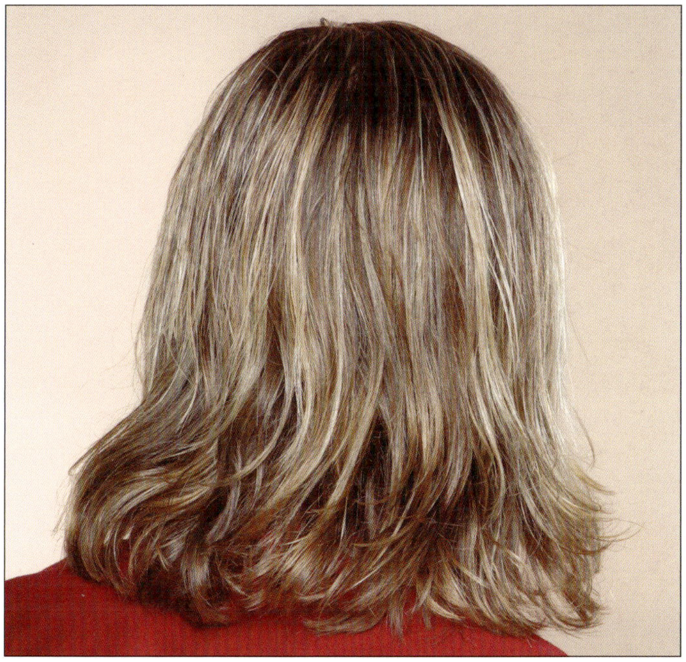

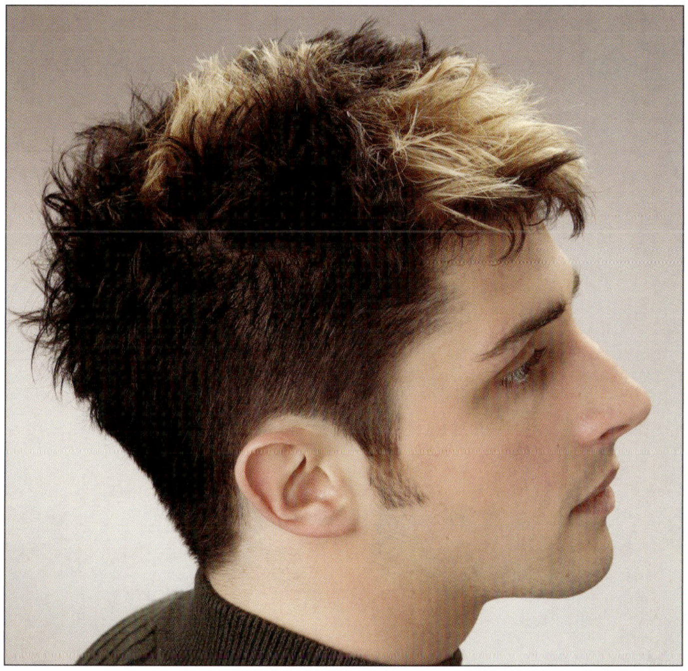

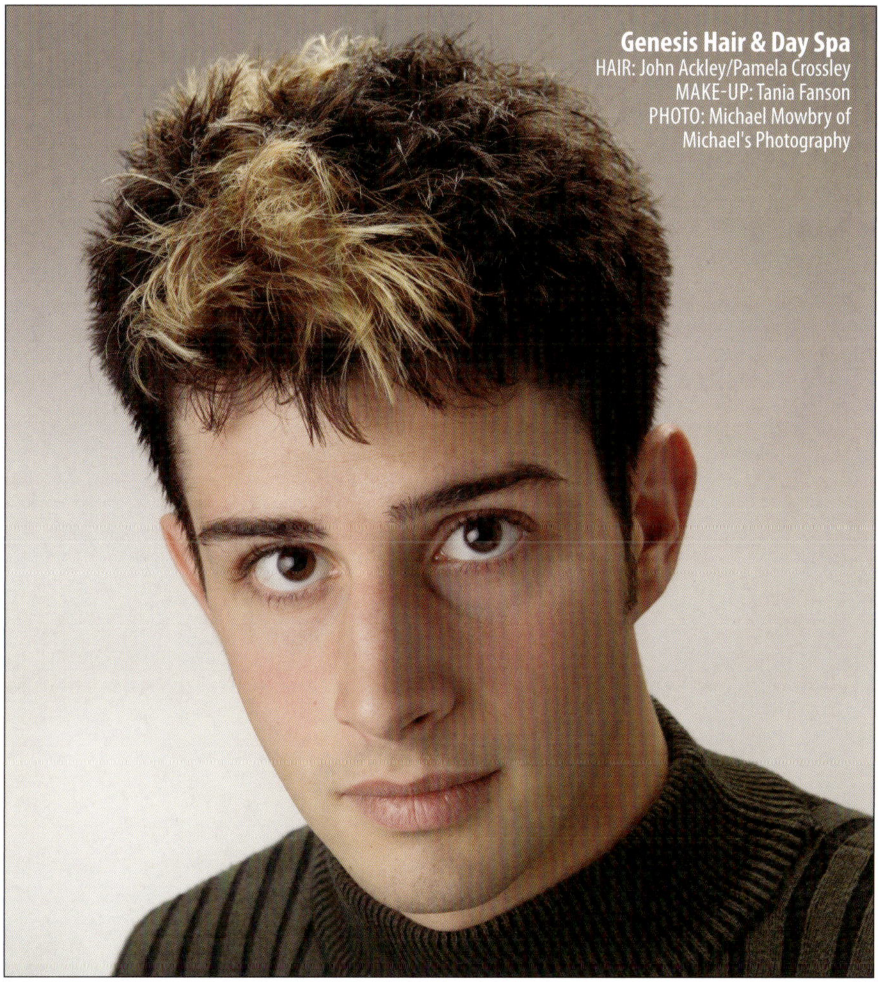

**Genesis Hair & Day Spa**
HAIR: John Ackley/Pamela Crossley
MAKE-UP: Tania Fanson
PHOTO: Michael Mowbry of Michael's Photography

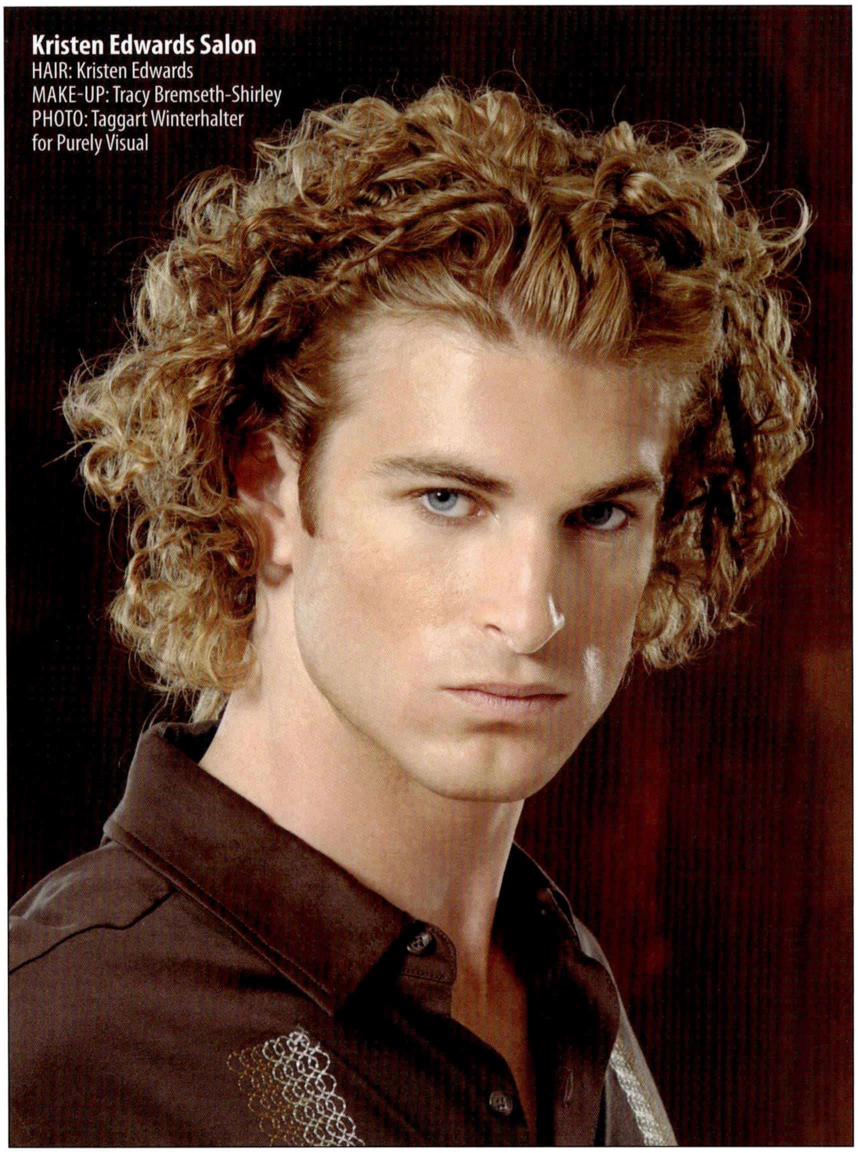

**Kristen Edwards Salon**
HAIR: Kristen Edwards
MAKE-UP: Tracy Bremseth-Shirley
PHOTO: Taggart Winterhalter
for Purely Visual

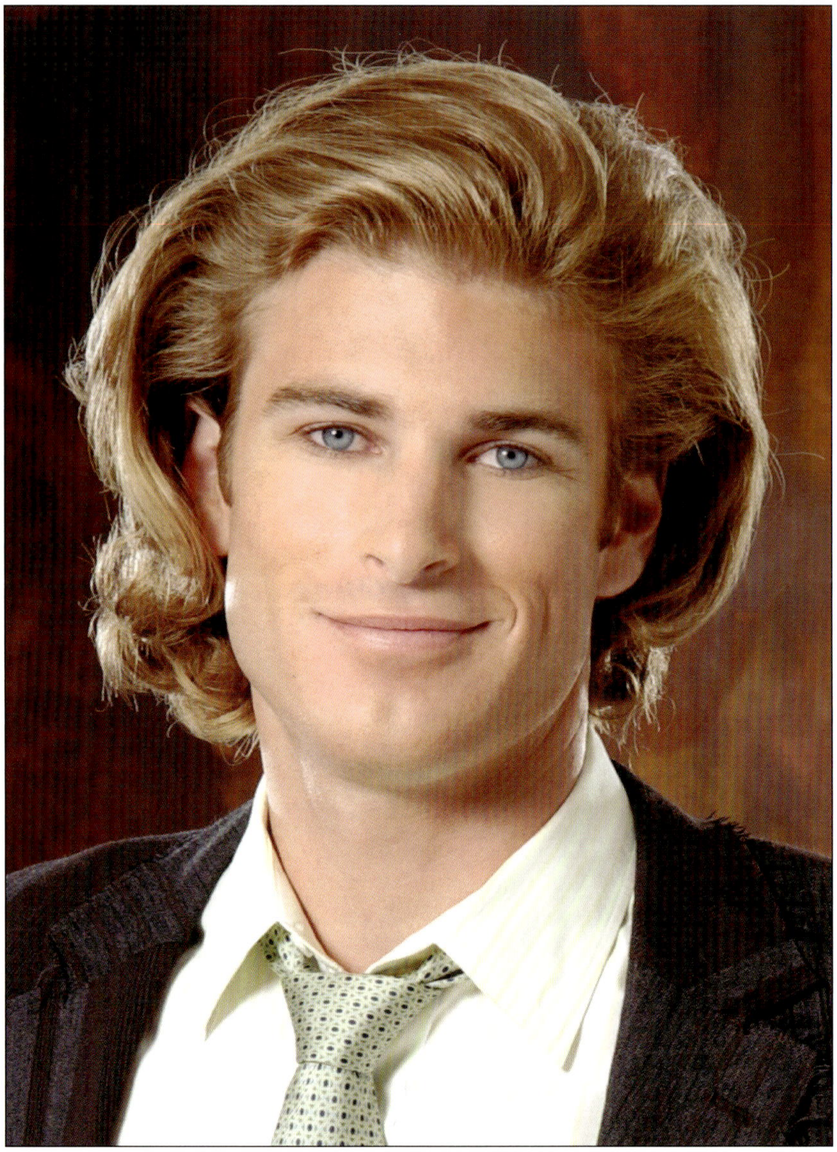

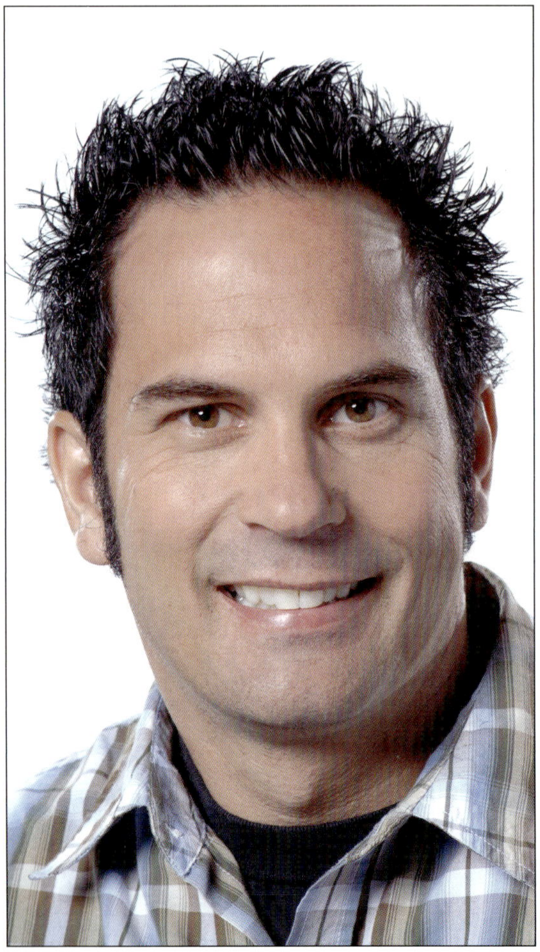

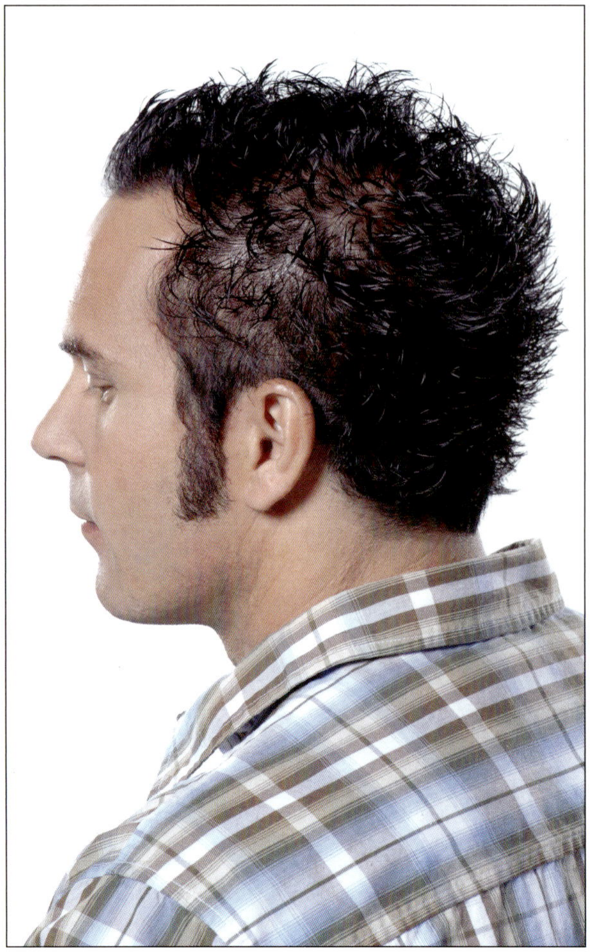

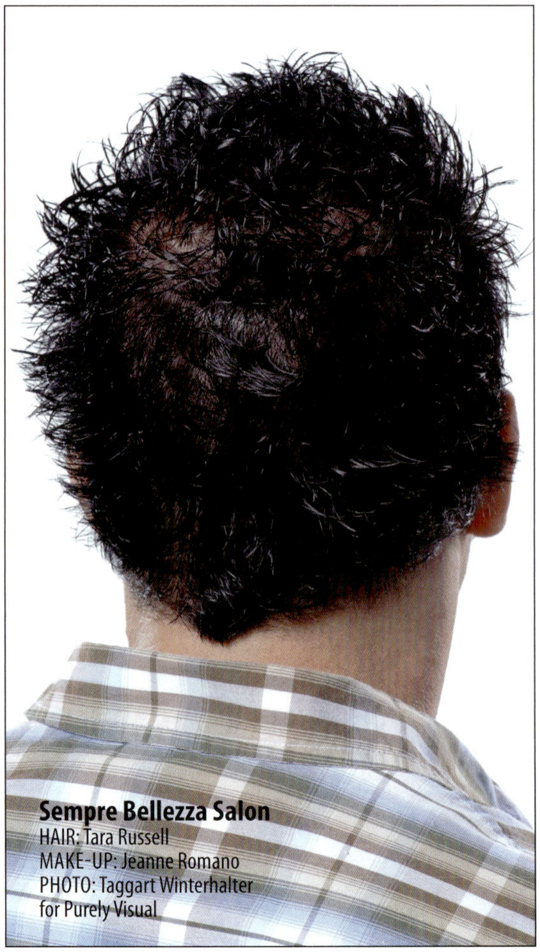

**Sempre Bellezza Salon**
HAIR: Tara Russell
MAKE-UP: Jeanne Romano
PHOTO: Taggart Winterhalter
for Purely Visual

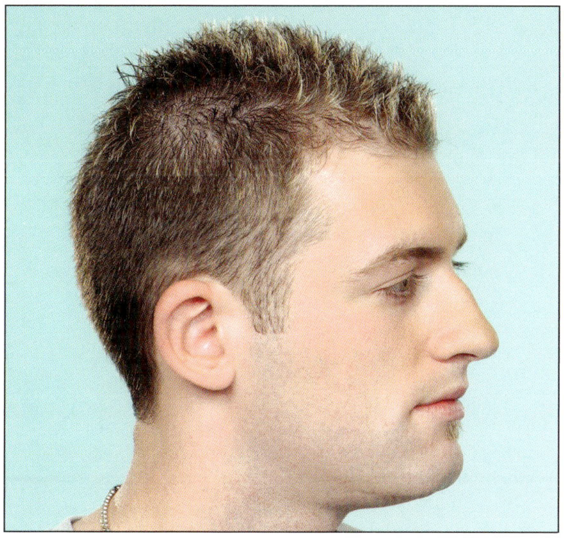

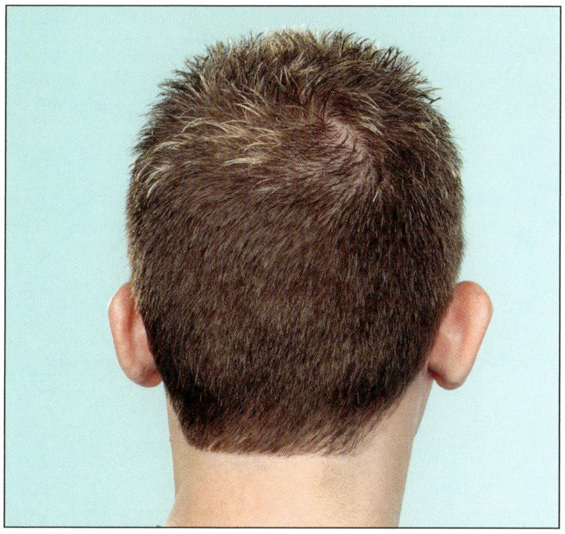

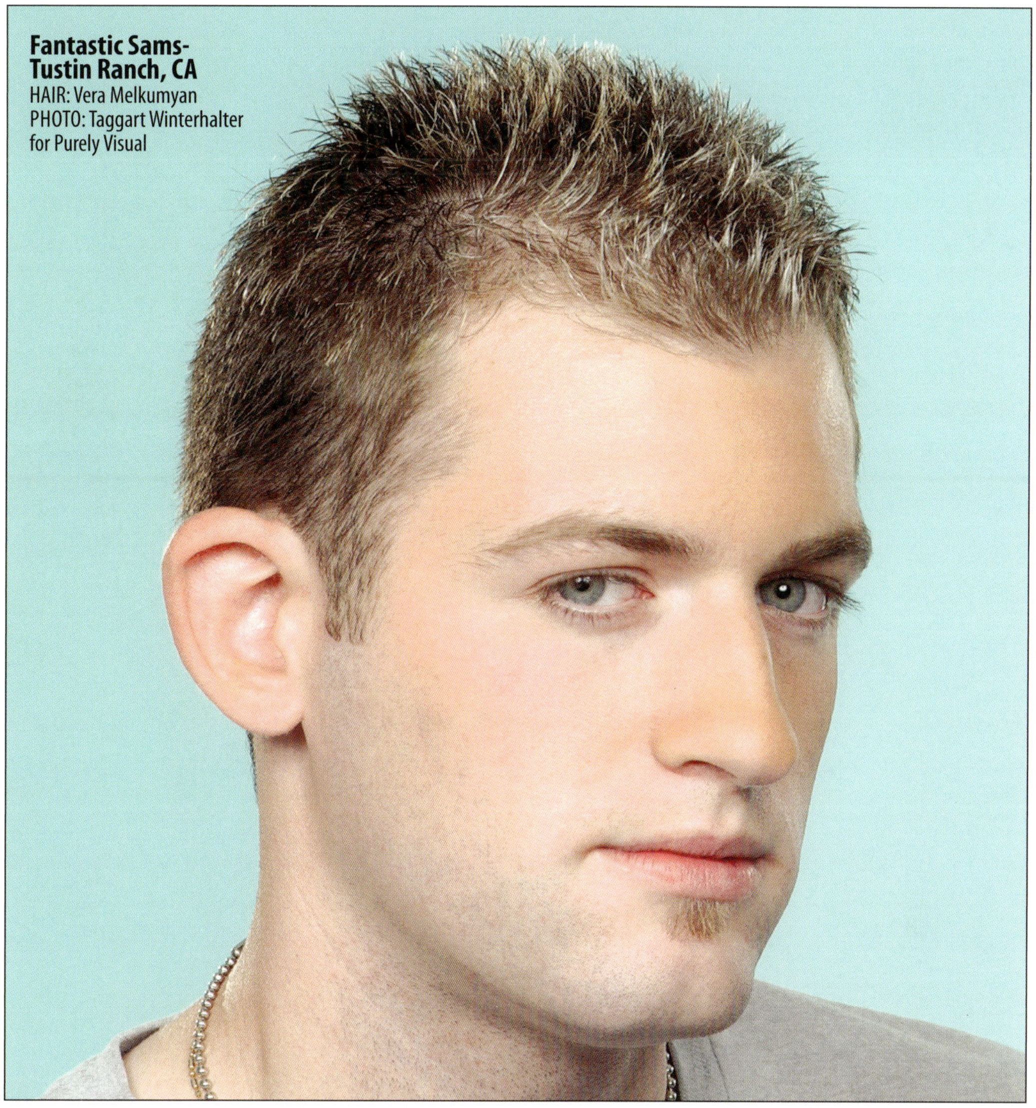

**Fantastic Sams-Tustin Ranch, CA**
HAIR: Vera Melkumyan
PHOTO: Taggart Winterhalter for Purely Visual

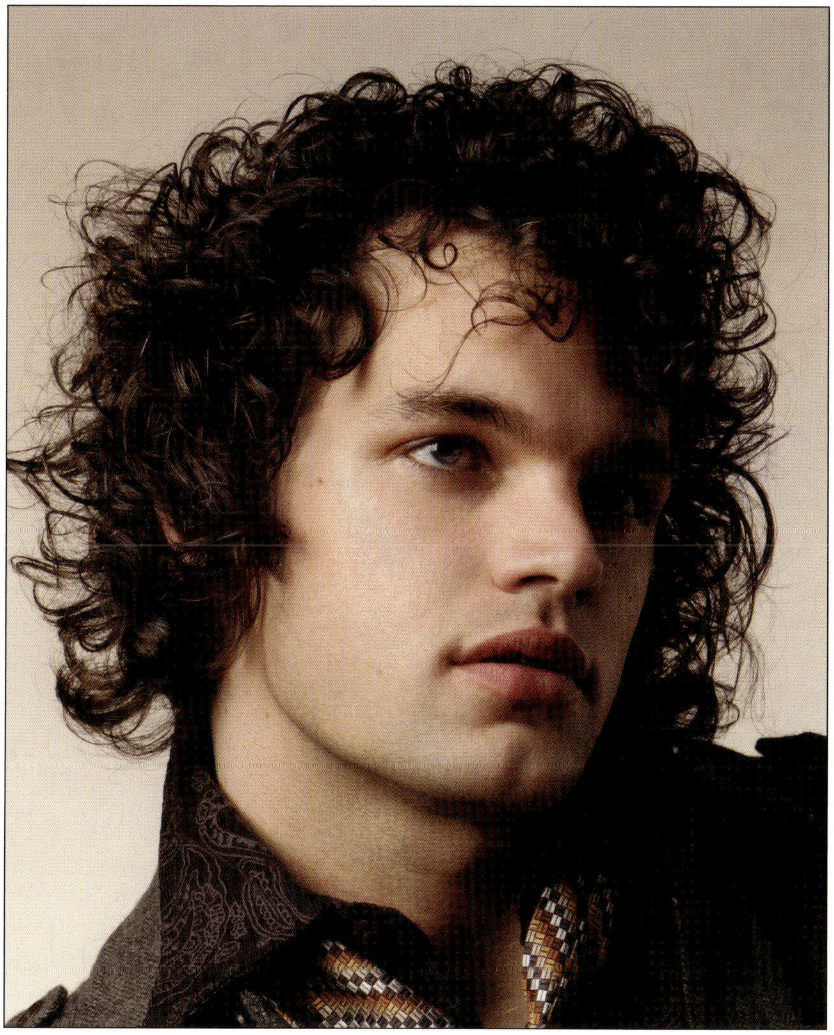

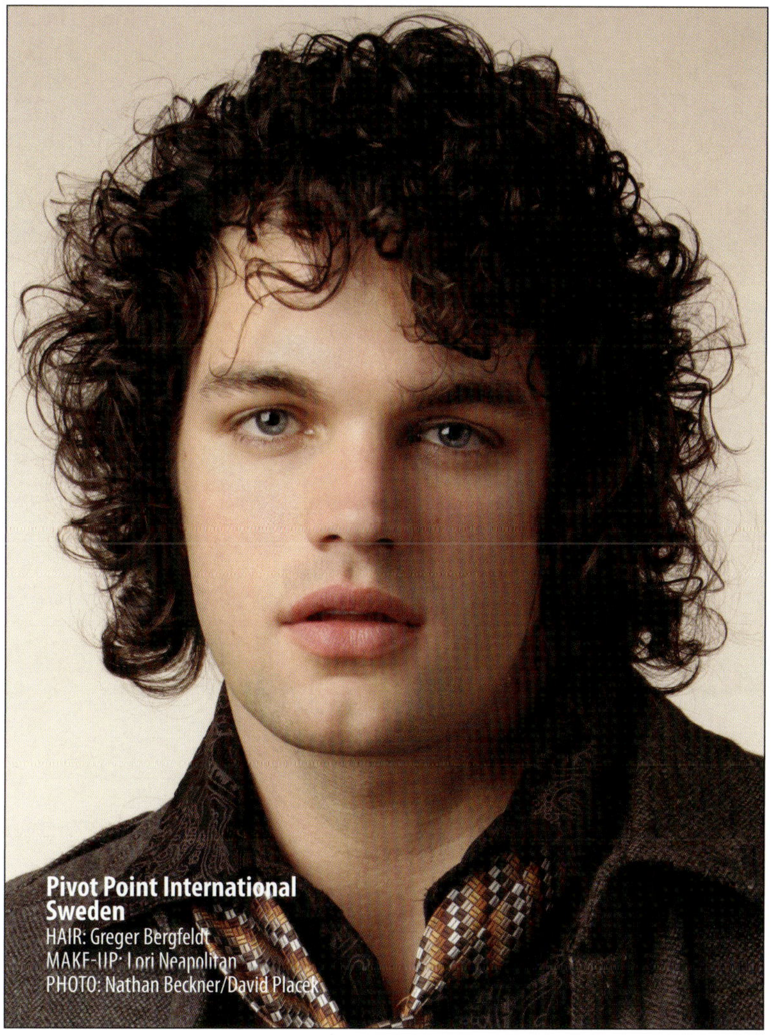

**Pivot Point International Sweden**
HAIR: Greger Bergfeldt
MAKE-UP: Lori Neapolitan
PHOTO: Nathan Beckner/David Placek

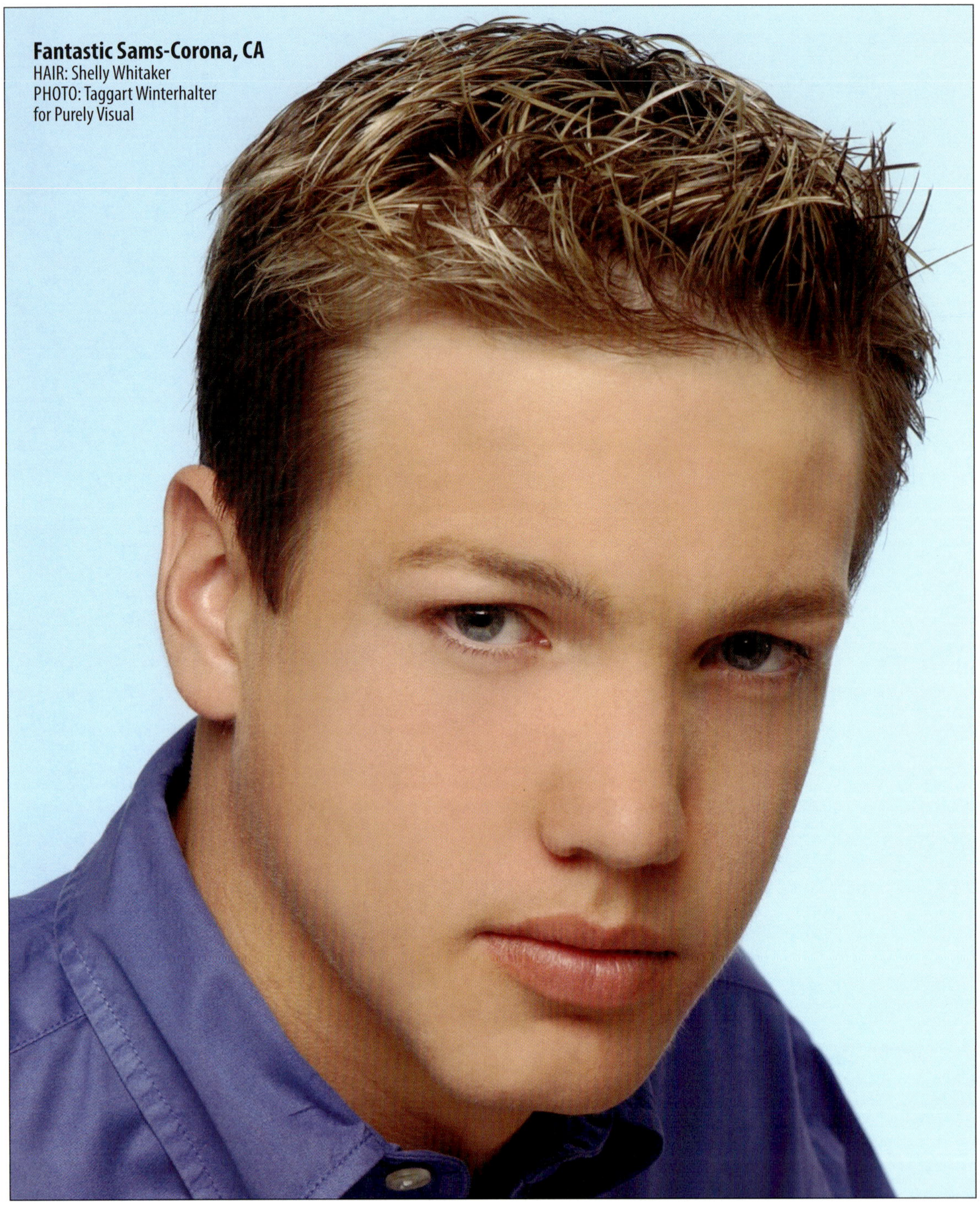
**Fantastic Sams-Corona, CA**
HAIR: Shelly Whitaker
PHOTO: Taggart Winterhalter
for Purely Visual

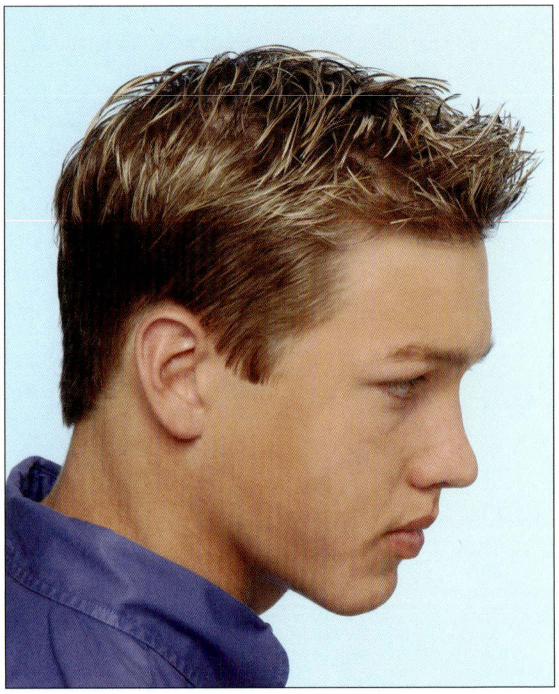

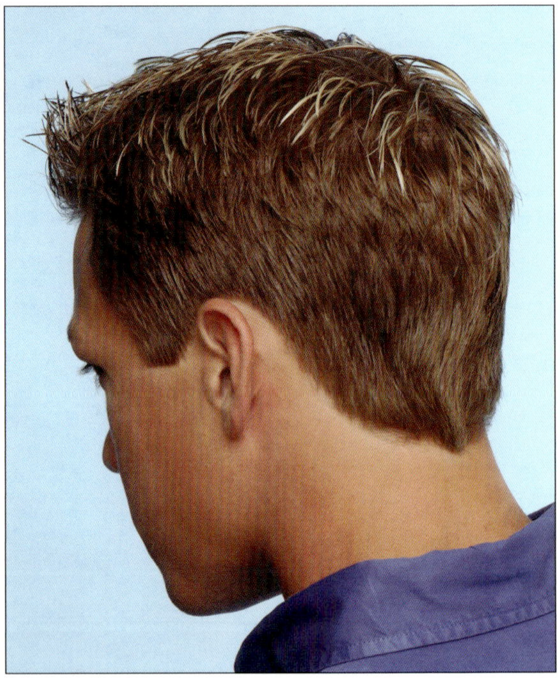

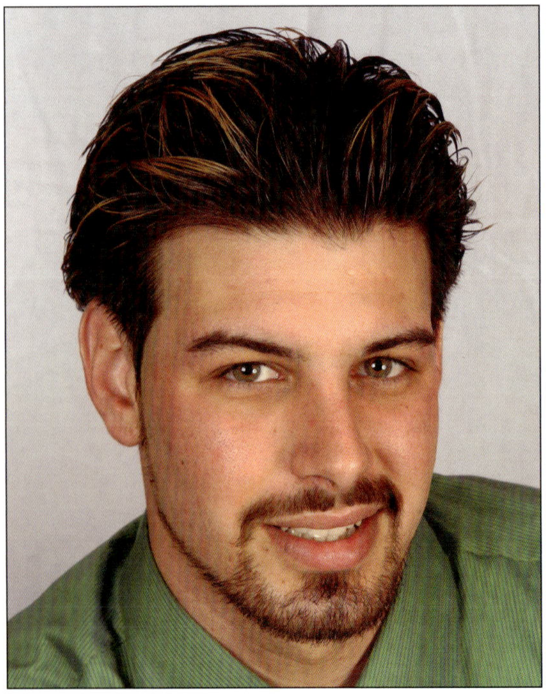

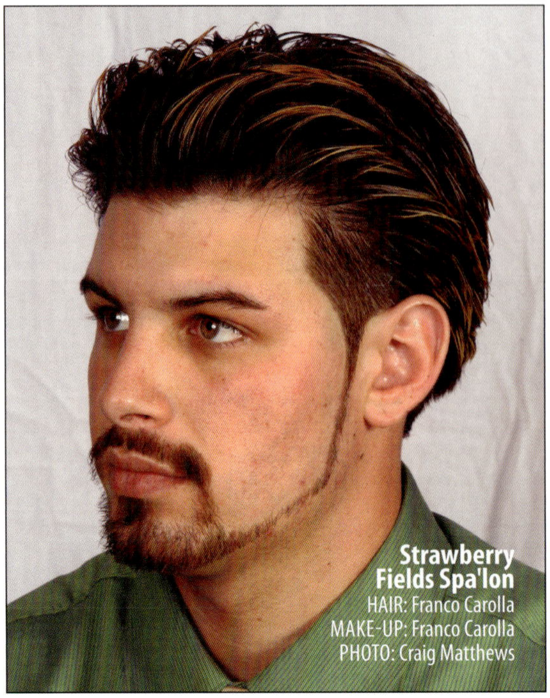
**Strawberry Fields Spa'lon**
HAIR: Franco Carolla
MAKE-UP: Franco Carolla
PHOTO: Craig Matthews

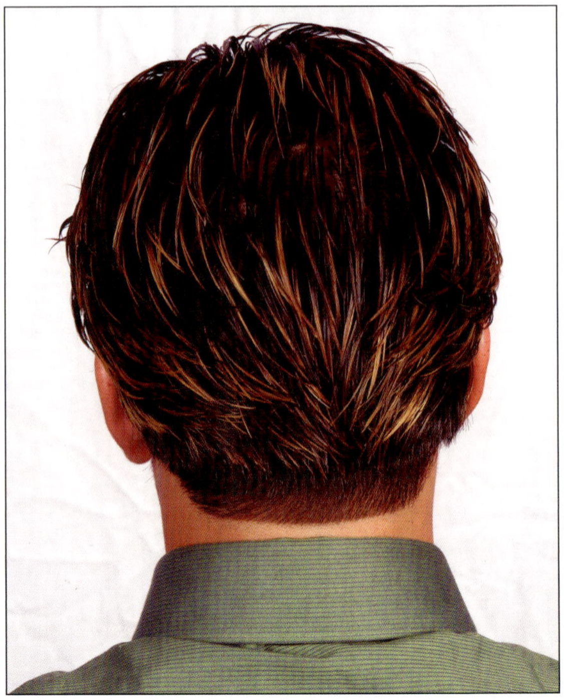

**Goldwell**
HAIR: Trend Zoom 06 Team

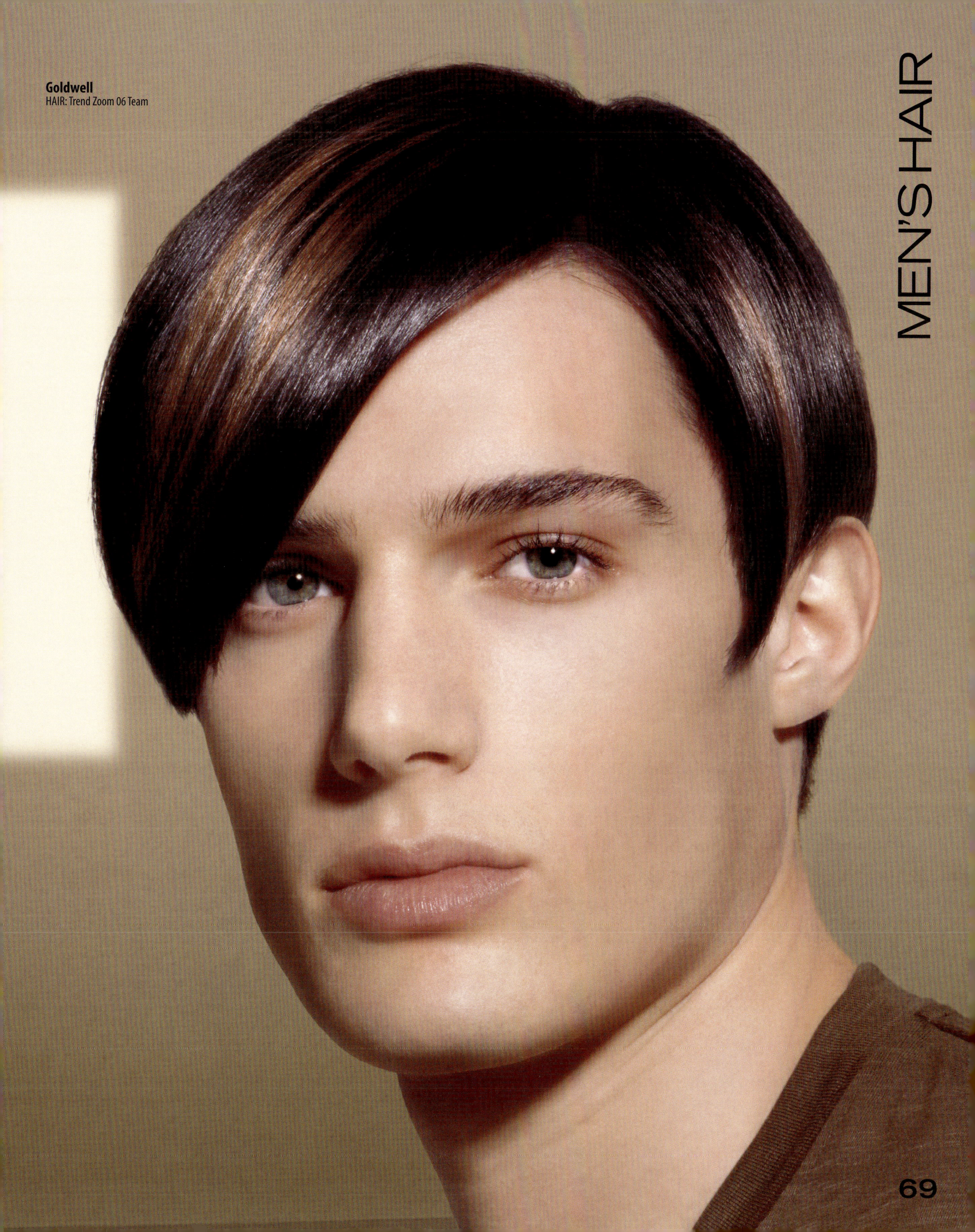

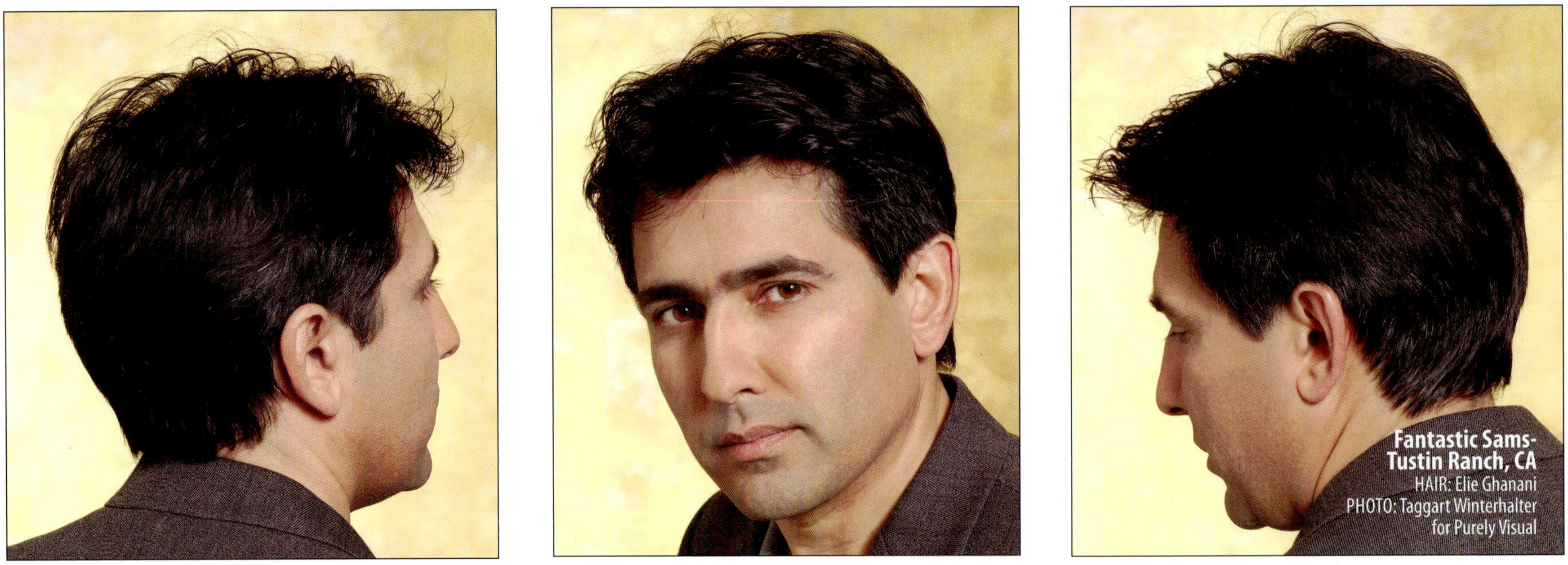

**Fantastic Sams-
Tustin Ranch, CA**
HAIR: Elie Ghanani
PHOTO: Taggart Winterhalter
for Purely Visual

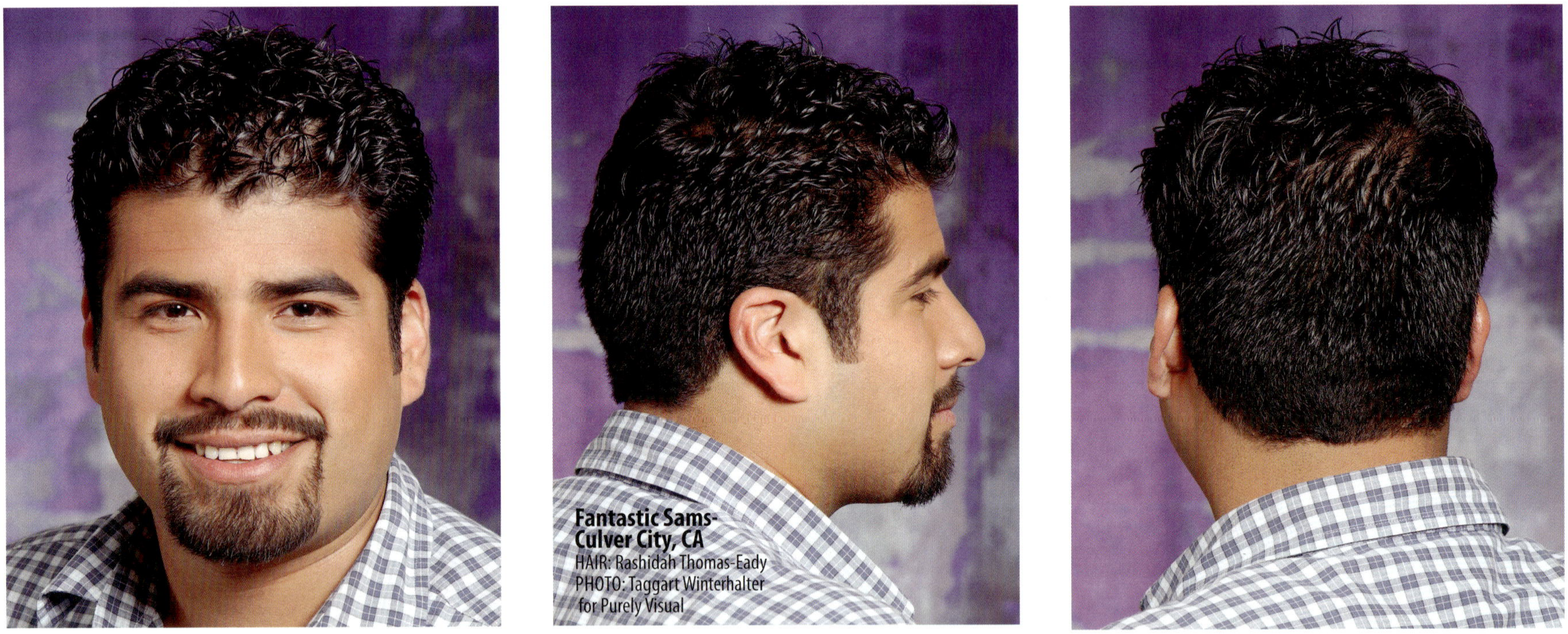

**Fantastic Sams-
Culver City, CA**
HAIR: Rashidah Thomas-Eady
PHOTO: Taggart Winterhalter
for Purely Visual

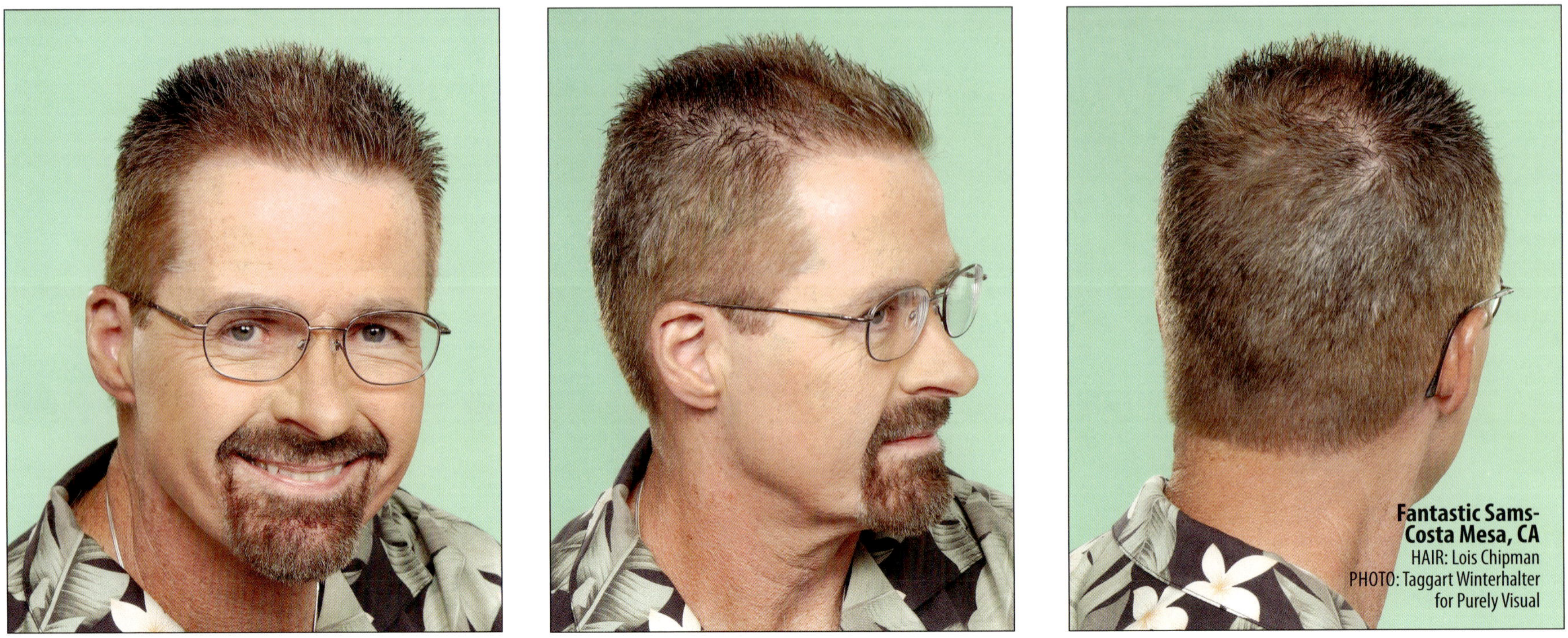

**Fantastic Sams-
Costa Mesa, CA**
HAIR: Lois Chipman
PHOTO: Taggart Winterhalter
for Purely Visual

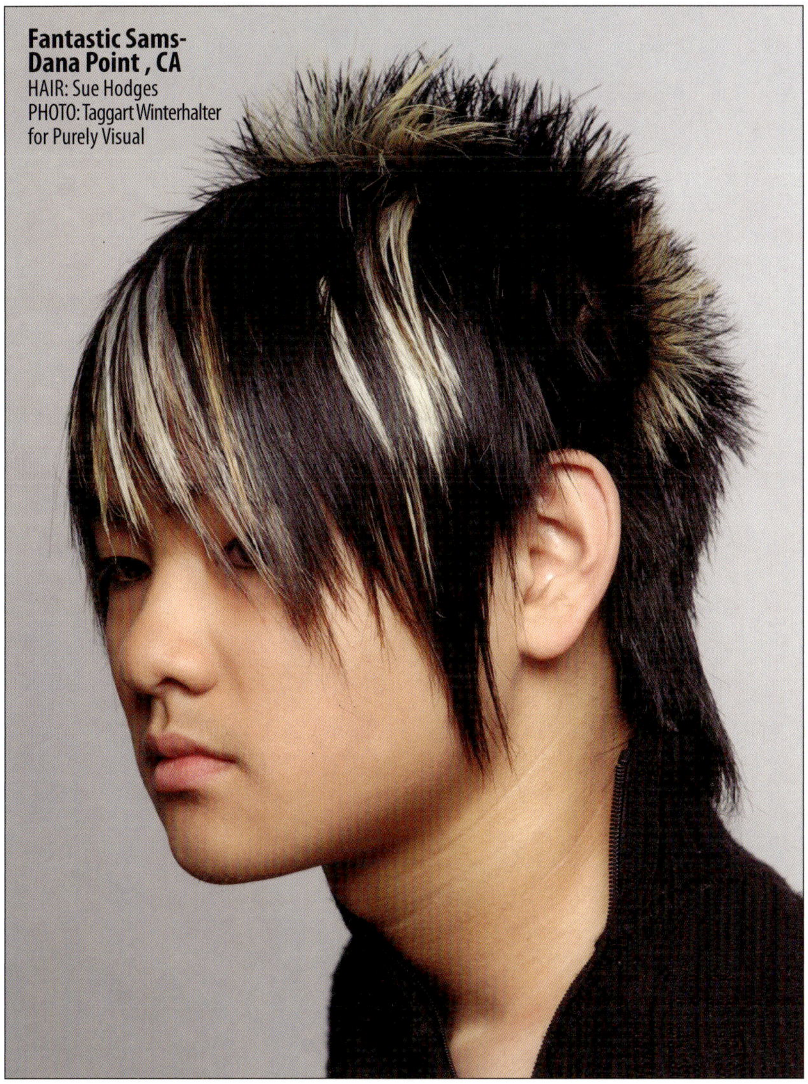

**Fantastic Sams-
Dana Point , CA**
HAIR: Sue Hodges
PHOTO: Taggart Winterhalter
for Purely Visual

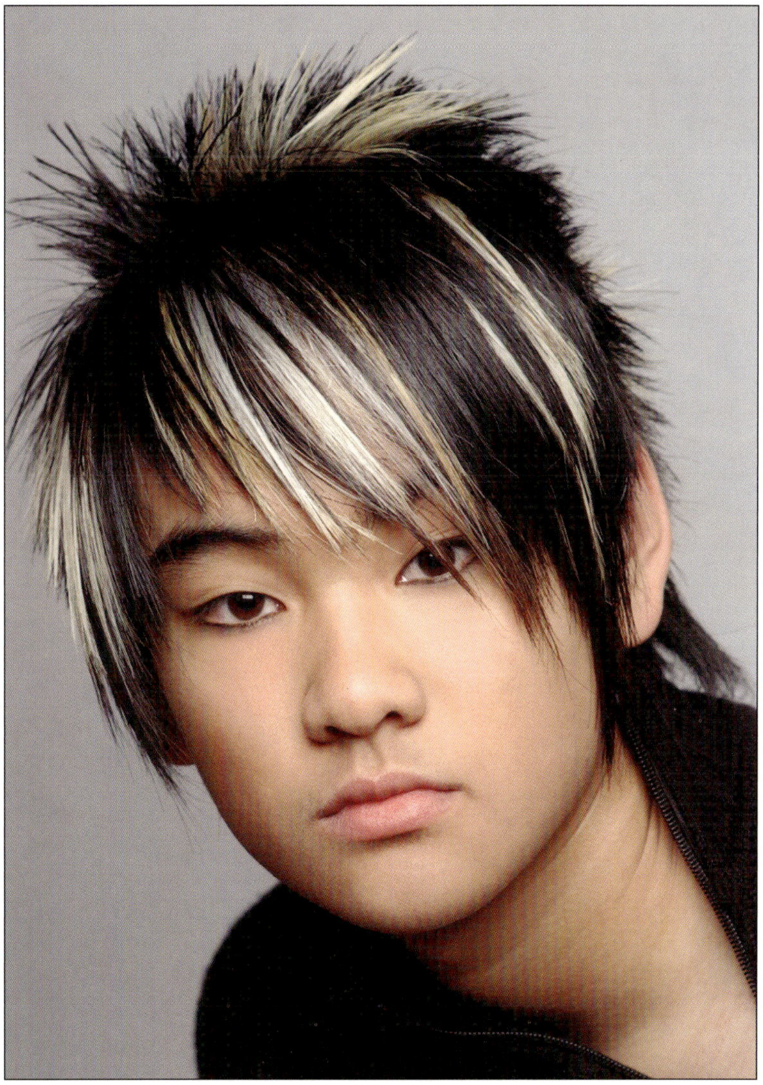

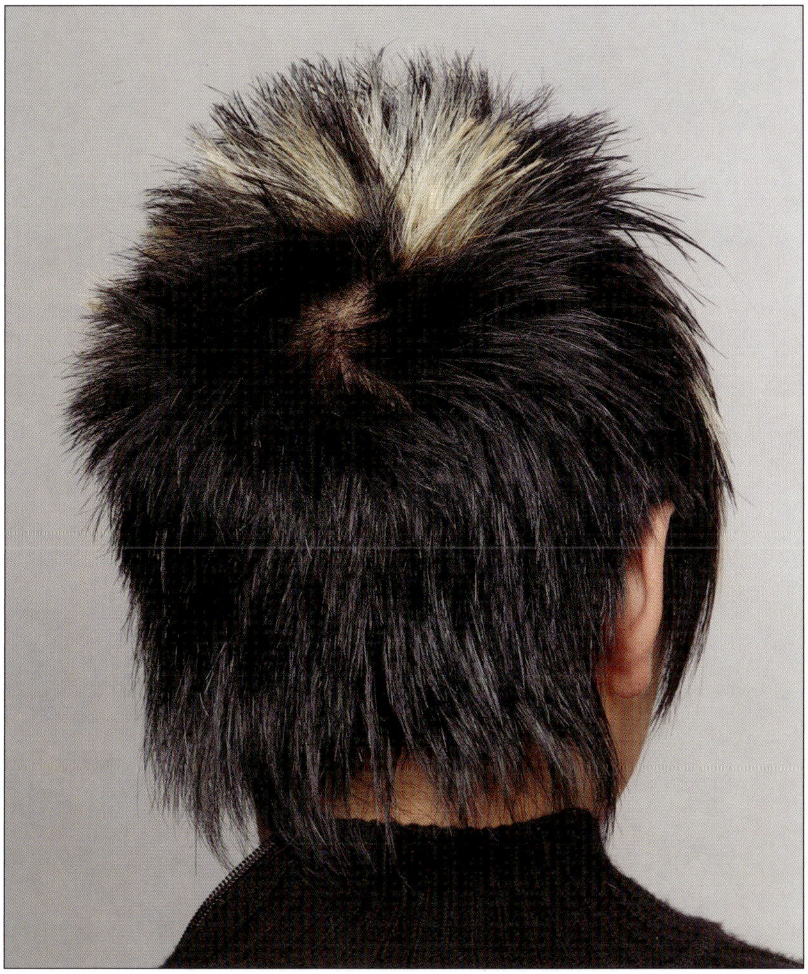

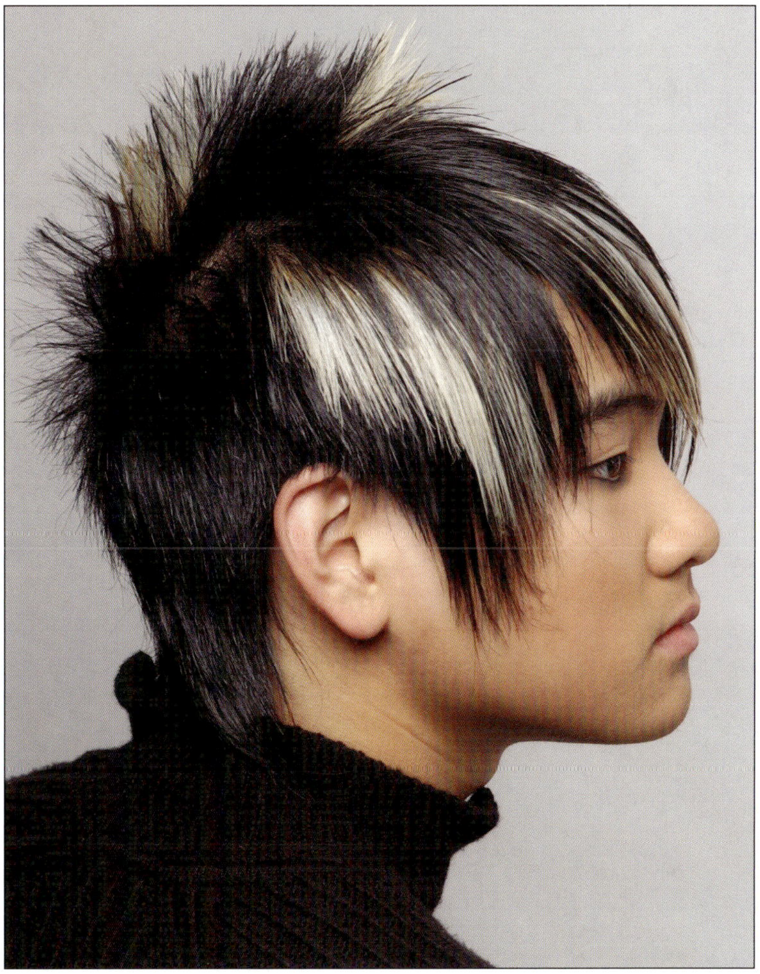

**Goldwell**
HAIR: Trend Zoom 06 Team

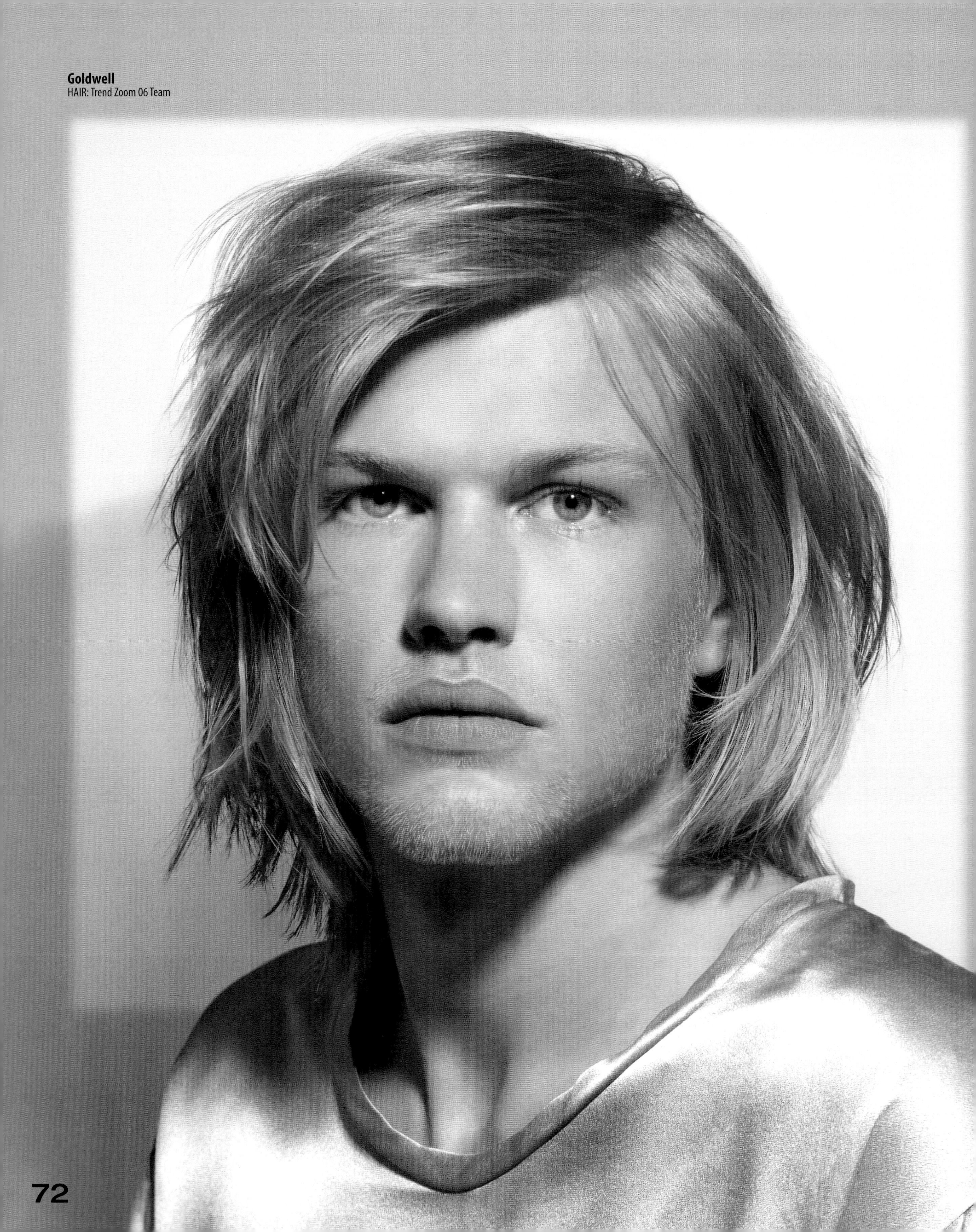

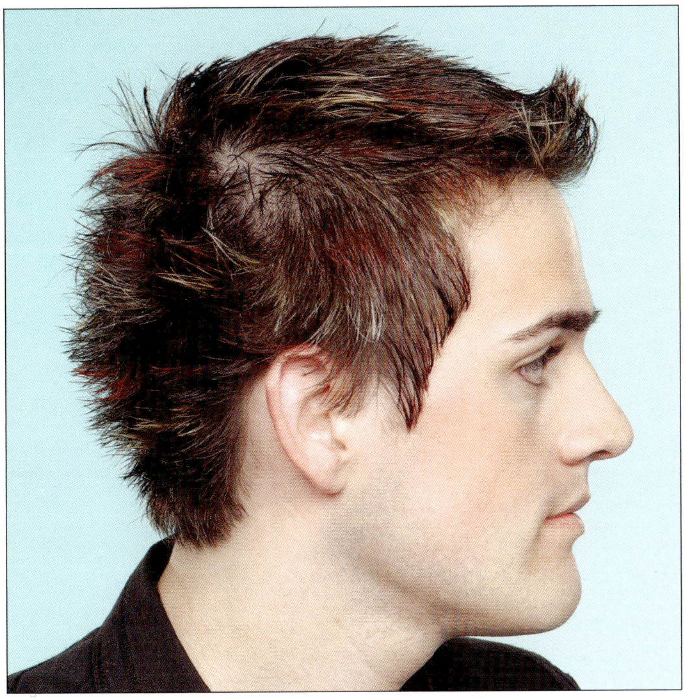

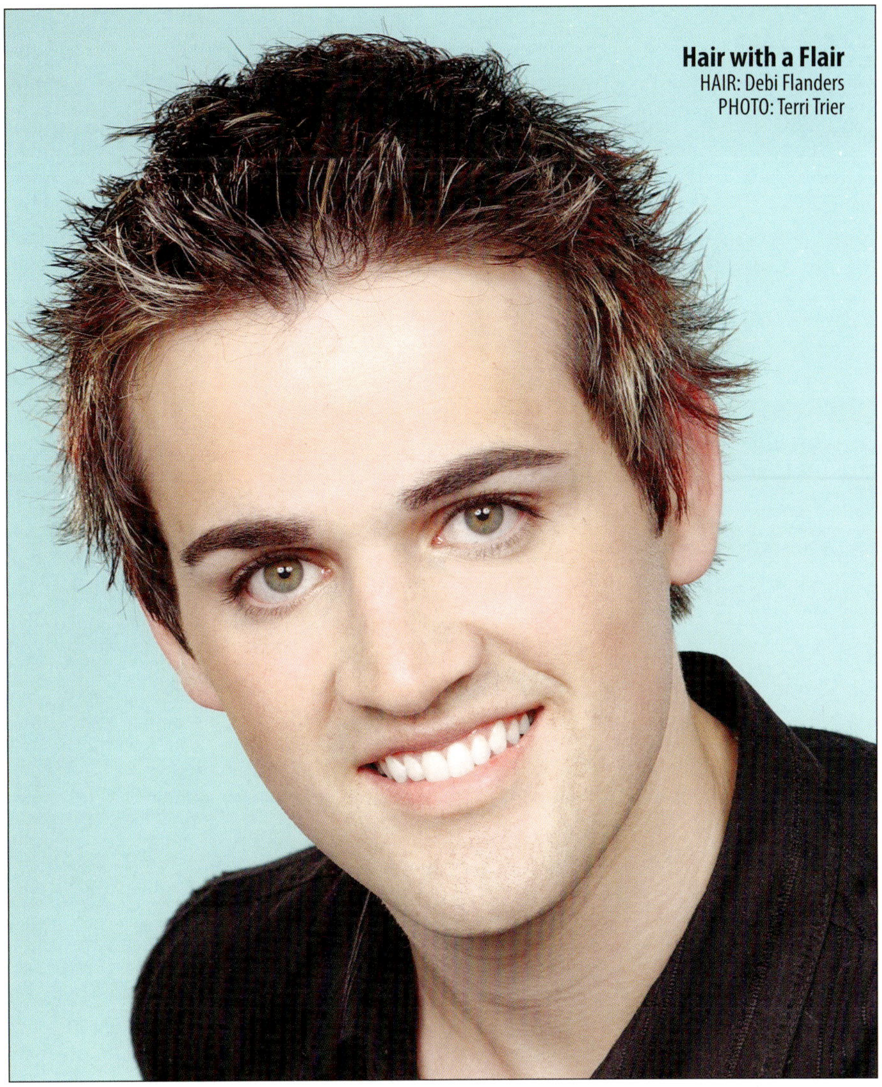

**Hair with a Flair**
HAIR: Debi Flanders
PHOTO: Terri Trier

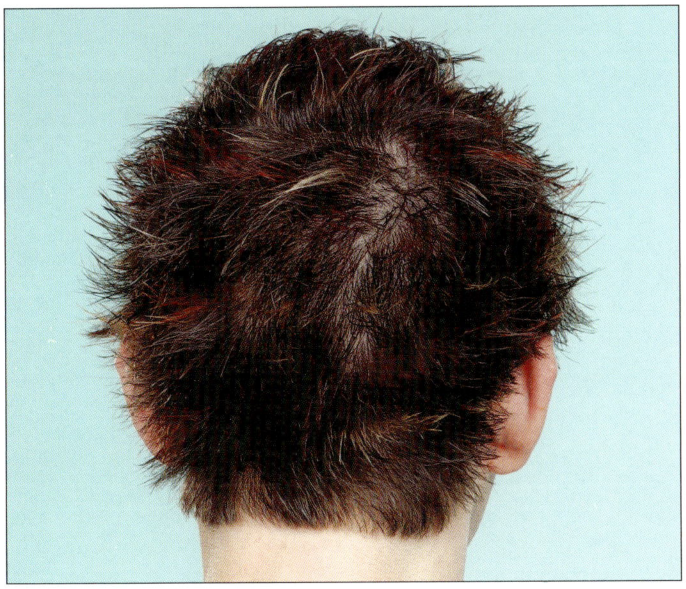

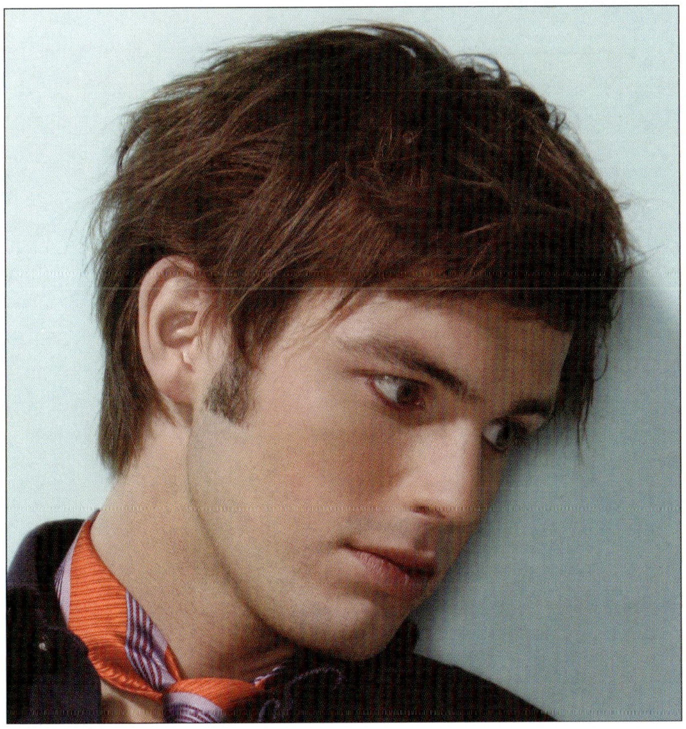

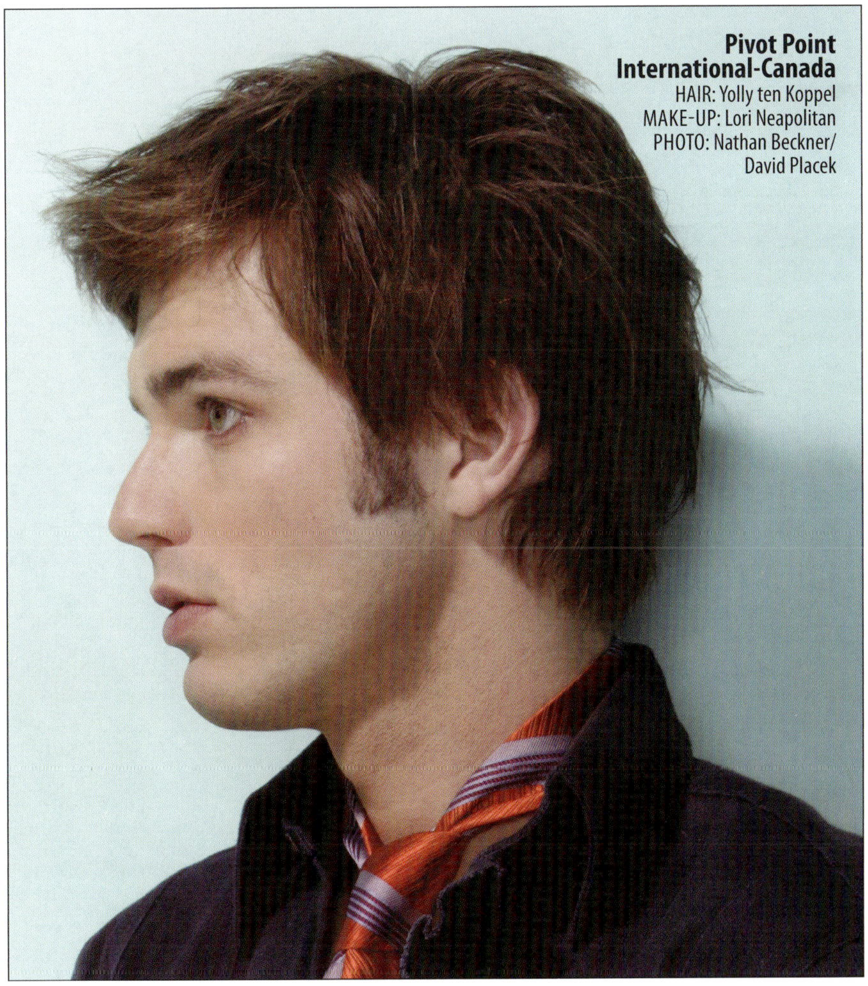

**Pivot Point International-Canada**
HAIR: Yolly ten Koppel
MAKE-UP: Lori Neapolitan
PHOTO: Nathan Beckner/ David Placek

**Genesis Hair & Day Spa**
HAIR: Amanda Atkinson
MAKE-UP: Tania Fanson
PHOTO: Michael Mowbry of Michael's Photography

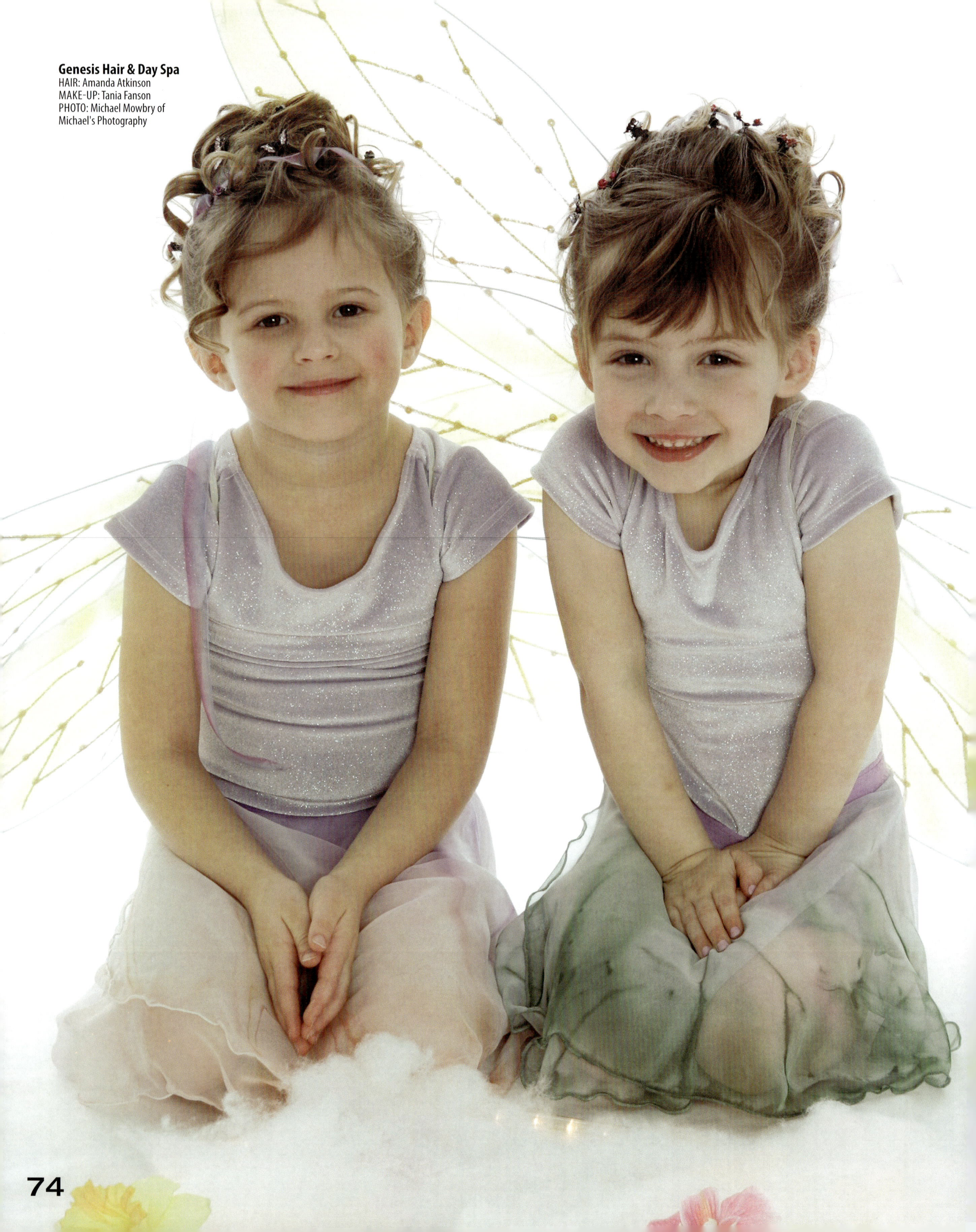

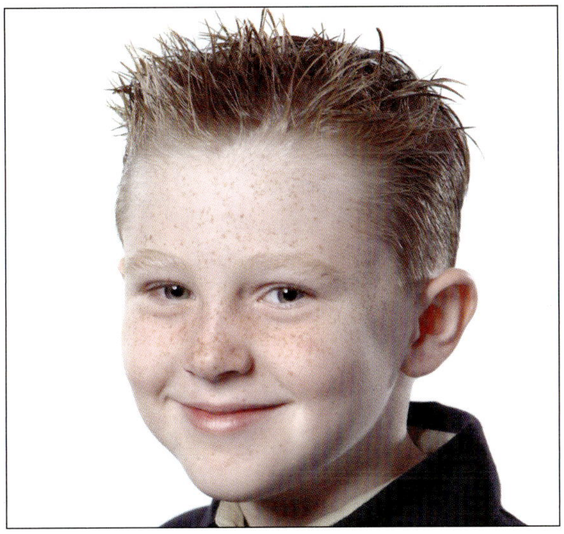

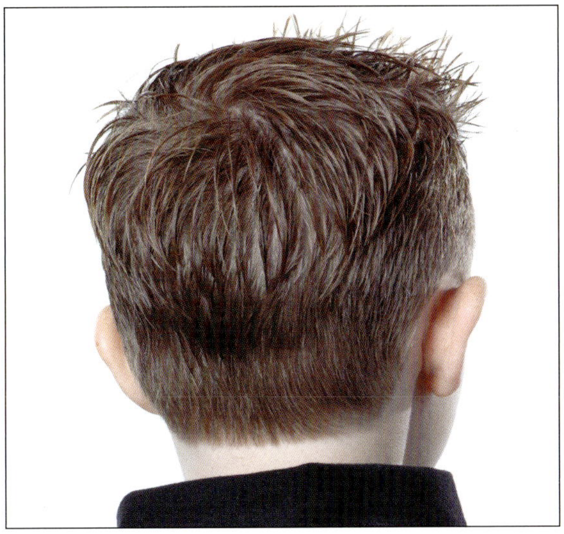

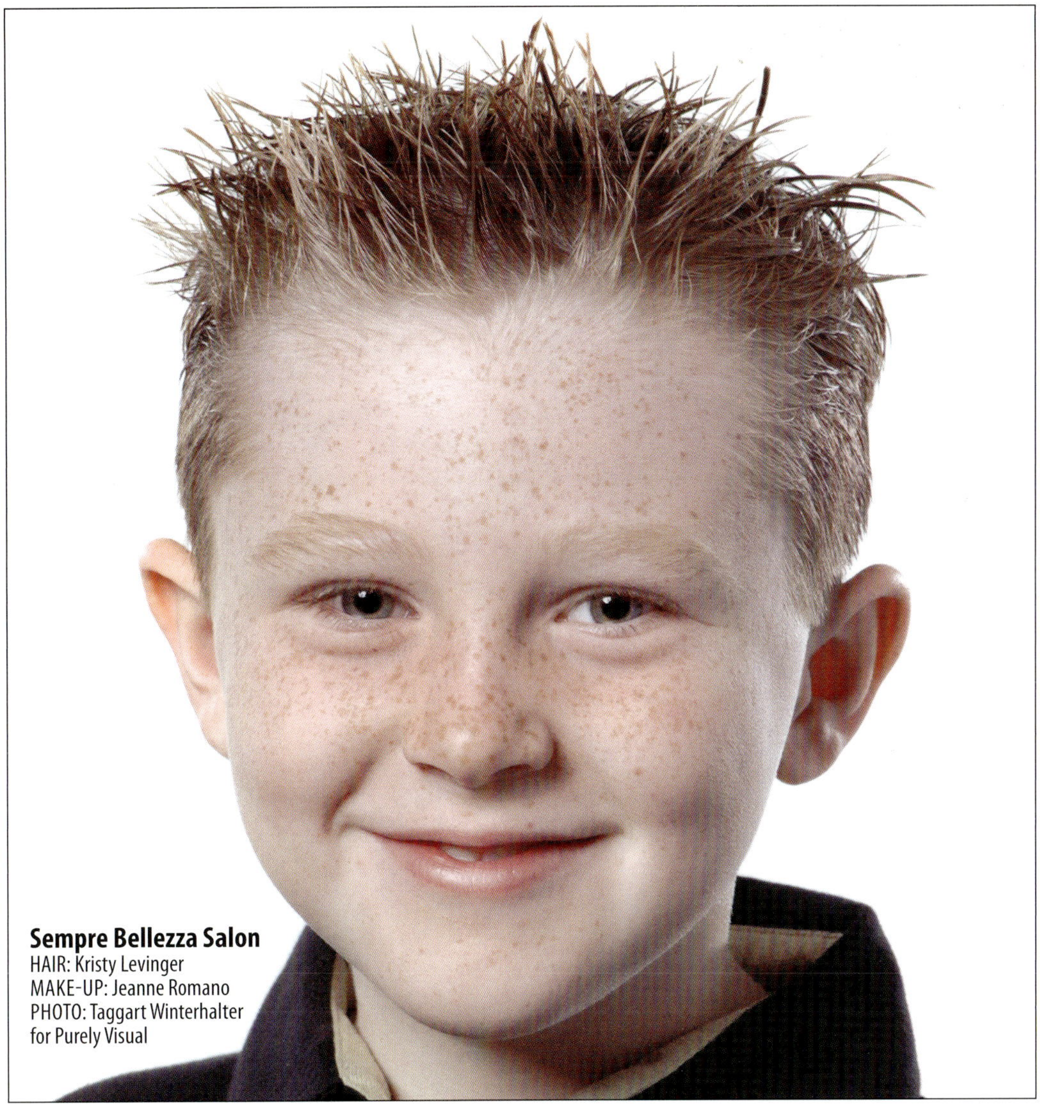

**Sempre Bellezza Salon**
HAIR: Kristy Levinger
MAKE-UP: Jeanne Romano
PHOTO: Taggart Winterhalter for Purely Visual

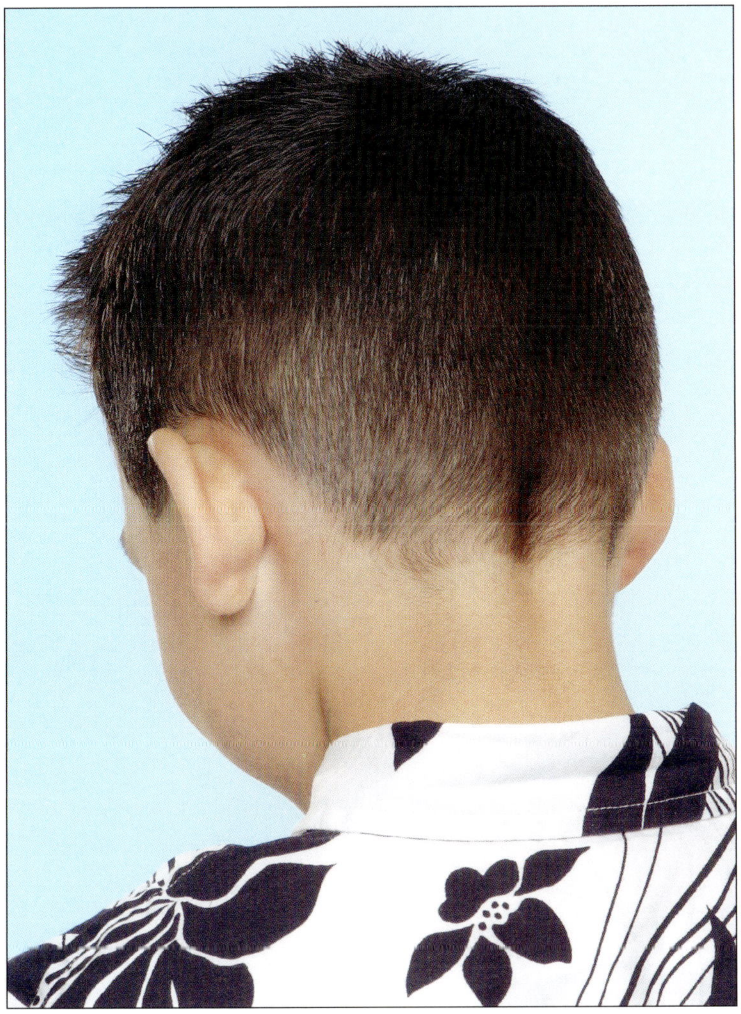

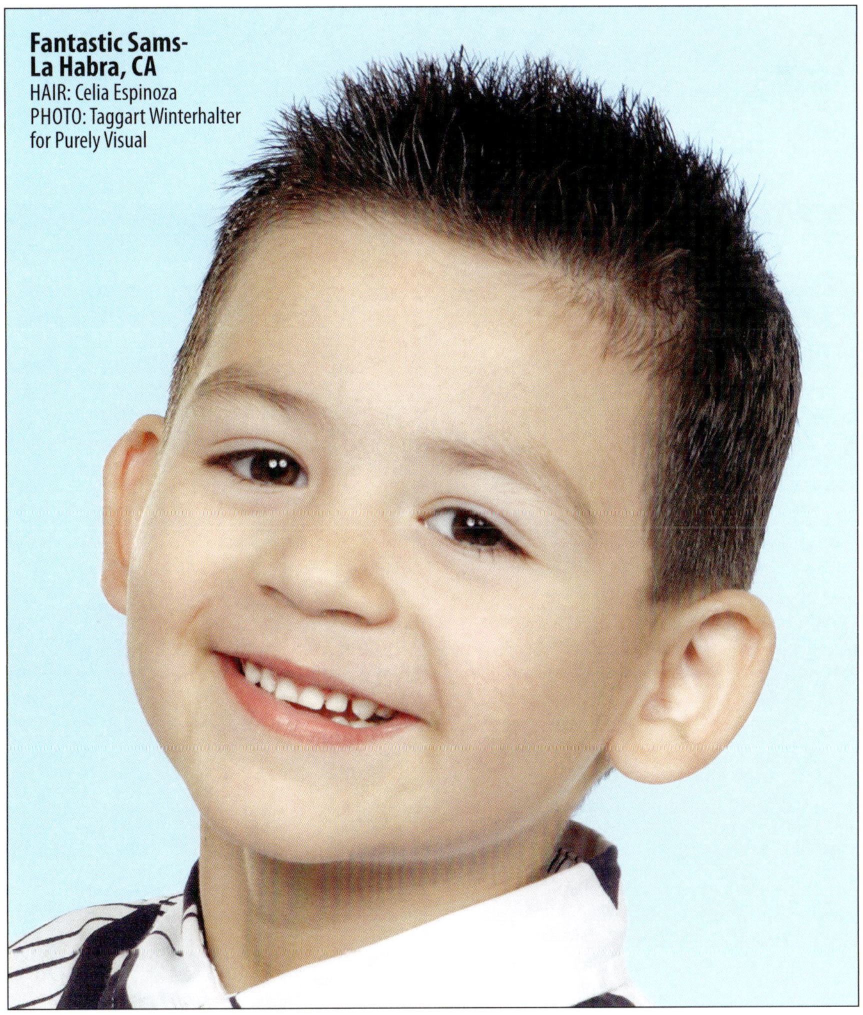

**Fantastic Sams-La Habra, CA**
HAIR: Celia Espinoza
PHOTO: Taggart Winterhalter for Purely Visual

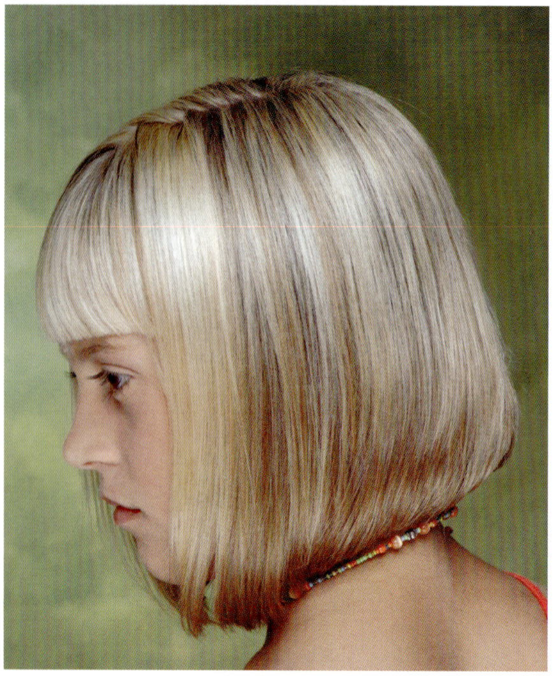

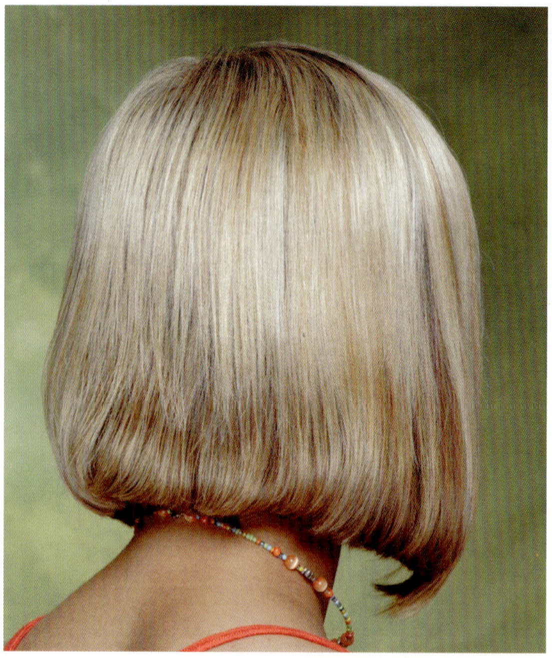

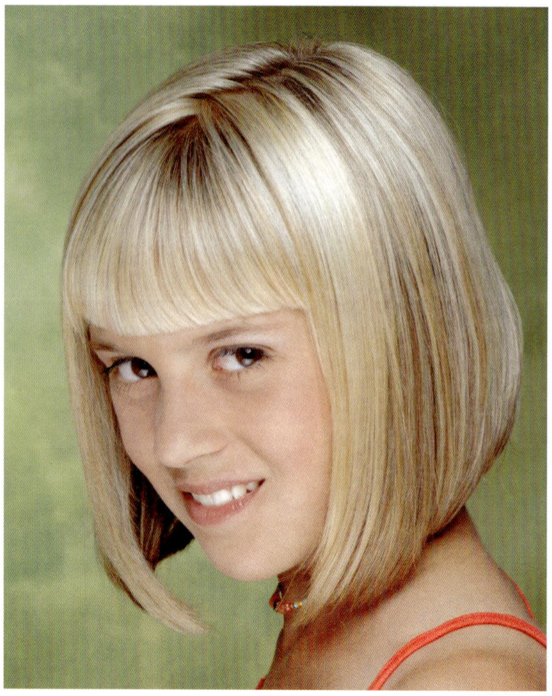

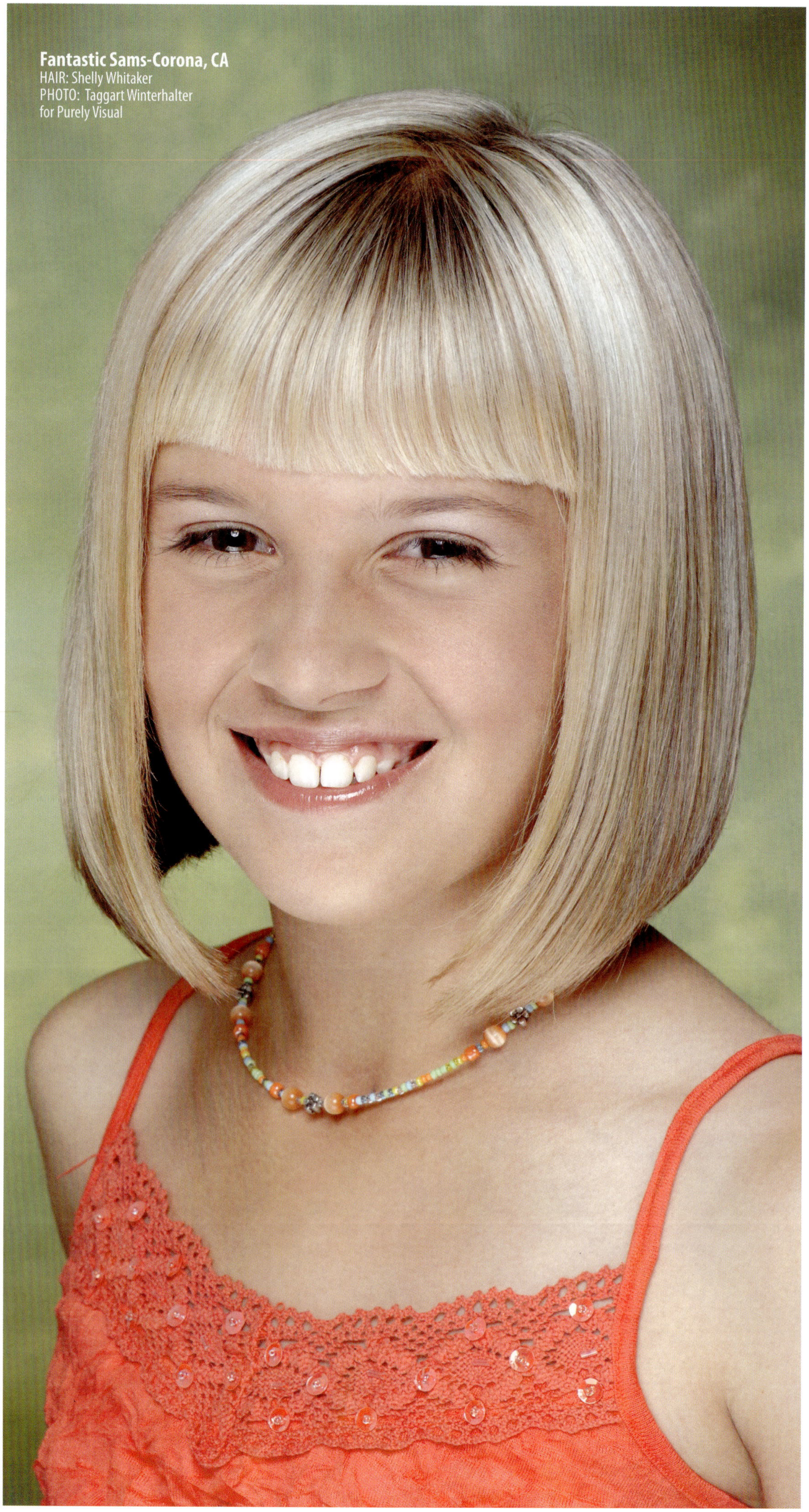

**Fantastic Sams-Corona, CA**
HAIR: Shelly Whitaker
PHOTO: Taggart Winterhalter
for Purely Visual

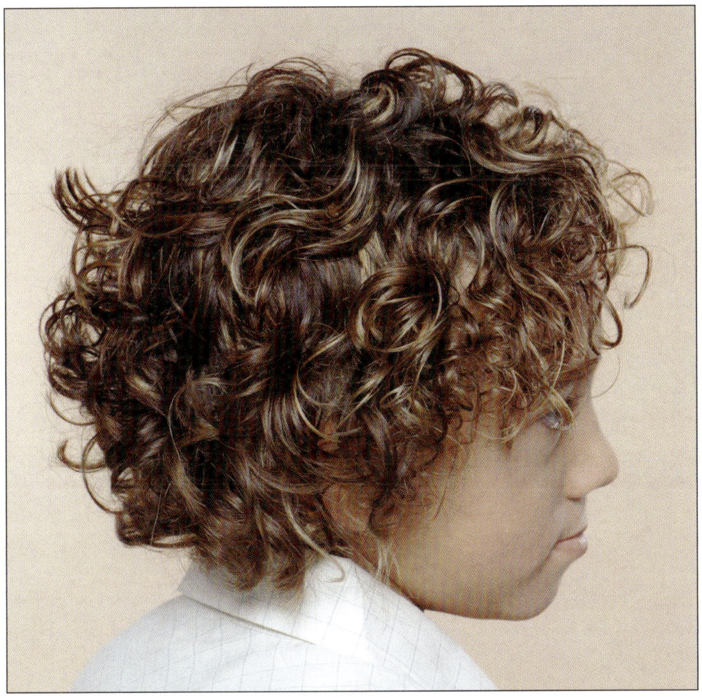

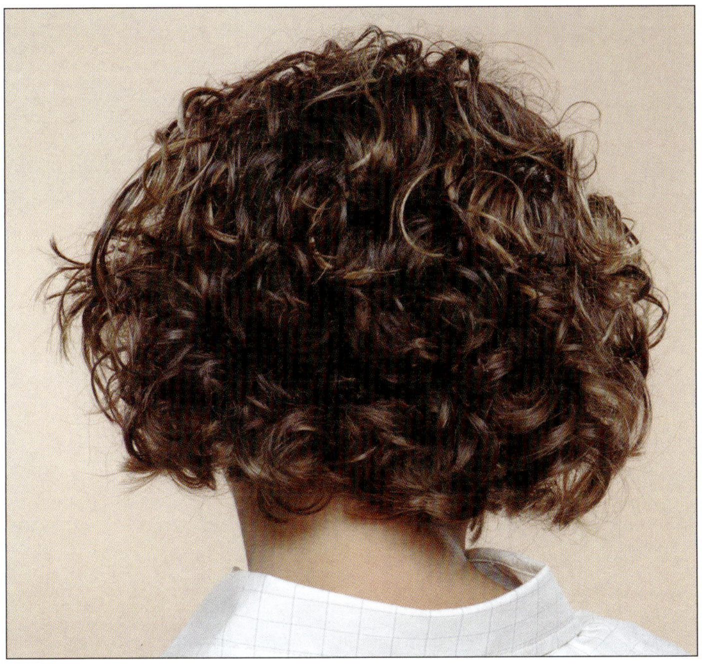

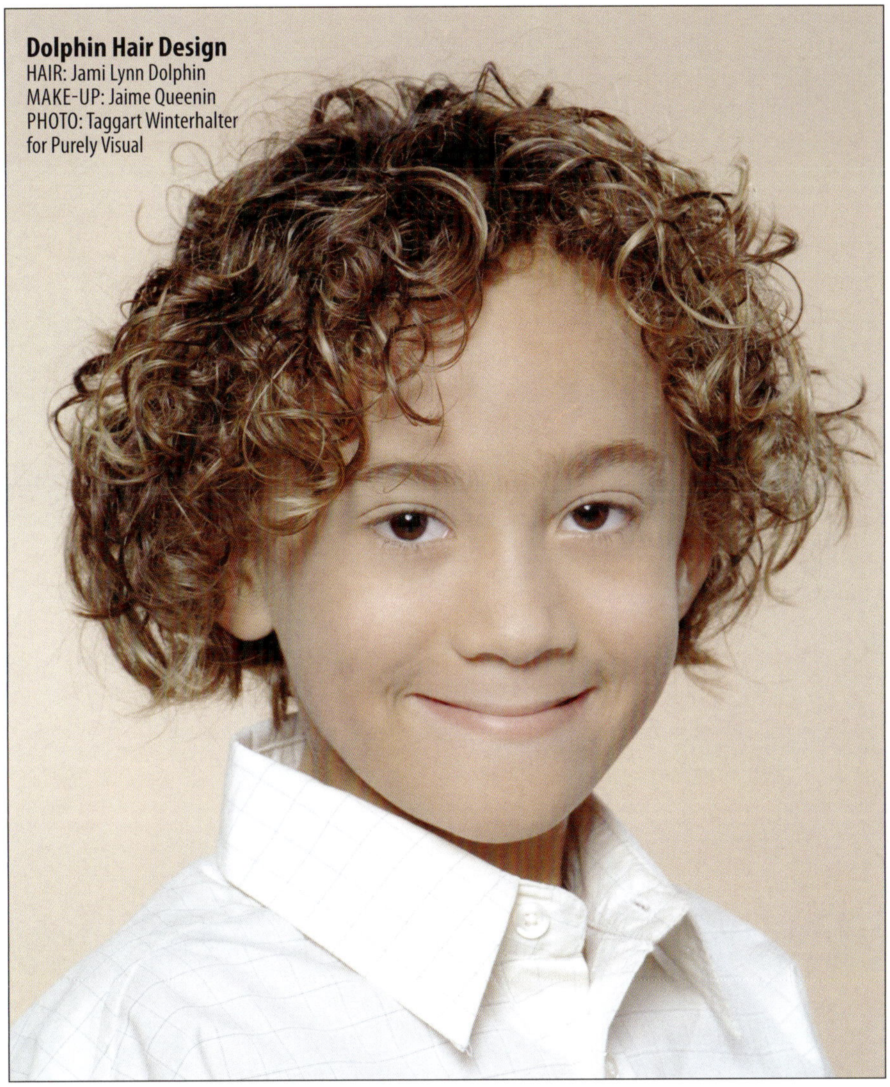

**Dolphin Hair Design**
HAIR: Jami Lynn Dolphin
MAKE-UP: Jaime Queenin
PHOTO: Taggart Winterhalter
for Purely Visual

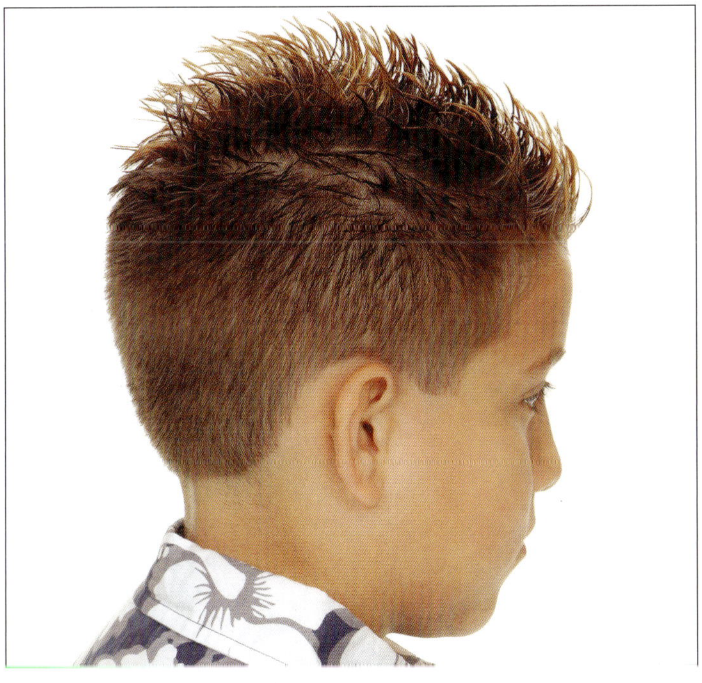

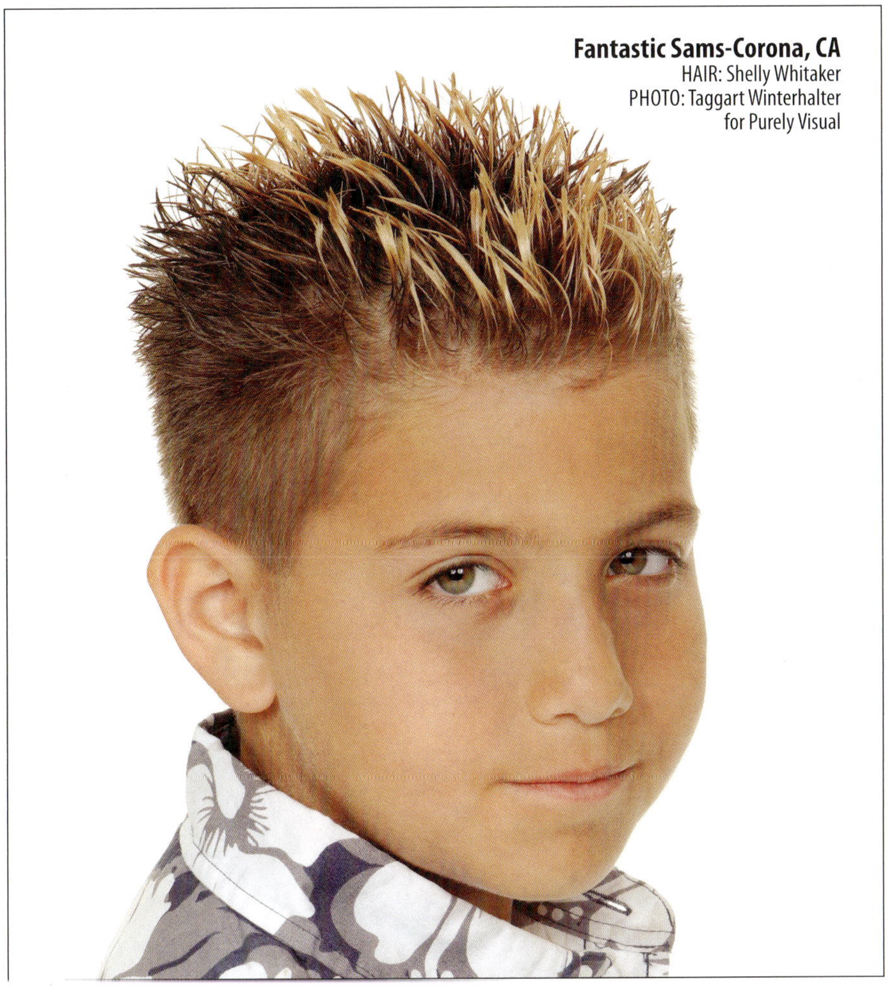

**Fantastic Sams-Corona, CA**
HAIR: Shelly Whitaker
PHOTO: Taggart Winterhalter
for Purely Visual

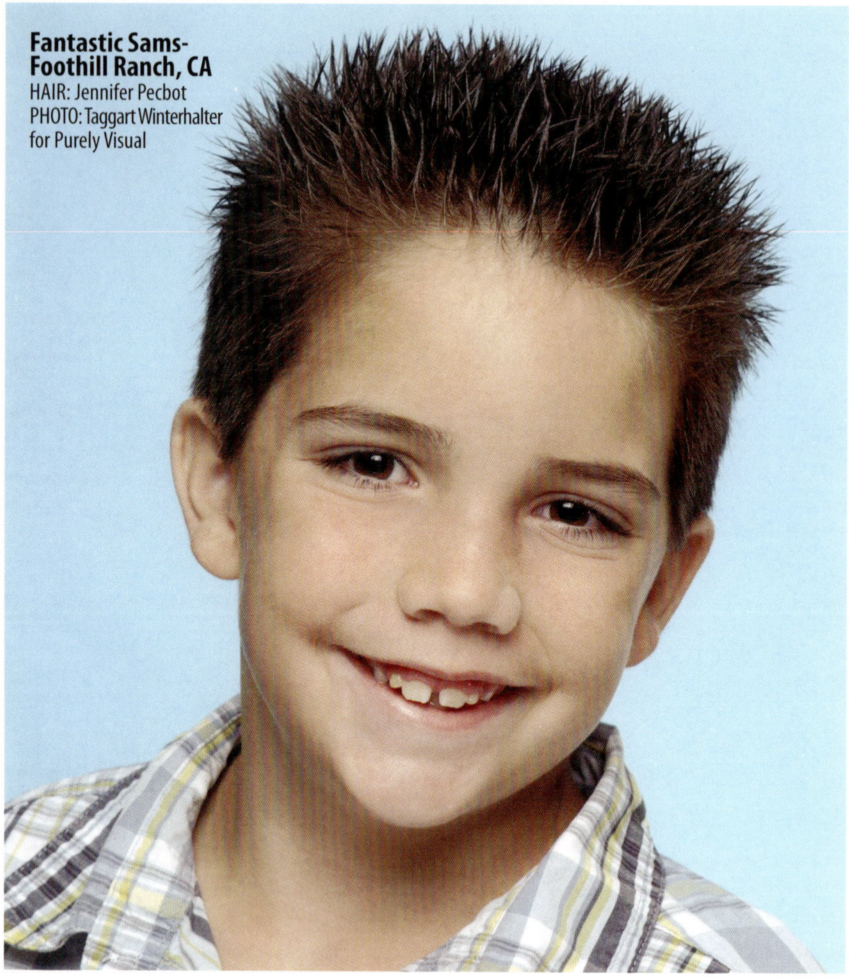

**Fantastic Sams-**
**Foothill Ranch, CA**
HAIR: Jennifer Pecbot
PHOTO: Taggart Winterhalter
for Purely Visual

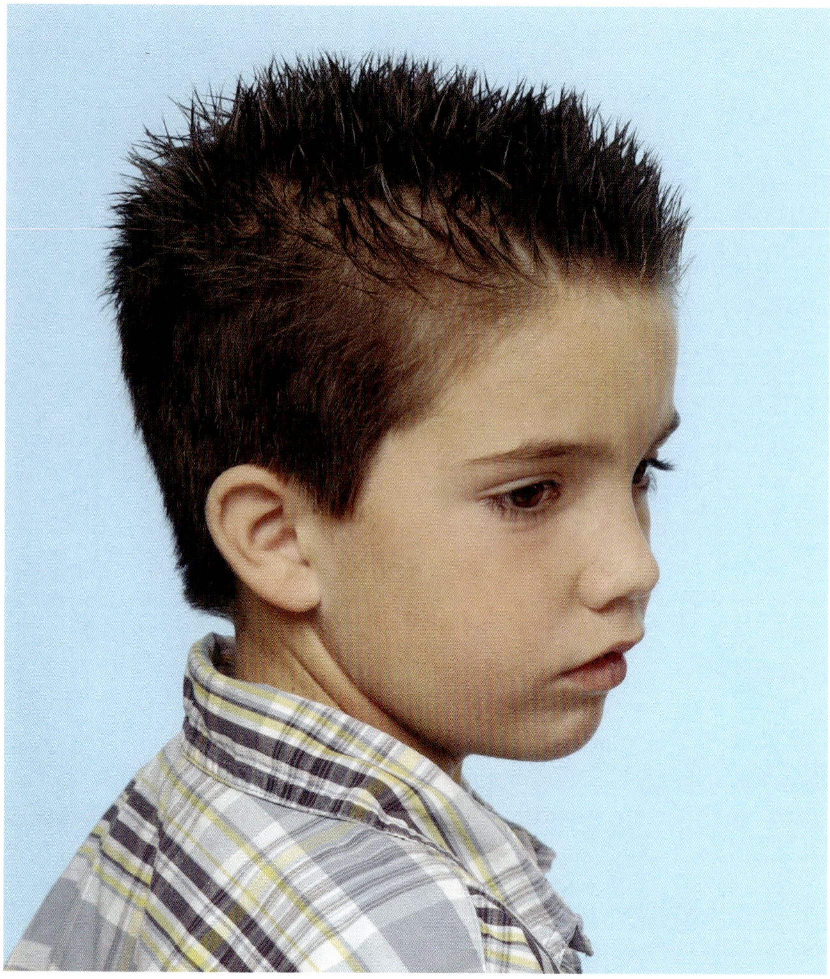

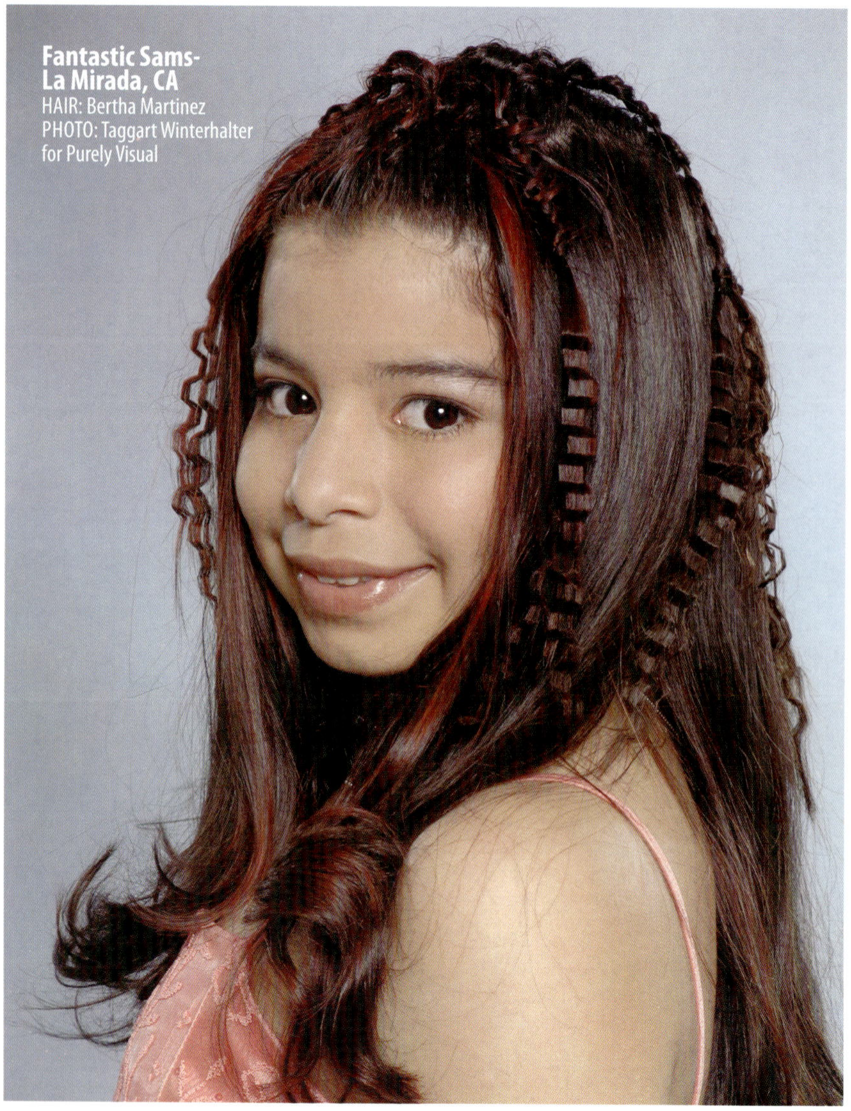

**Fantastic Sams-**
**La Mirada, CA**
HAIR: Bertha Martinez
PHOTO: Taggart Winterhalter
for Purely Visual

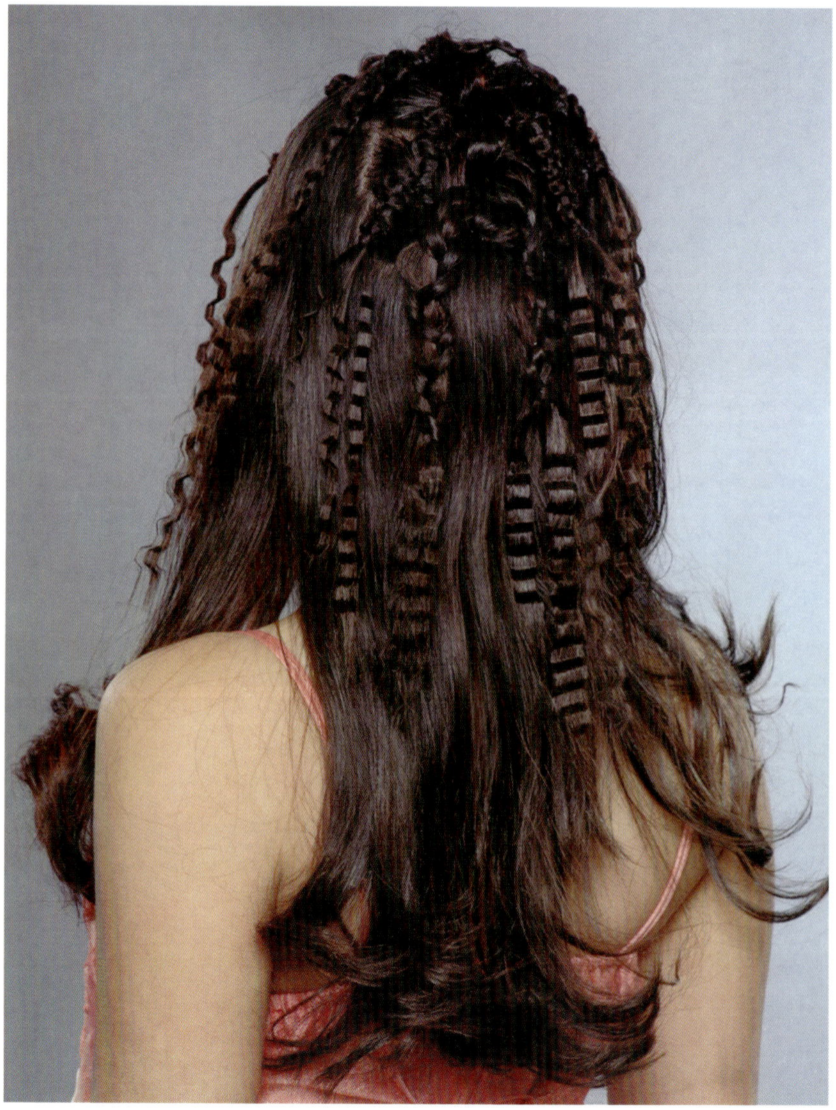

**Fantastic Sams-Foothill Ranch, CA**
HAIR: Jennifer Pecbot
PHOTO: Taggart Winterhalter for Purely Visual



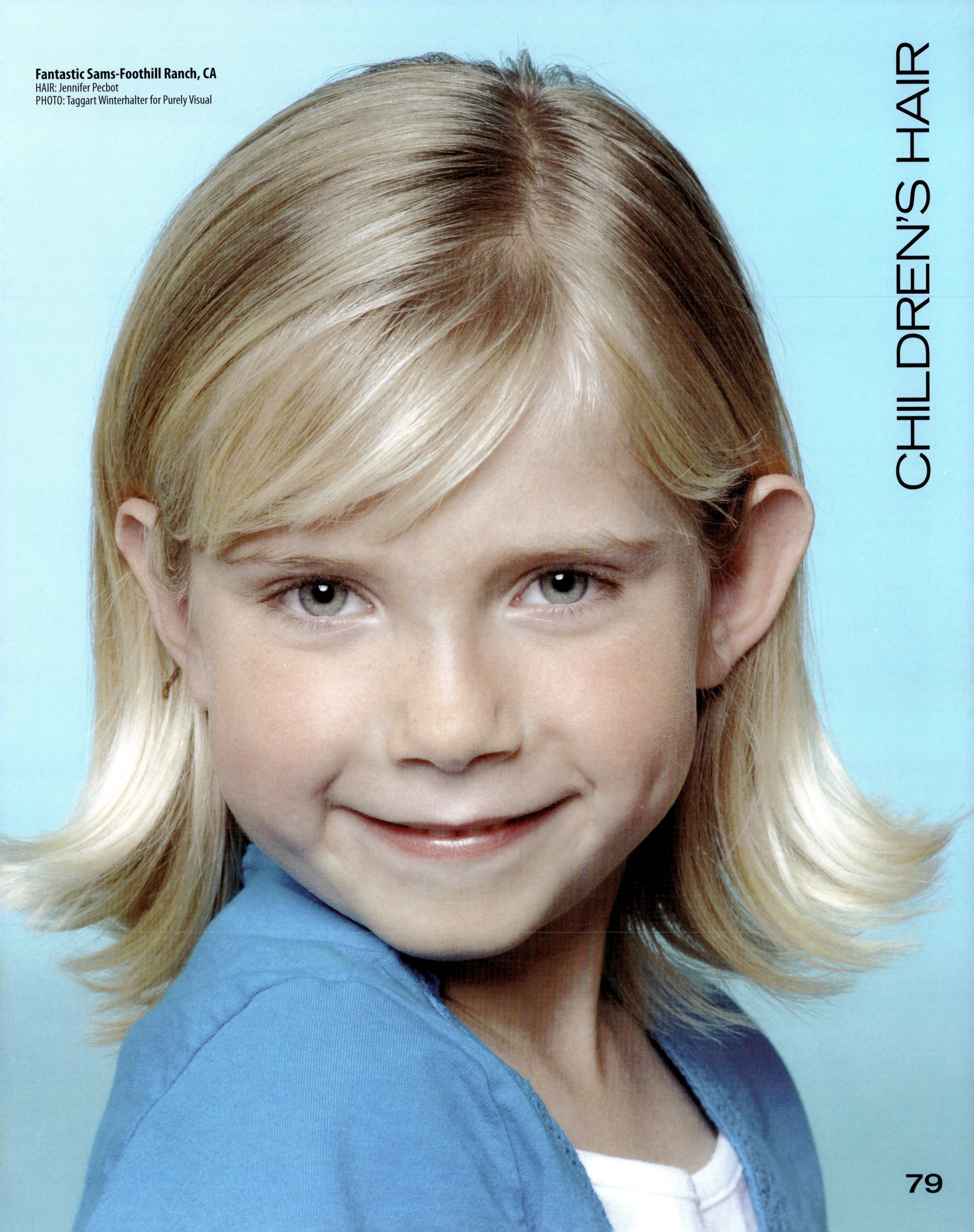

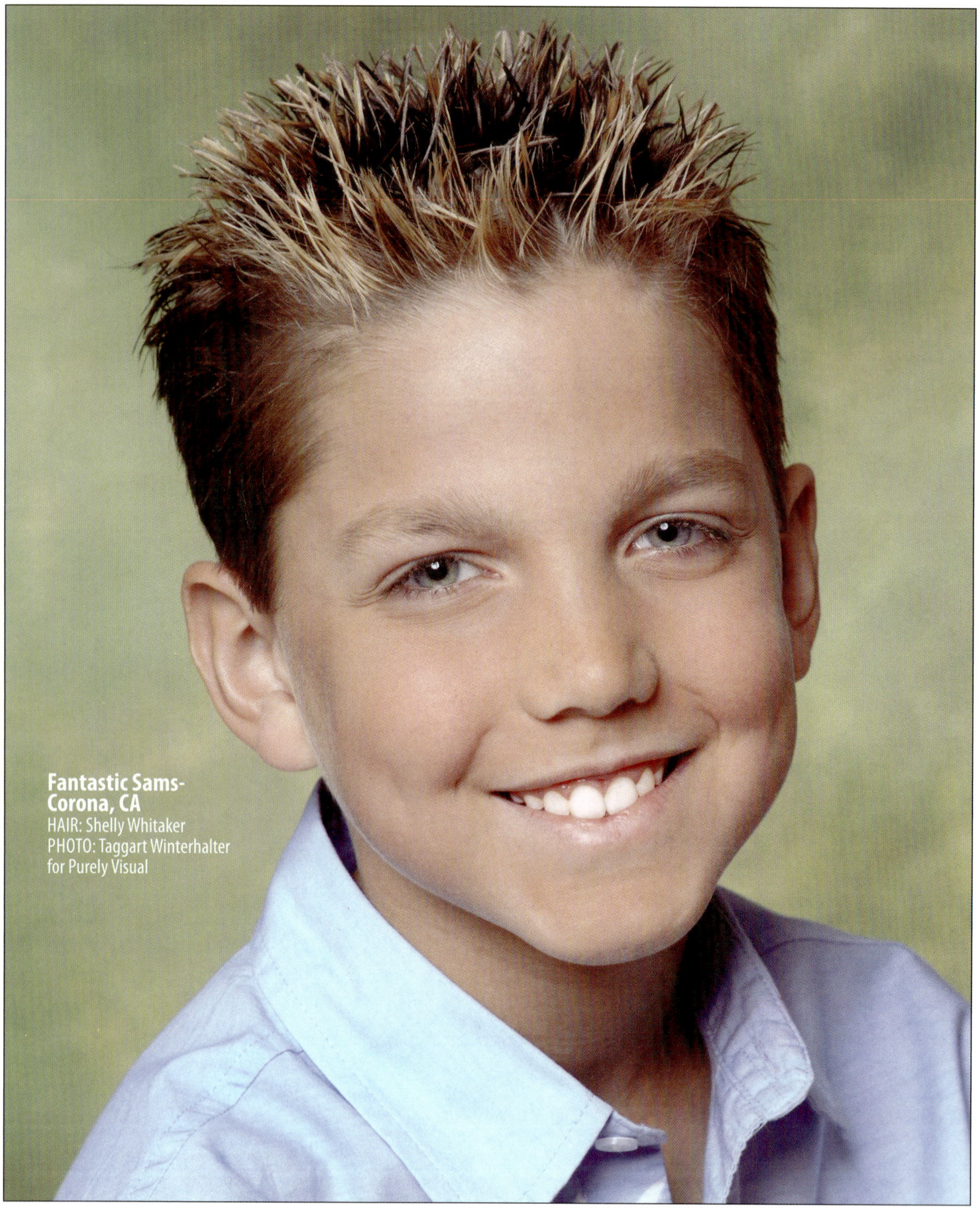

**Fantastic Sams-**
**Corona, CA**
HAIR: Shelly Whitaker
PHOTO: Taggart Winterhalter
for Purely Visual

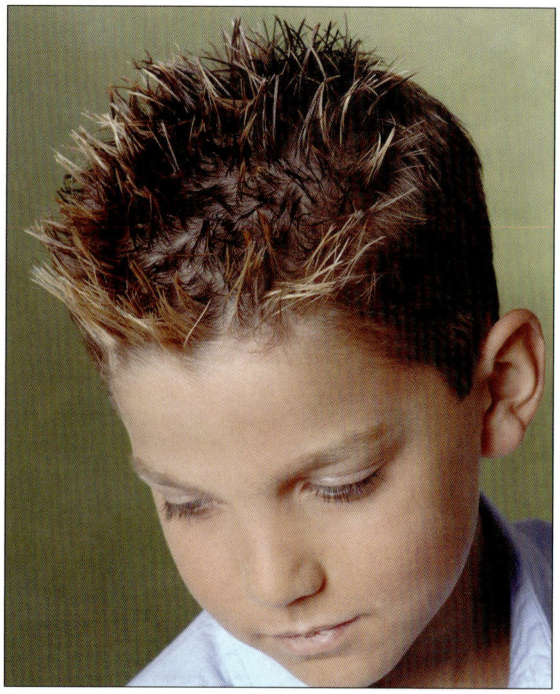

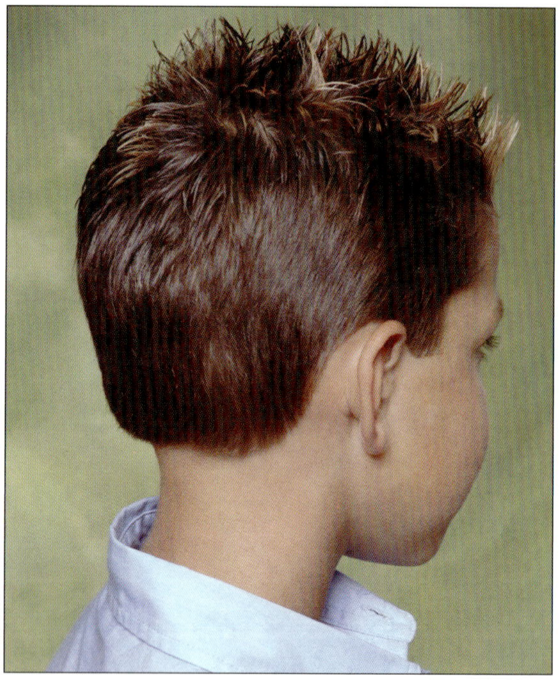

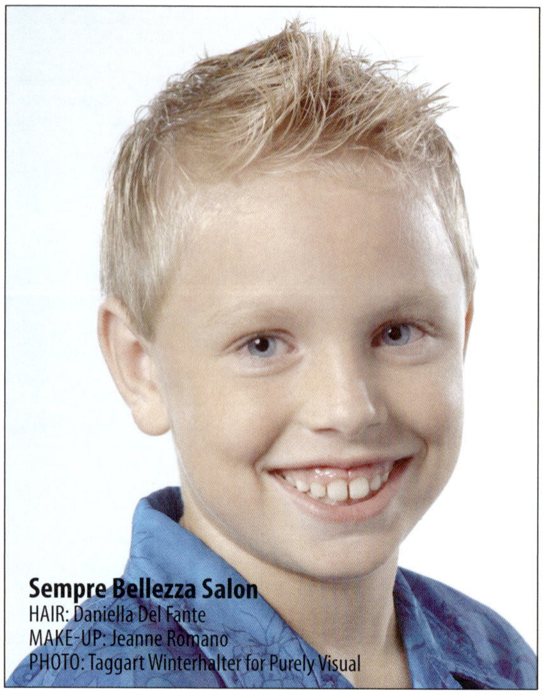

**Sempre Bellezza Salon**
HAIR: Daniella Del Fante
MAKE-UP: Jeanne Romano
PHOTO: Taggart Winterhalter for Purely Visual

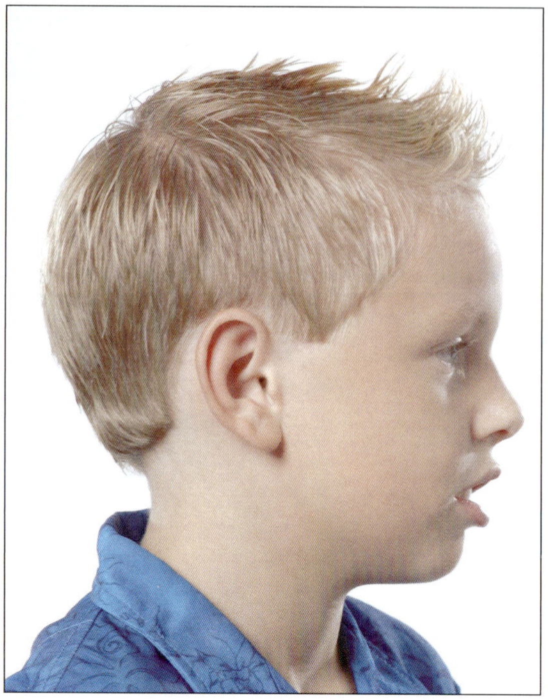

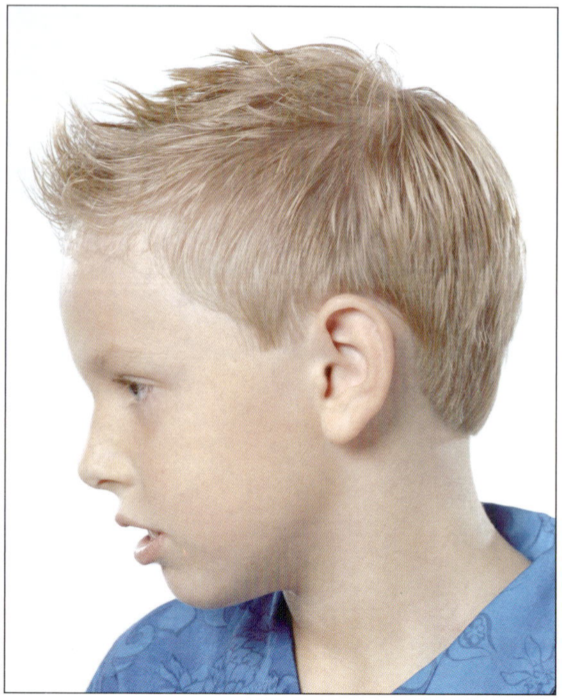

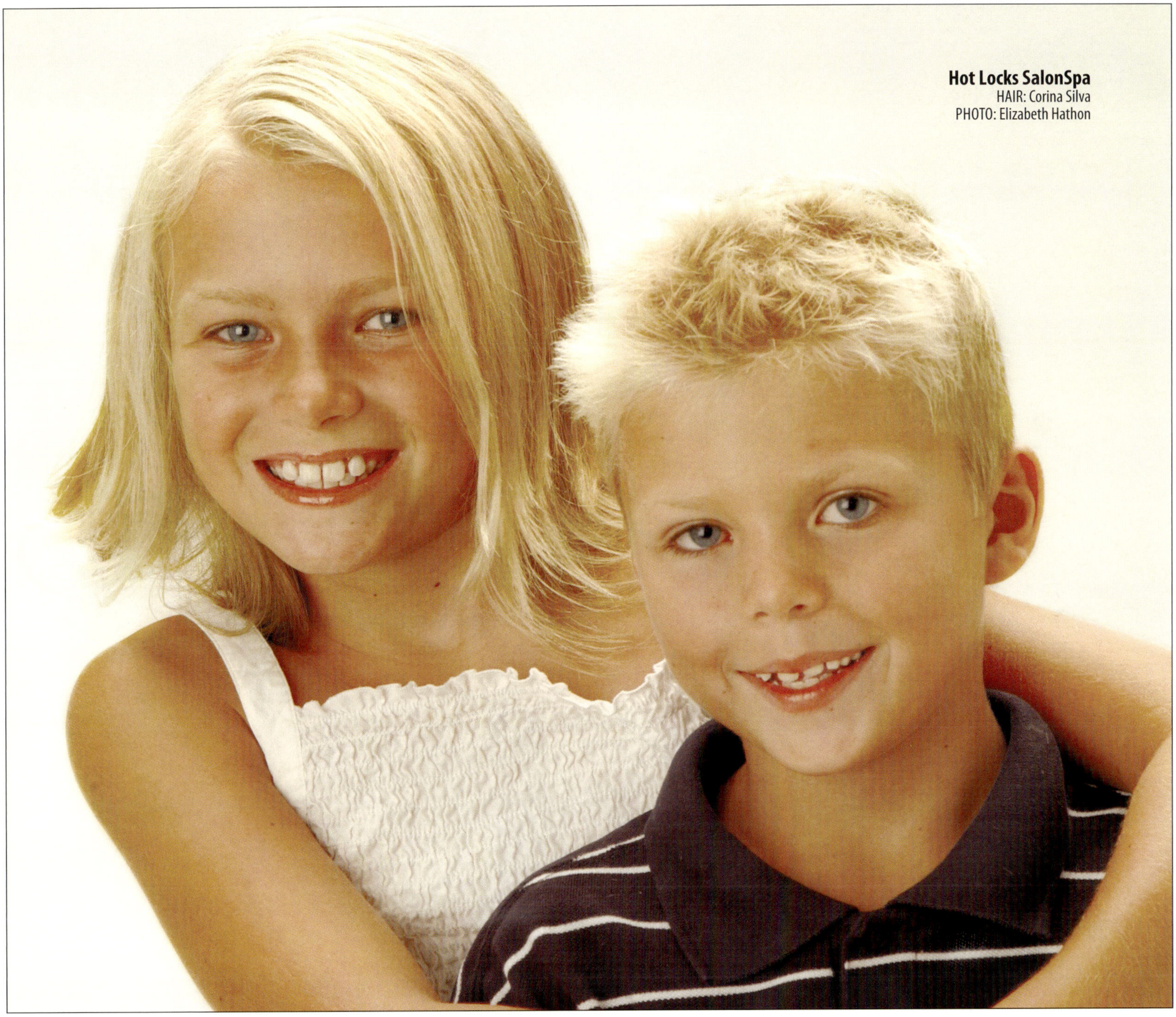

**Hot Locks SalonSpa**
HAIR: Corina Silva
PHOTO: Elizabeth Hathon

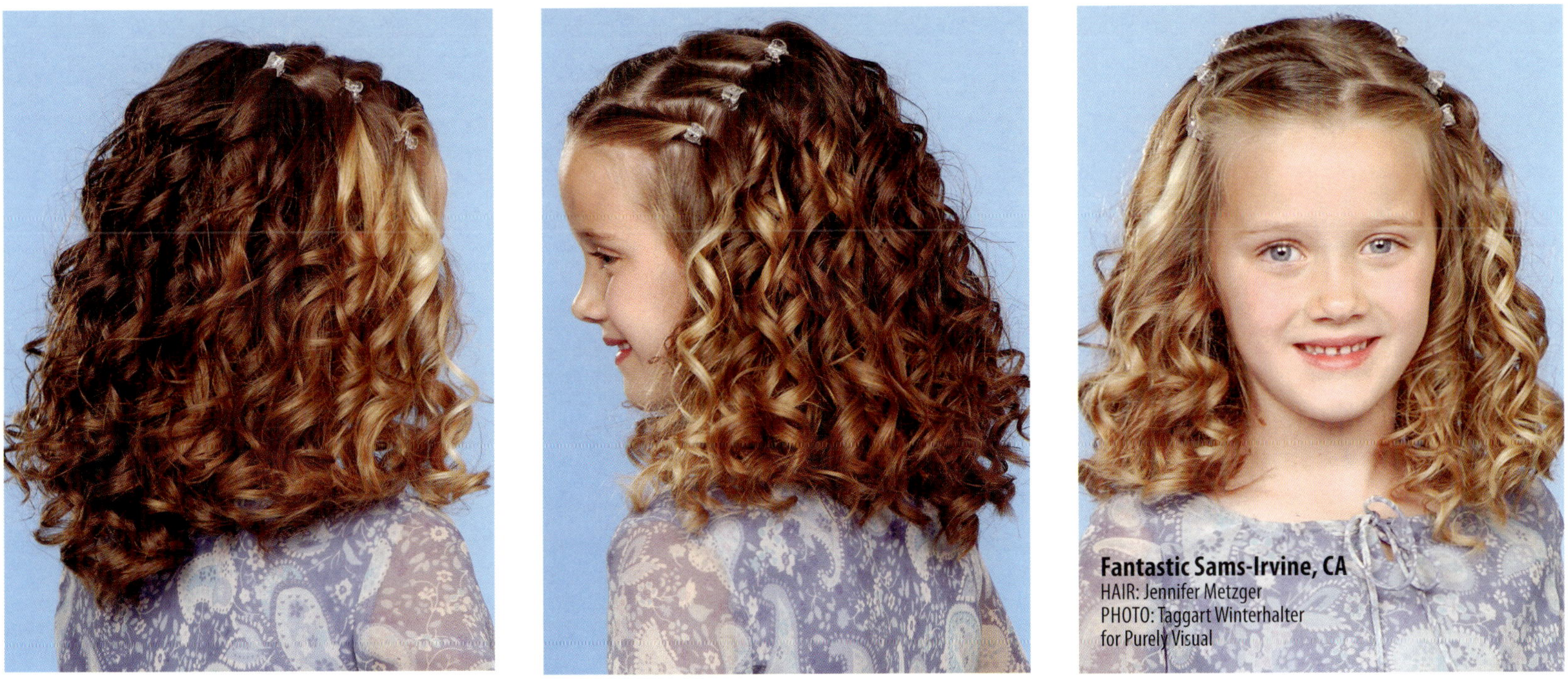

**Fantastic Sams-Irvine, CA**
HAIR: Jennifer Metzger
PHOTO: Taggart Winterhalter for Purely Visual

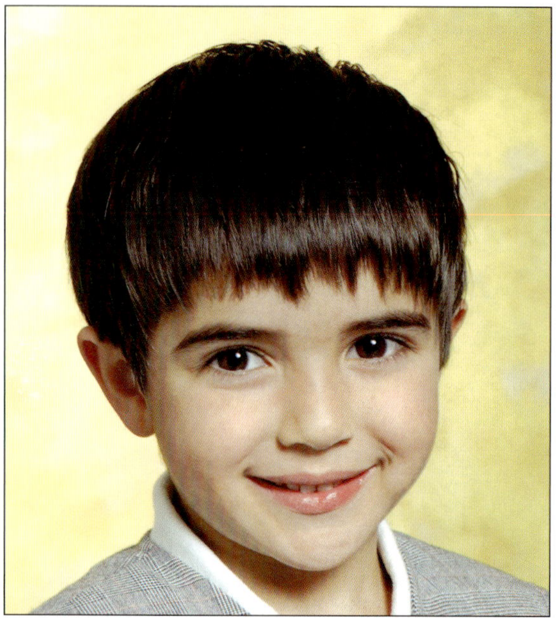

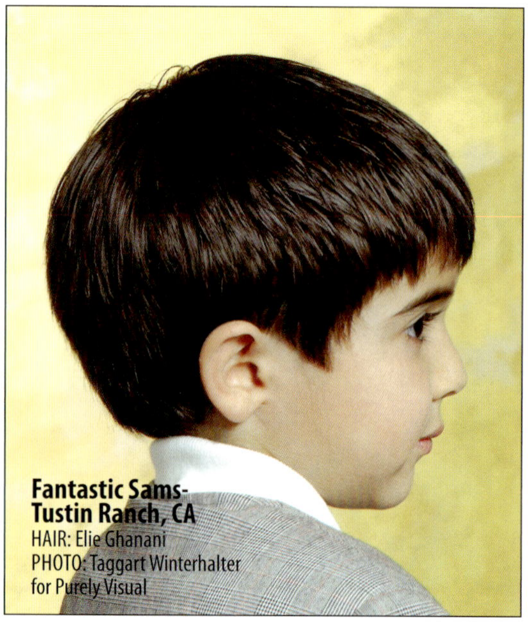

**Fantastic Sams-**
**Tustin Ranch, CA**
HAIR: Elie Ghanani
PHOTO: Taggart Winterhalter
for Purely Visual

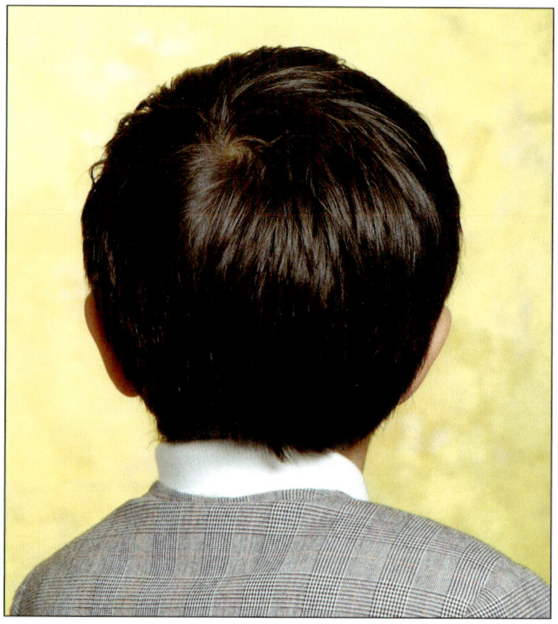

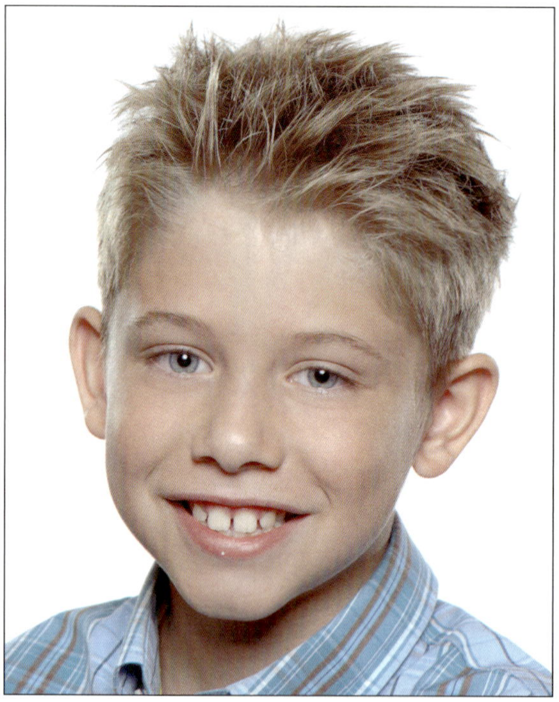

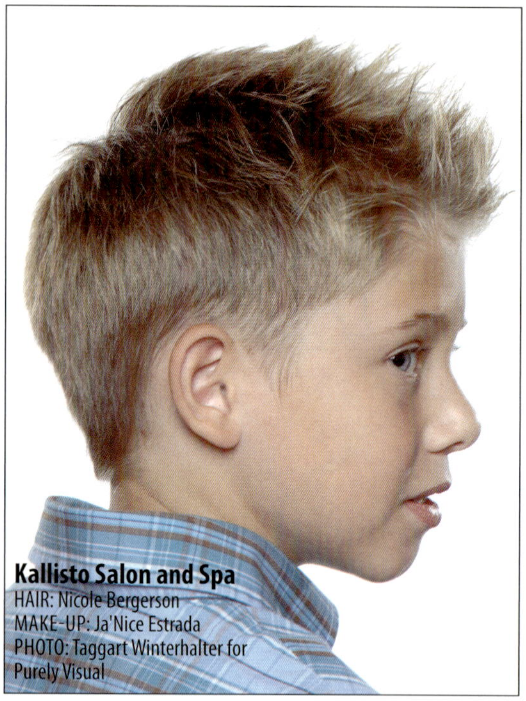

**Kallisto Salon and Spa**
HAIR: Nicole Bergerson
MAKE-UP: Ja'Nice Estrada
PHOTO: Taggart Winterhalter for
Purely Visual

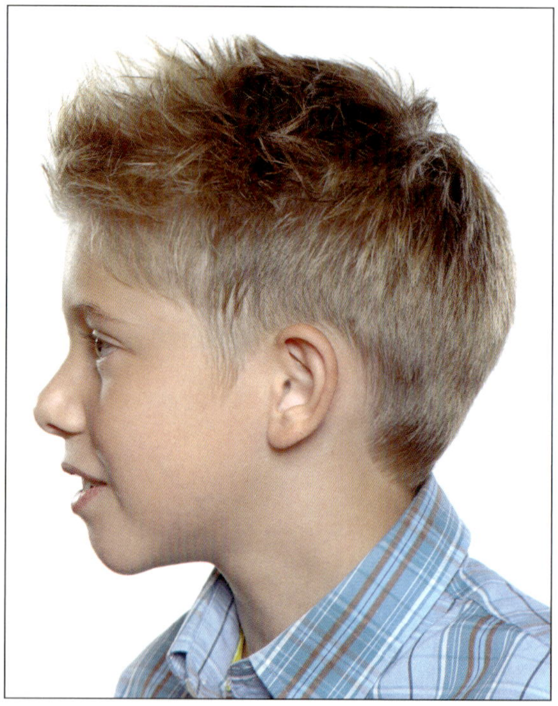

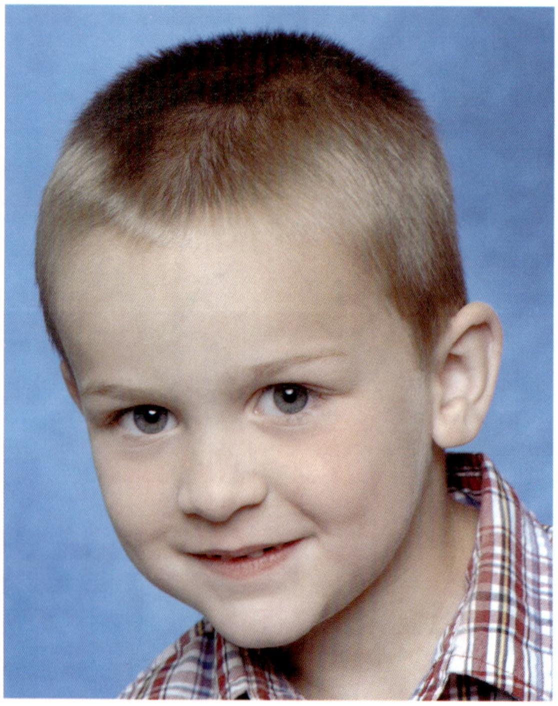

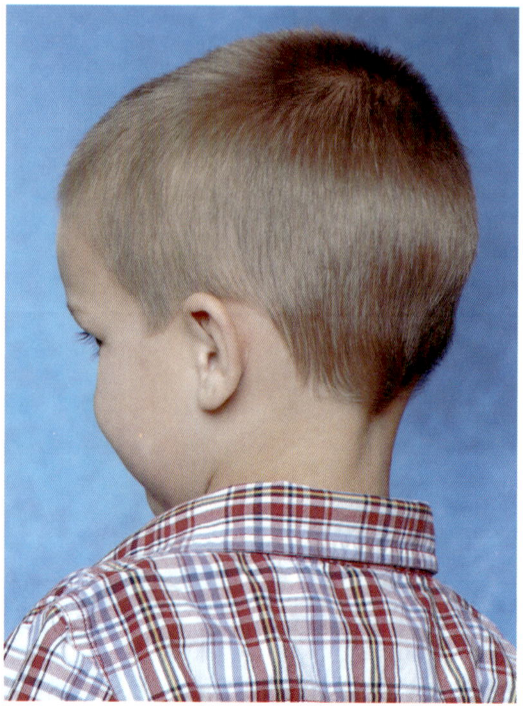

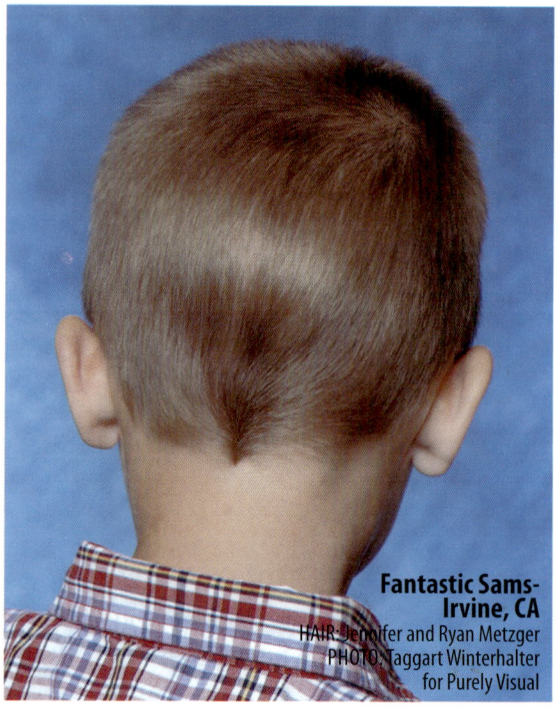

**Fantastic Sams-**
**Irvine, CA**
HAIR: Jennifer and Ryan Metzger
PHOTO: Taggart Winterhalter
for Purely Visual

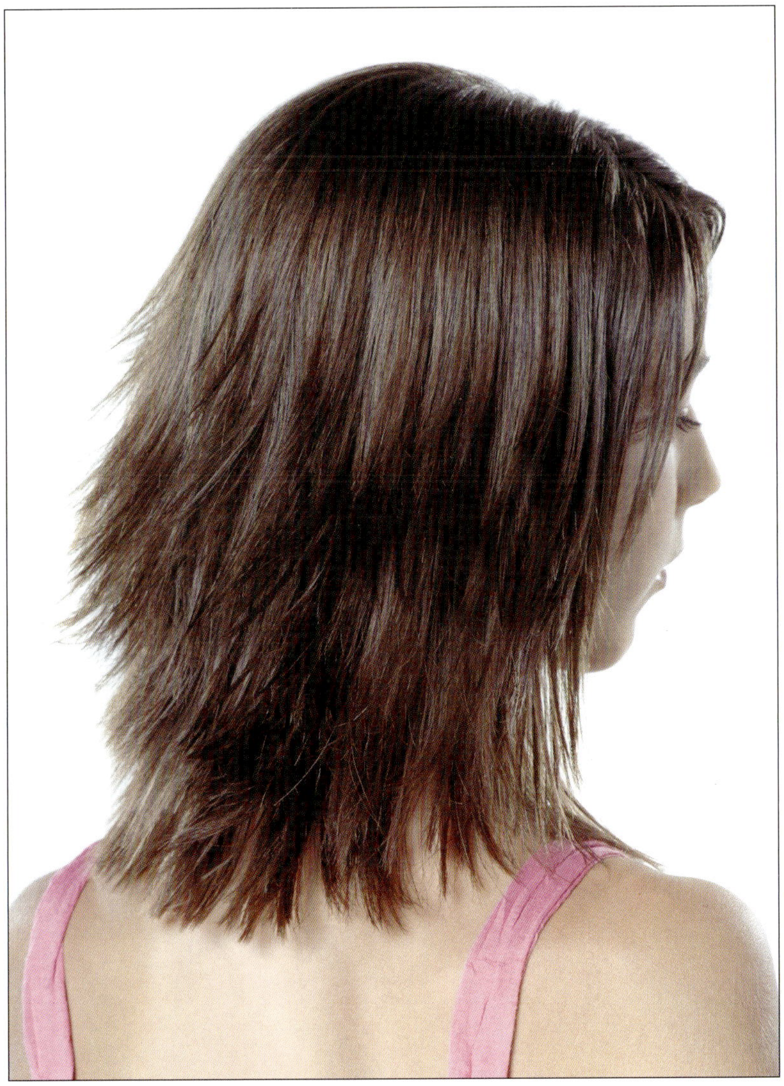

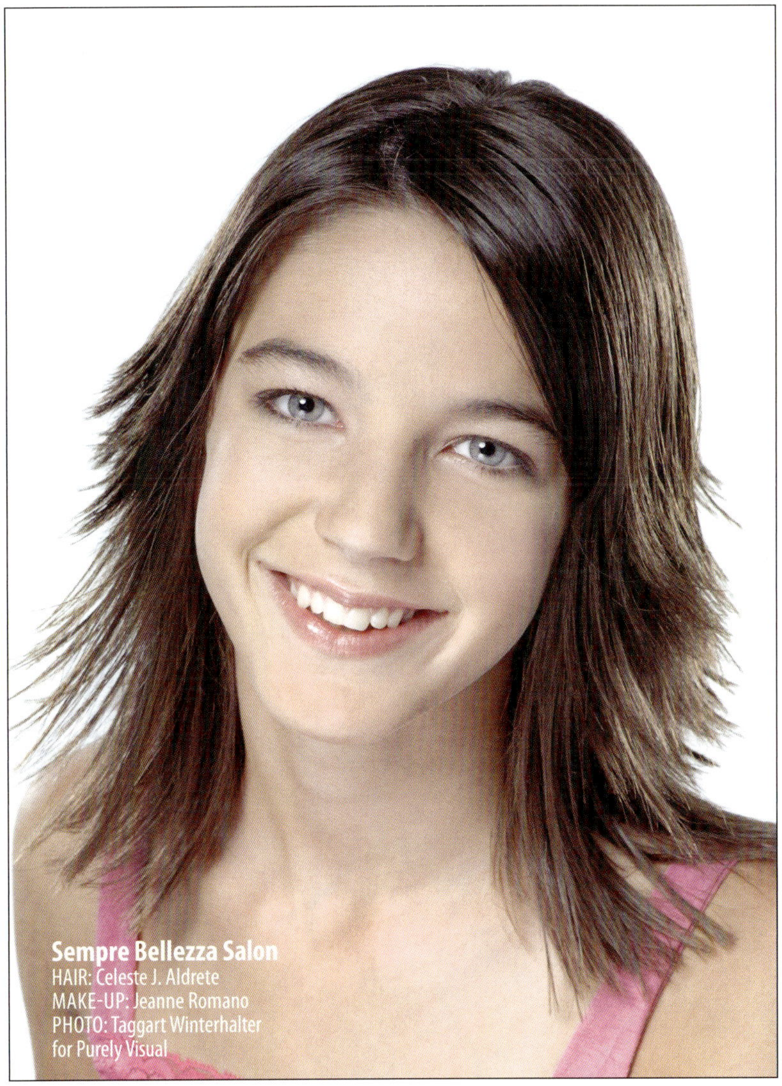

**Sempre Bellezza Salon**
HAIR: Celeste J. Aldrete
MAKE-UP: Jeanne Romano
PHOTO: Taggart Winterhalter
for Purely Visual

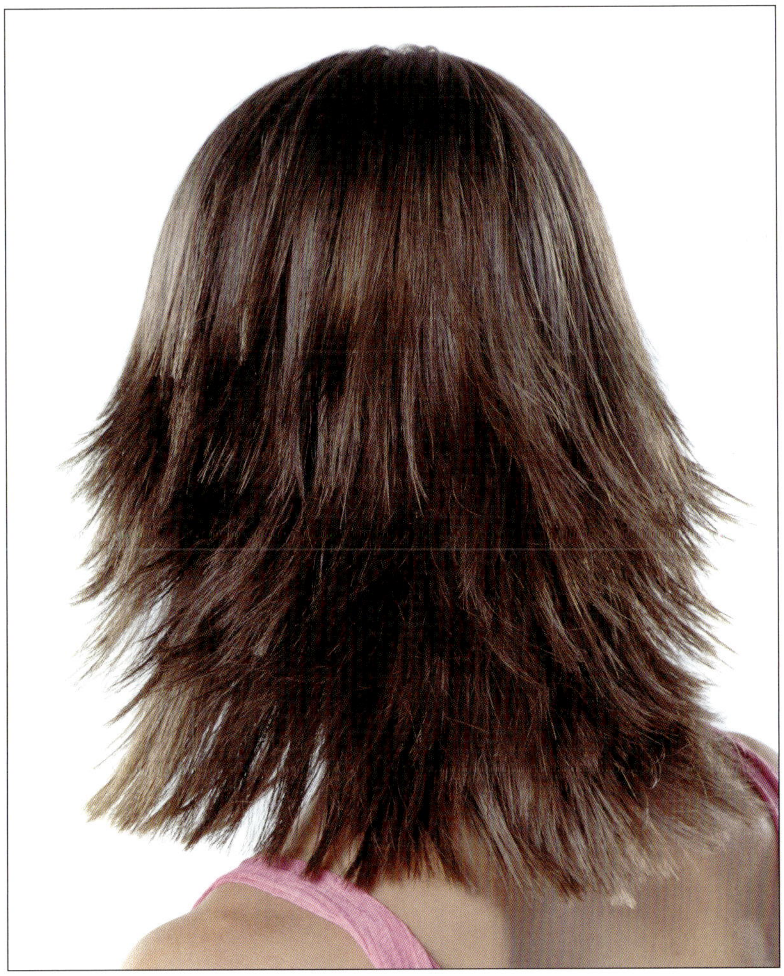

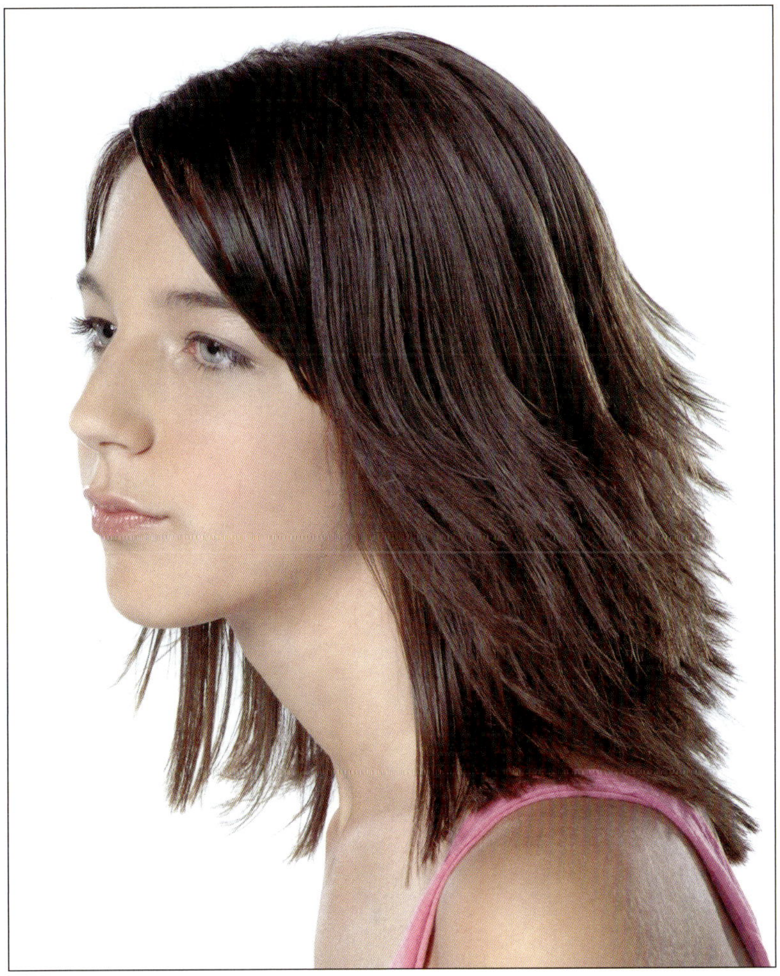

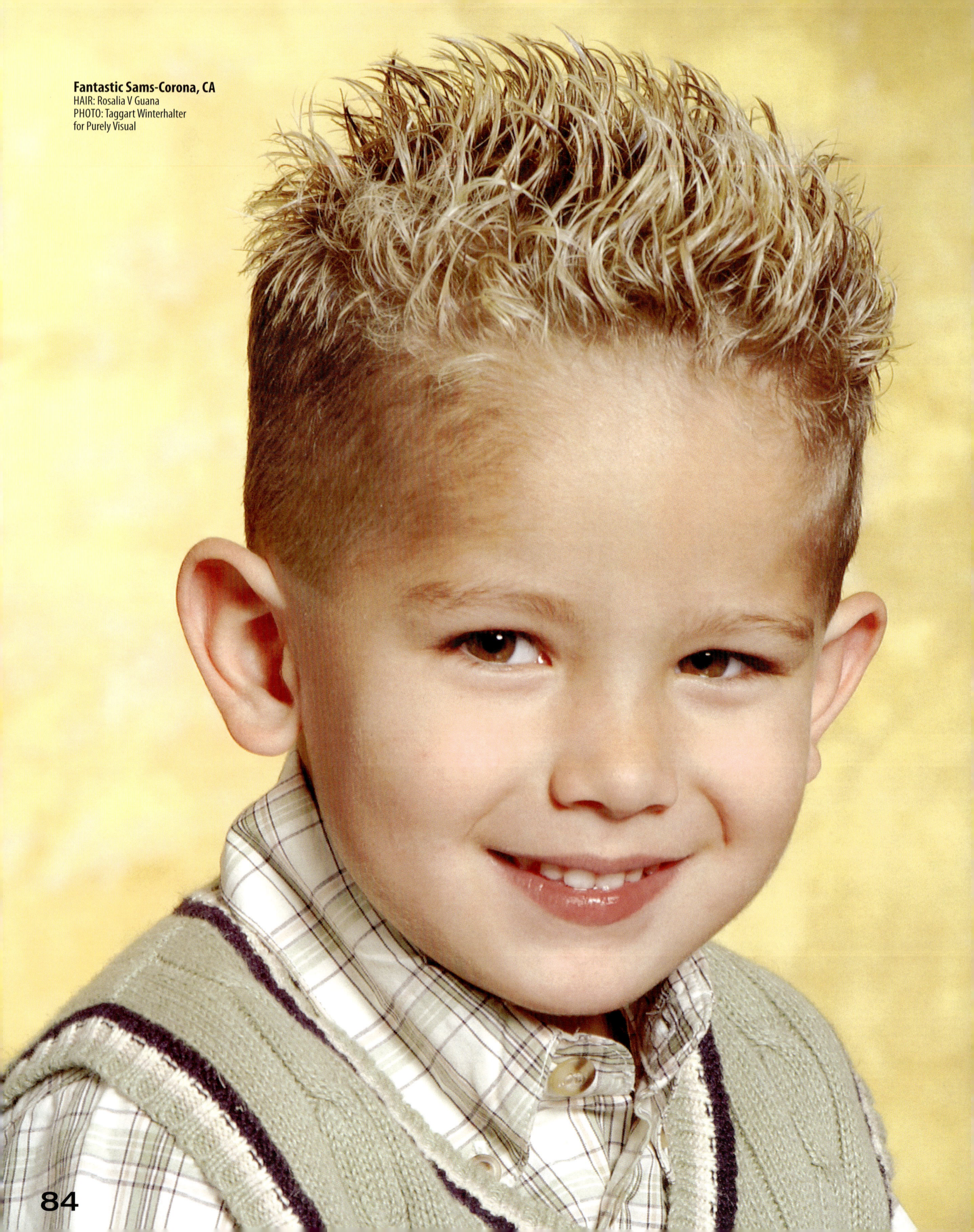

**Fantastic Sams-Corona, CA**
HAIR: Rosalia V Guana
PHOTO: Taggart Winterhalter
for Purely Visual

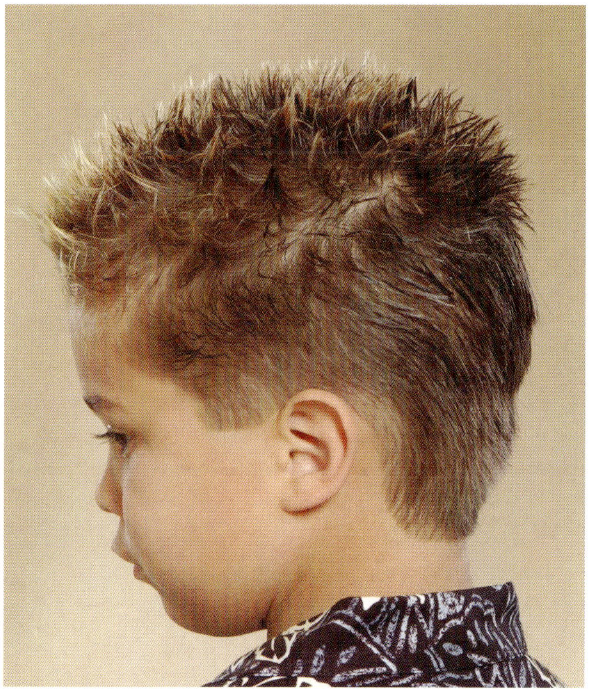

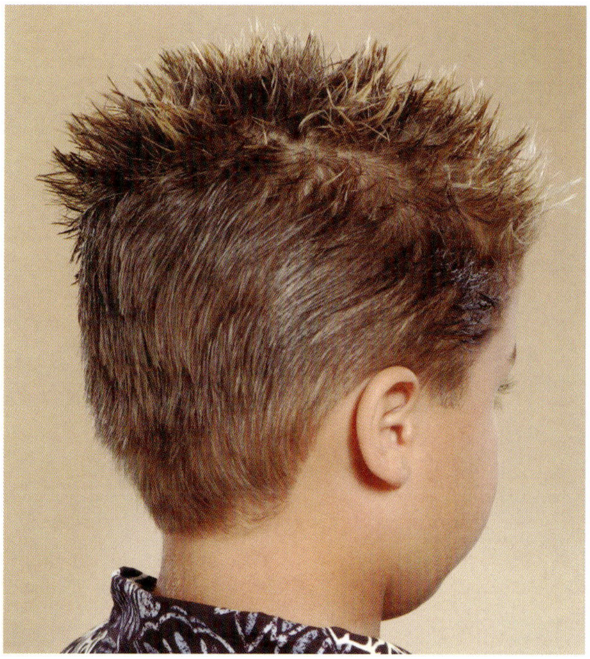

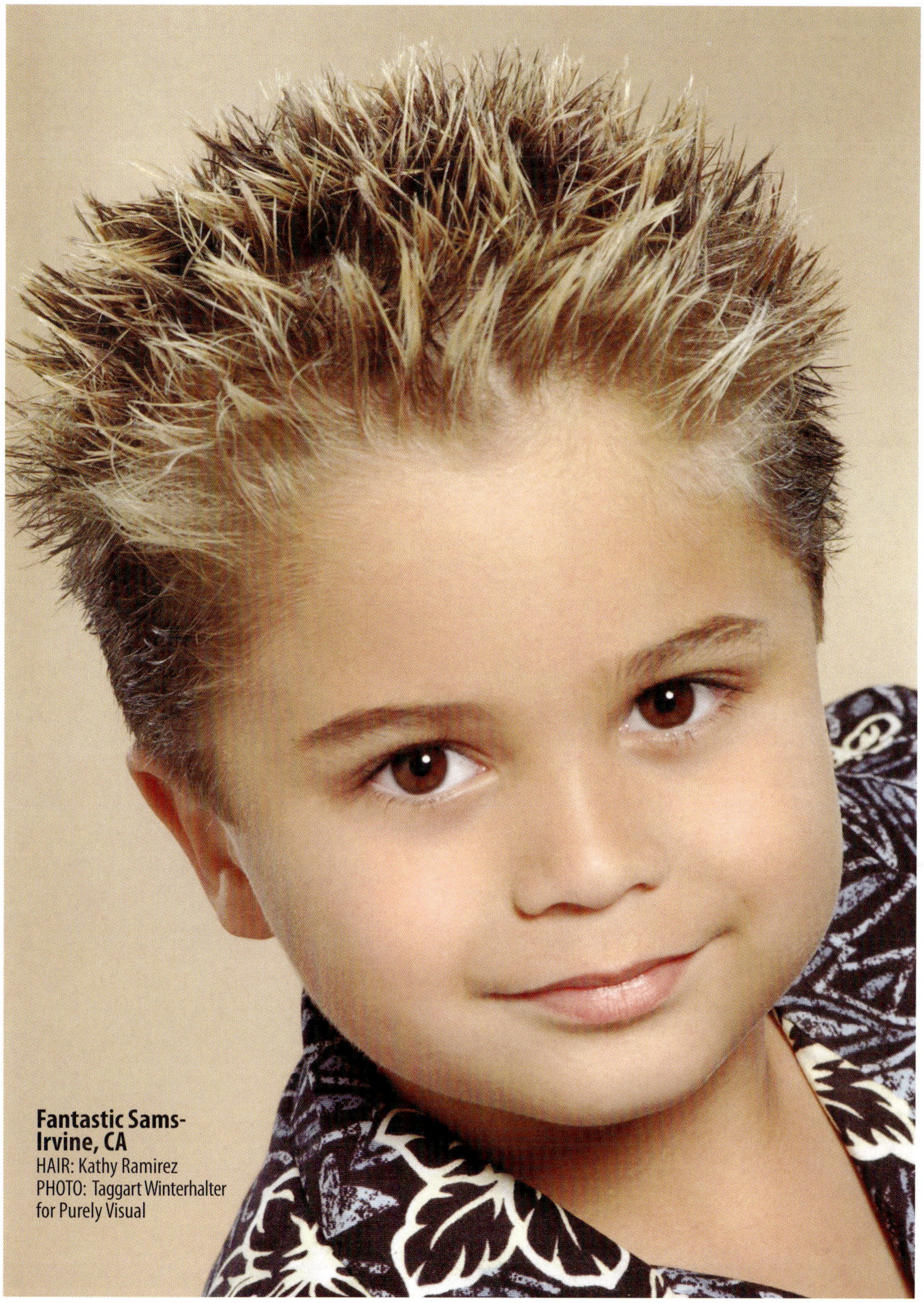

**Fantastic Sams-
Irvine, CA**
HAIR: Kathy Ramirez
PHOTO: Taggart Winterhalter
for Purely Visual

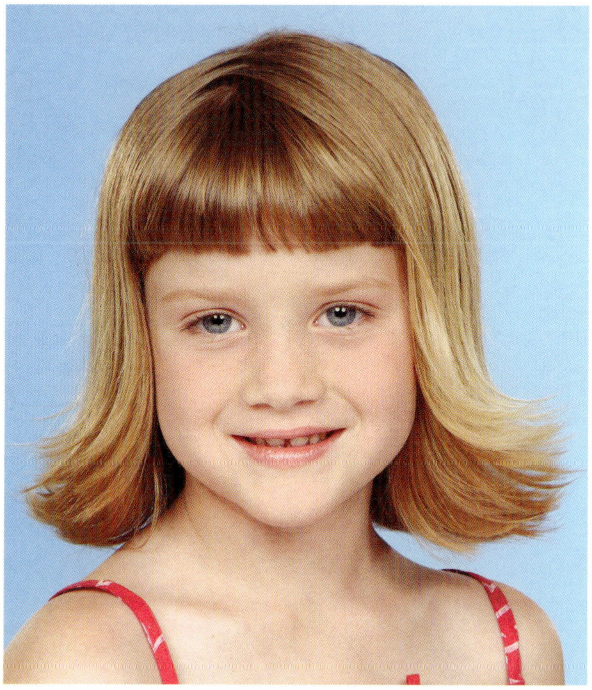

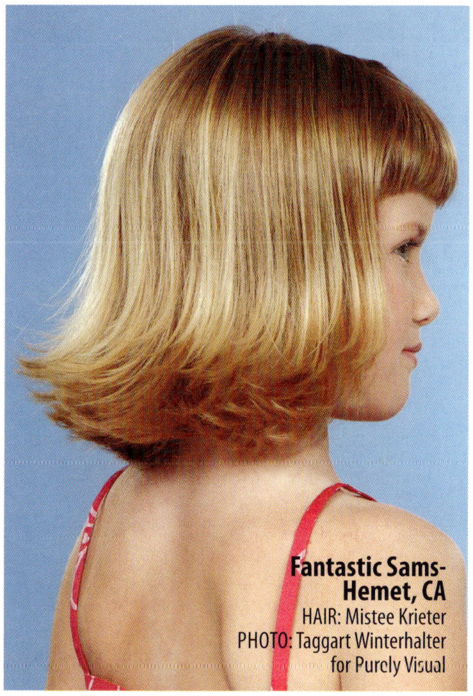

**Fantastic Sams-
Hemet, CA**
HAIR: Mistee Krieter
PHOTO: Taggart Winterhalter
for Purely Visual

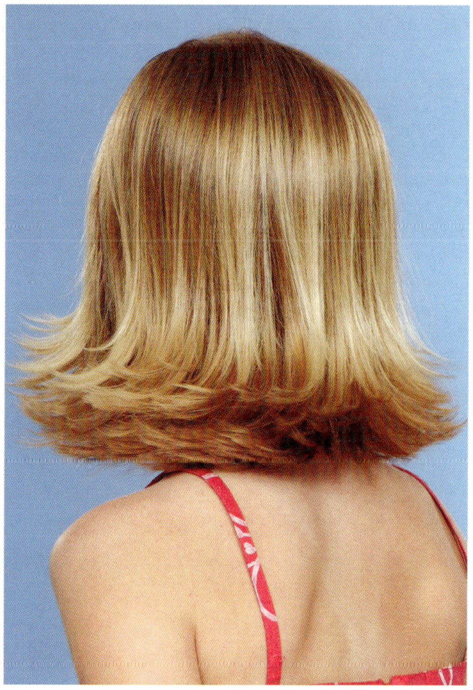

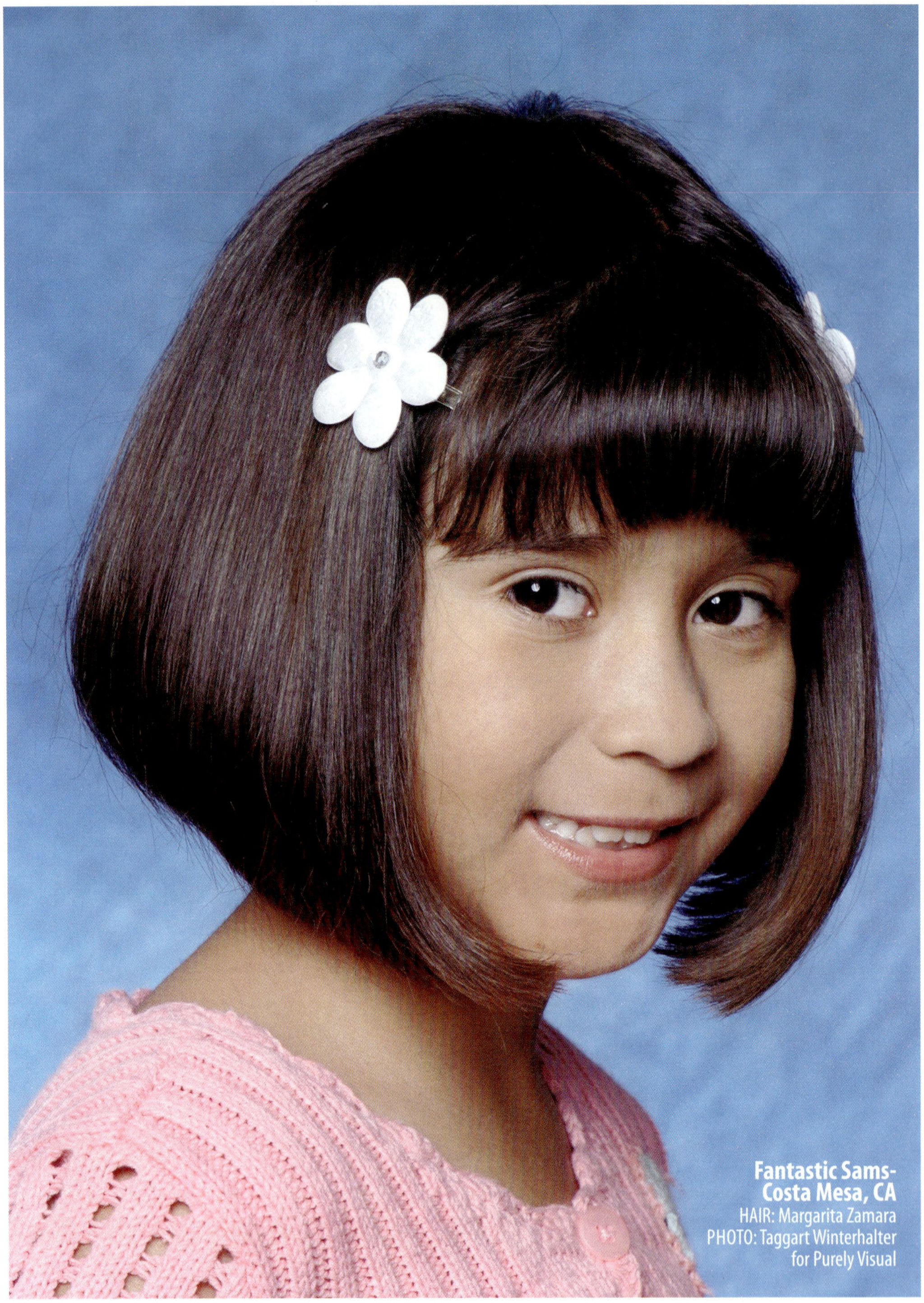

**Fantastic Sams-**
**Costa Mesa, CA**
HAIR: Margarita Zamara
PHOTO: Taggart Winterhalter
for Purely Visual

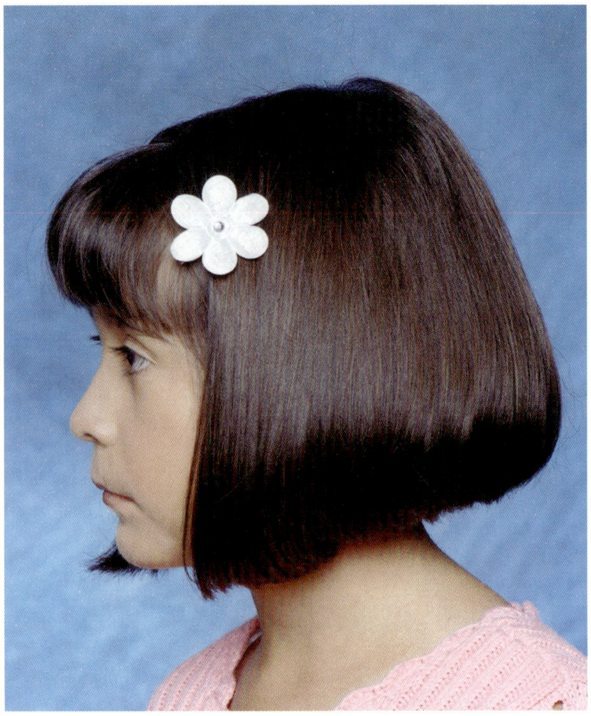

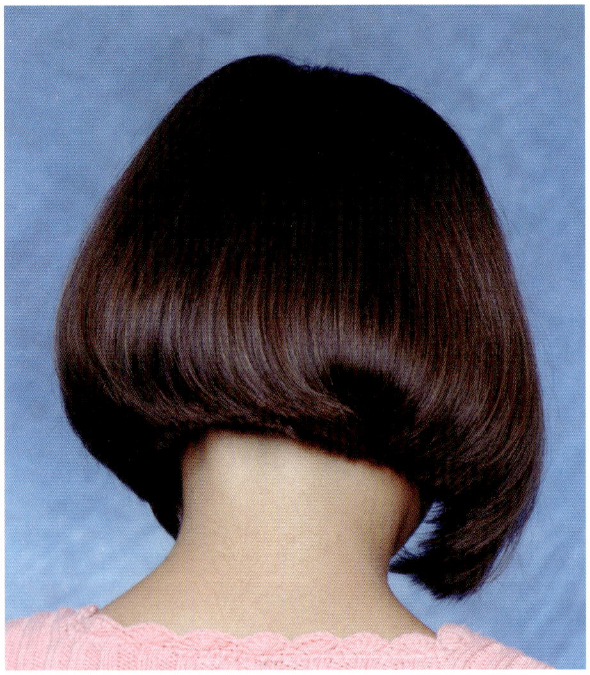

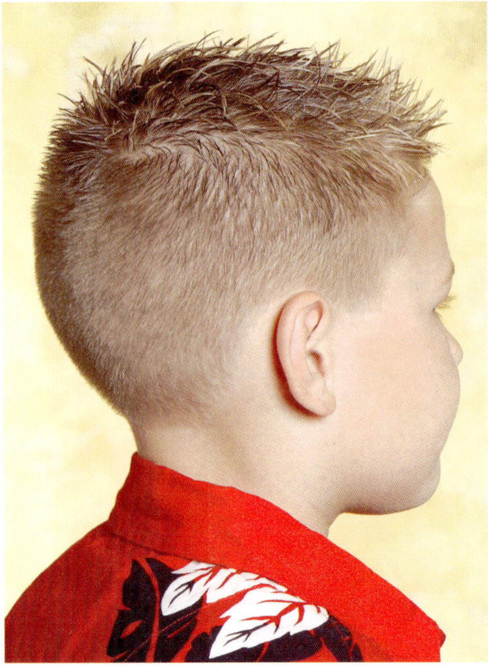

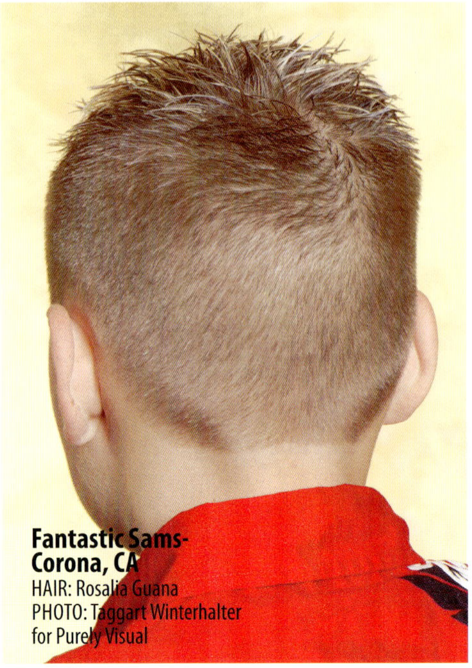

**Fantastic Sams-**
**Corona, CA**
HAIR: Rosalia Guana
PHOTO: Taggart Winterhalter
for Purely Visual

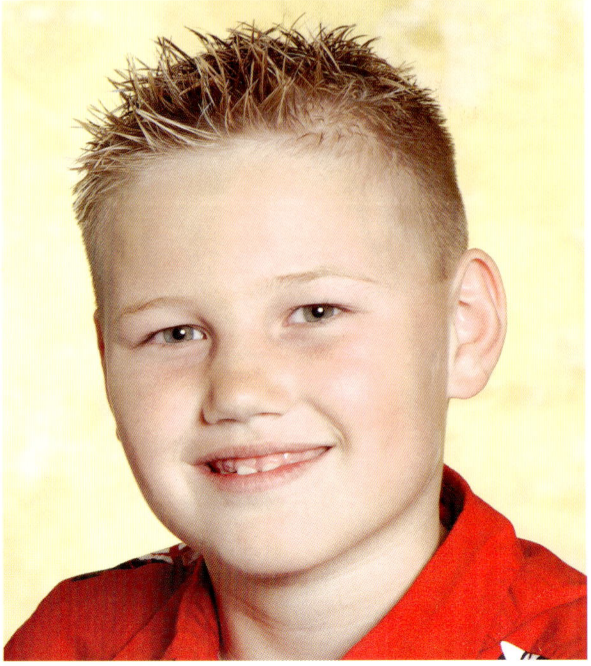

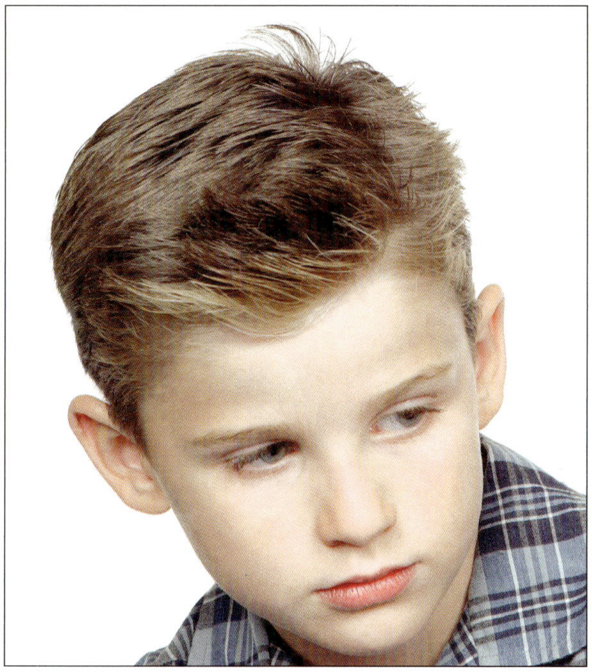

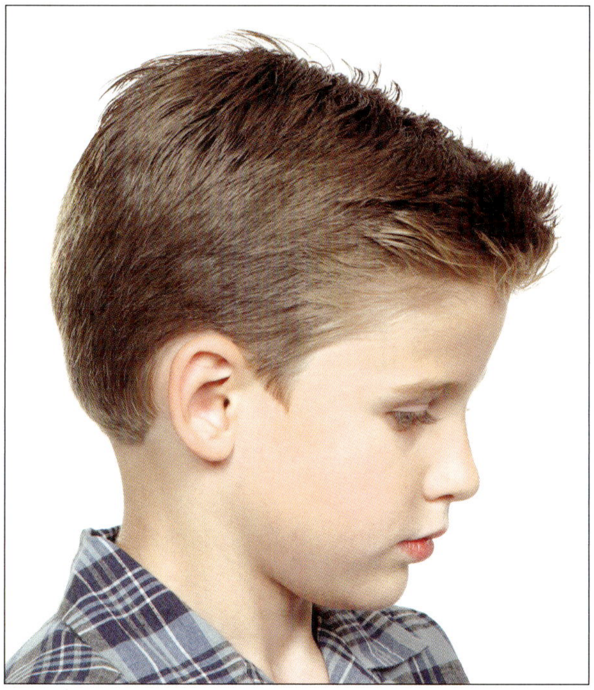

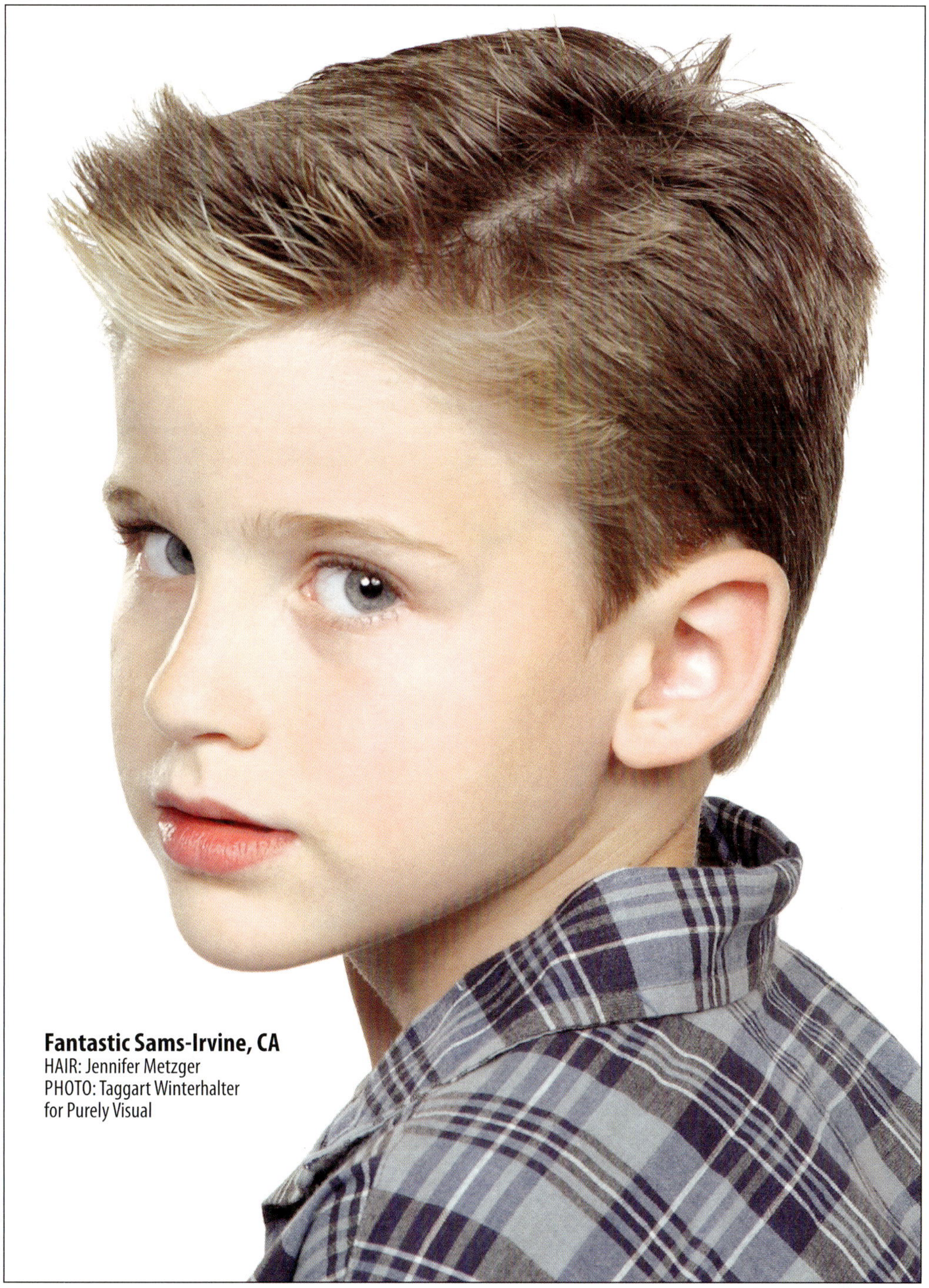

**Fantastic Sams-Irvine, CA**
HAIR: Jennifer Metzger
PHOTO: Taggart Winterhalter for Purely Visual

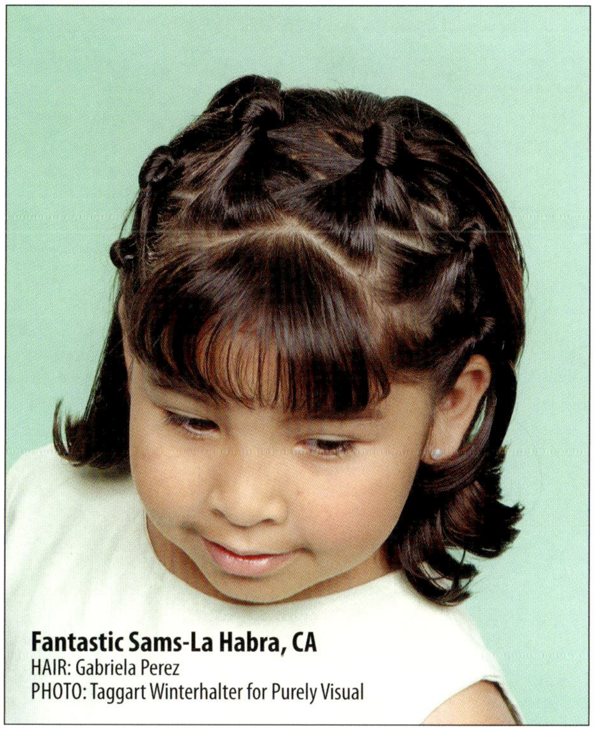

**Fantastic Sams-La Habra, CA**
HAIR: Gabriela Perez
PHOTO: Taggart Winterhalter for Purely Visual

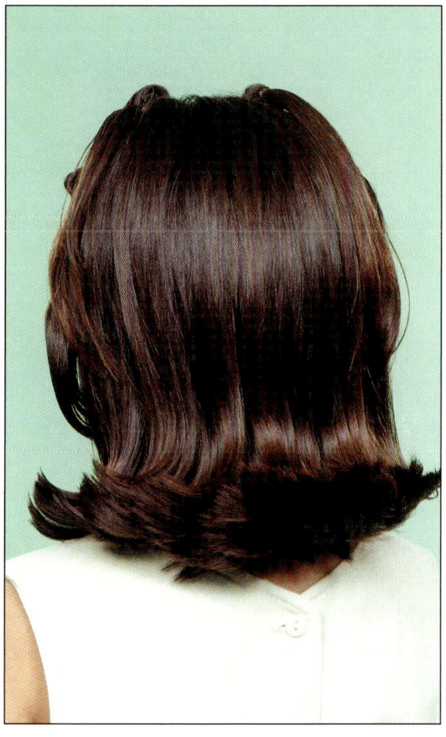

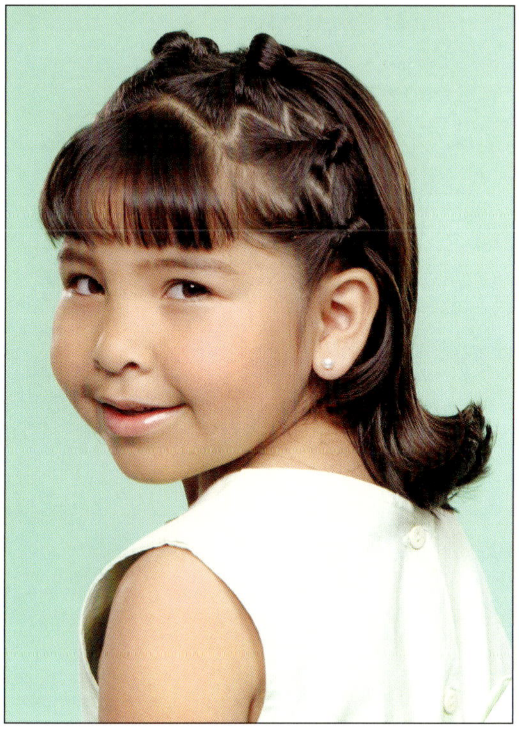

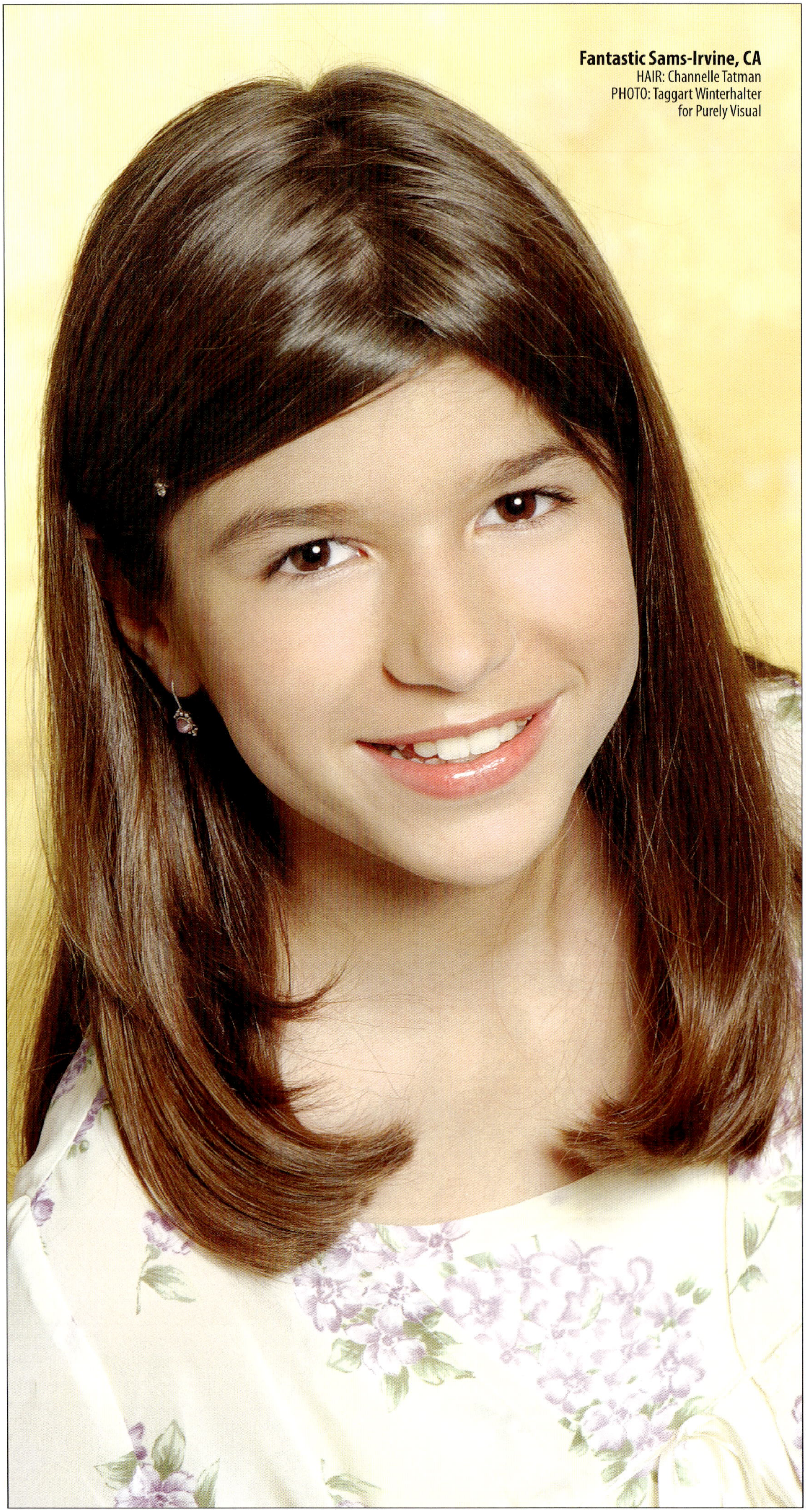

**Fantastic Sams-Irvine, CA**
HAIR: Channelle Tatman
PHOTO: Taggart Winterhalter
for Purely Visual

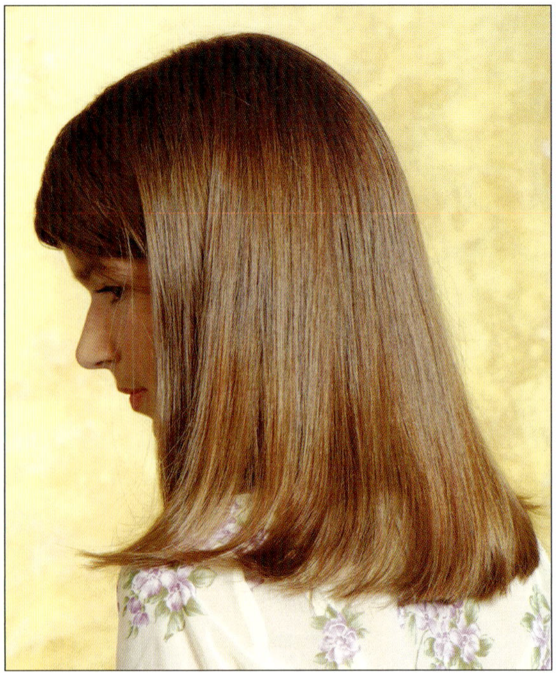

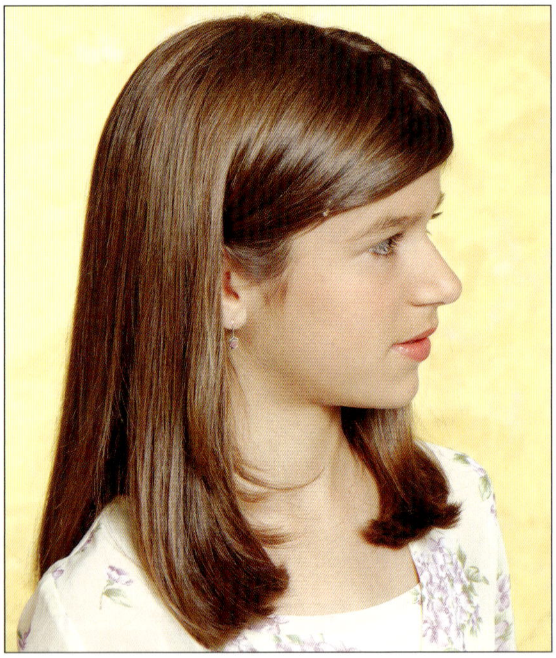

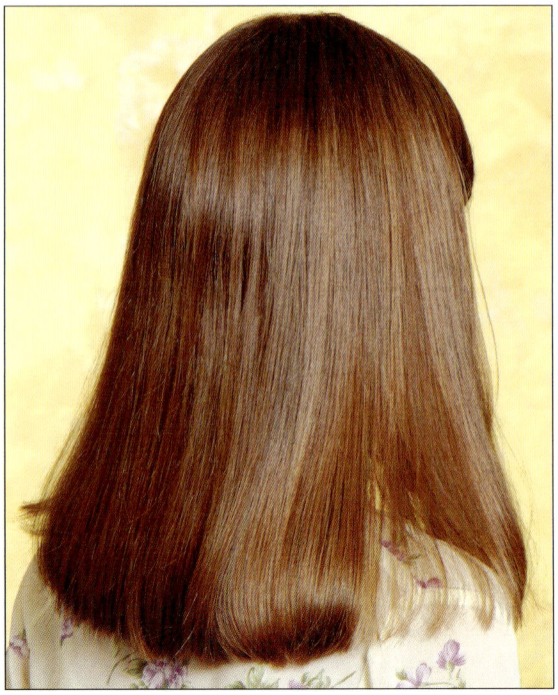

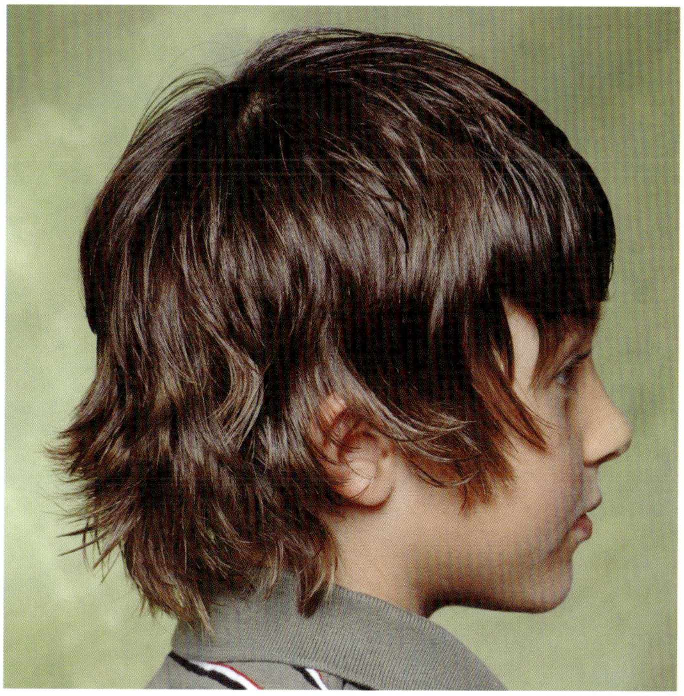

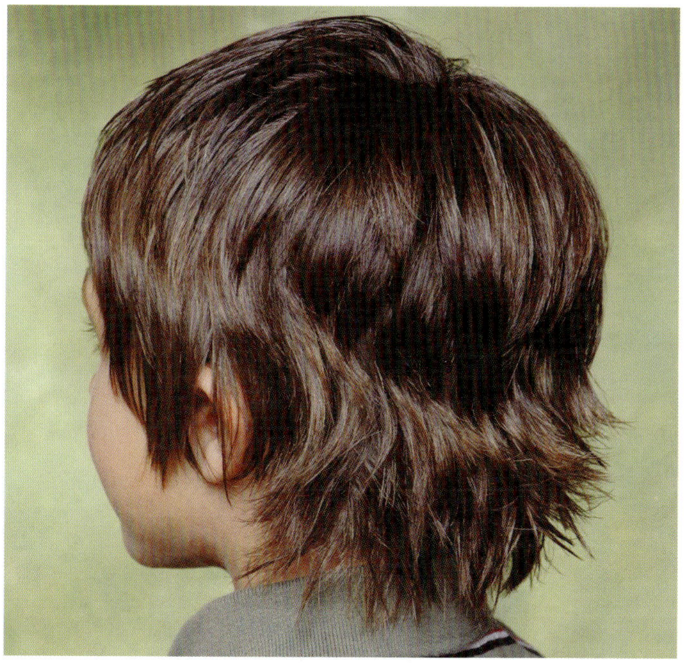

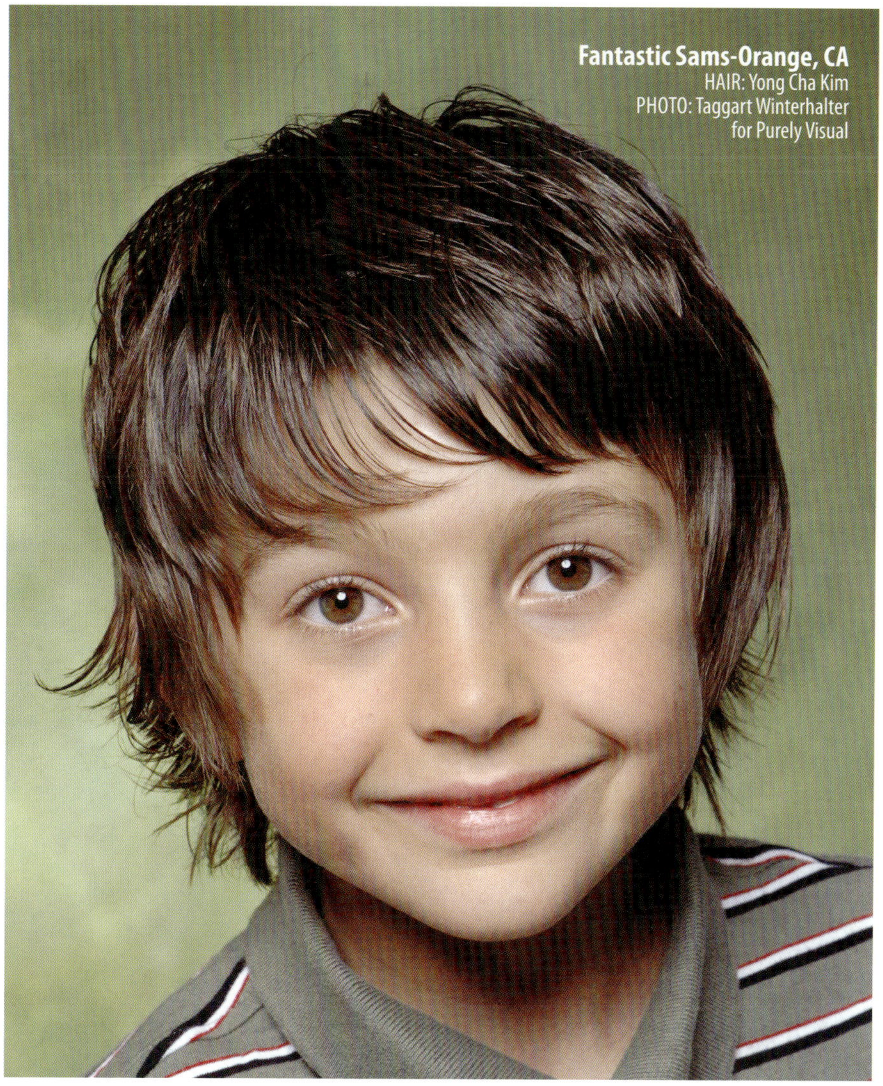

**Fantastic Sams-Orange, CA**
HAIR: Yong Cha Kim
PHOTO: Taggart Winterhalter for Purely Visual

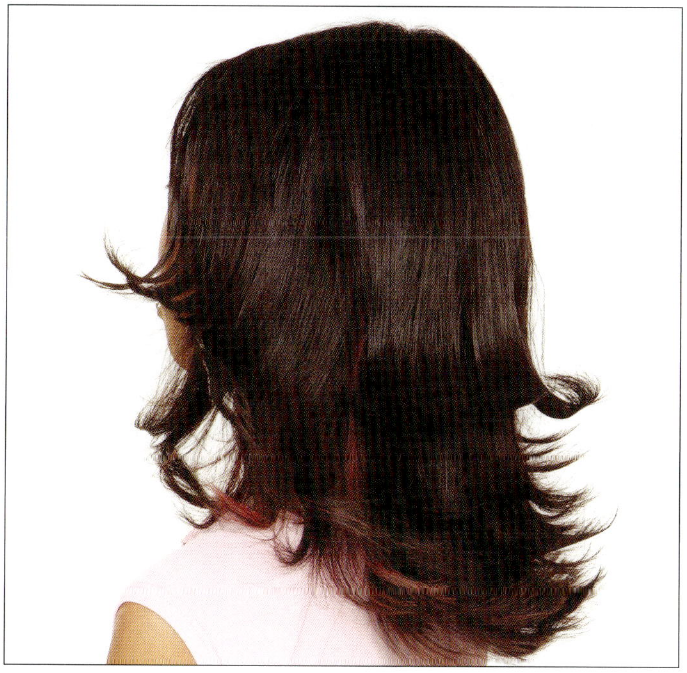

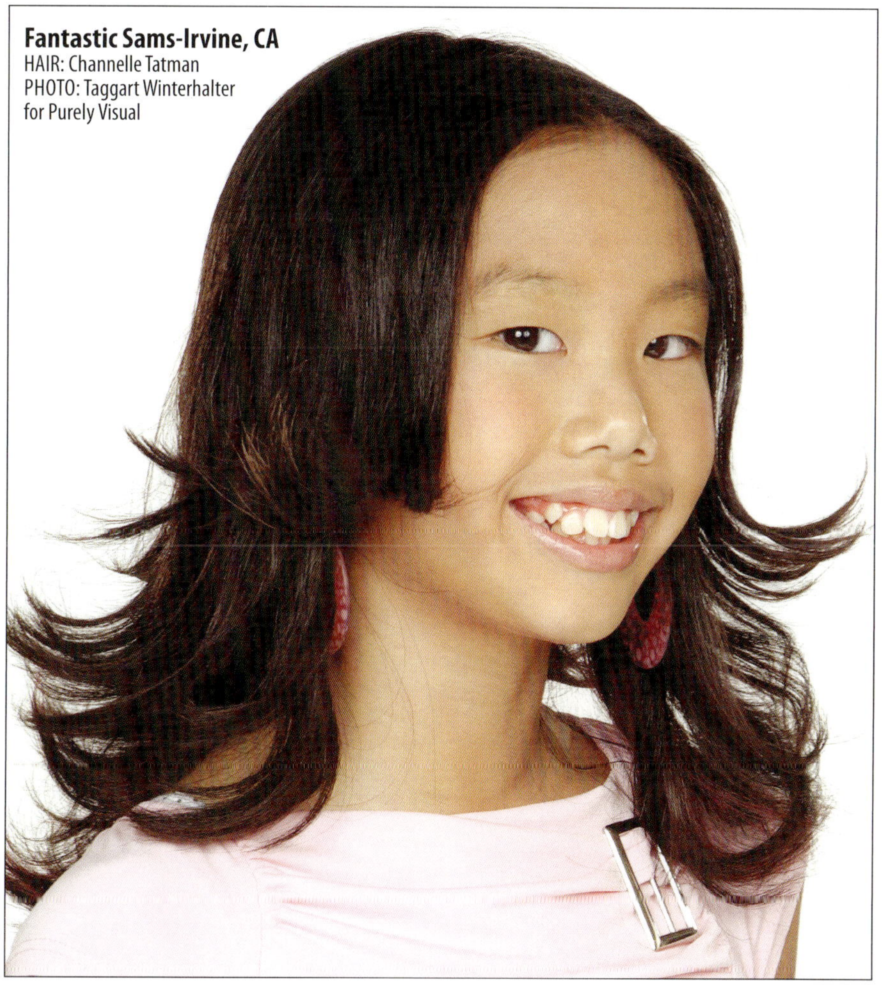

**Fantastic Sams-Irvine, CA**
HAIR: Channelle Tatman
PHOTO: Taggart Winterhalter for Purely Visual

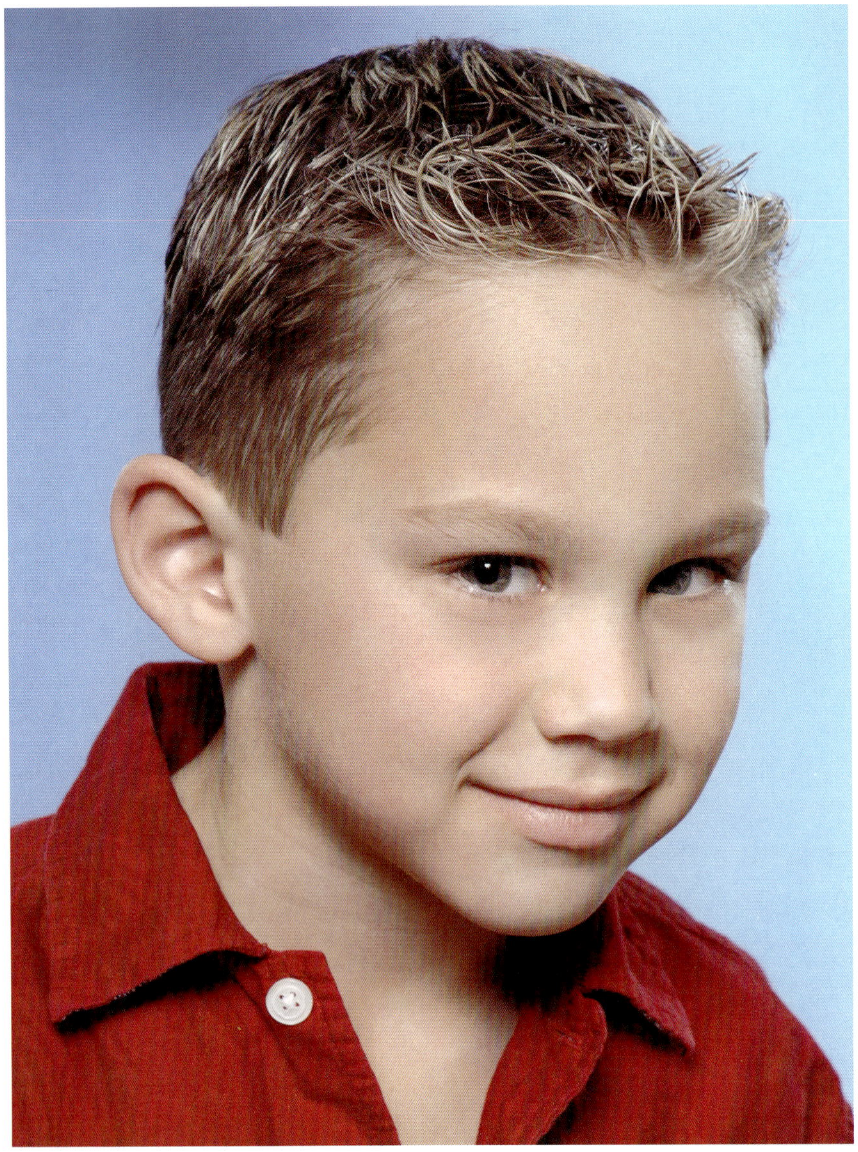

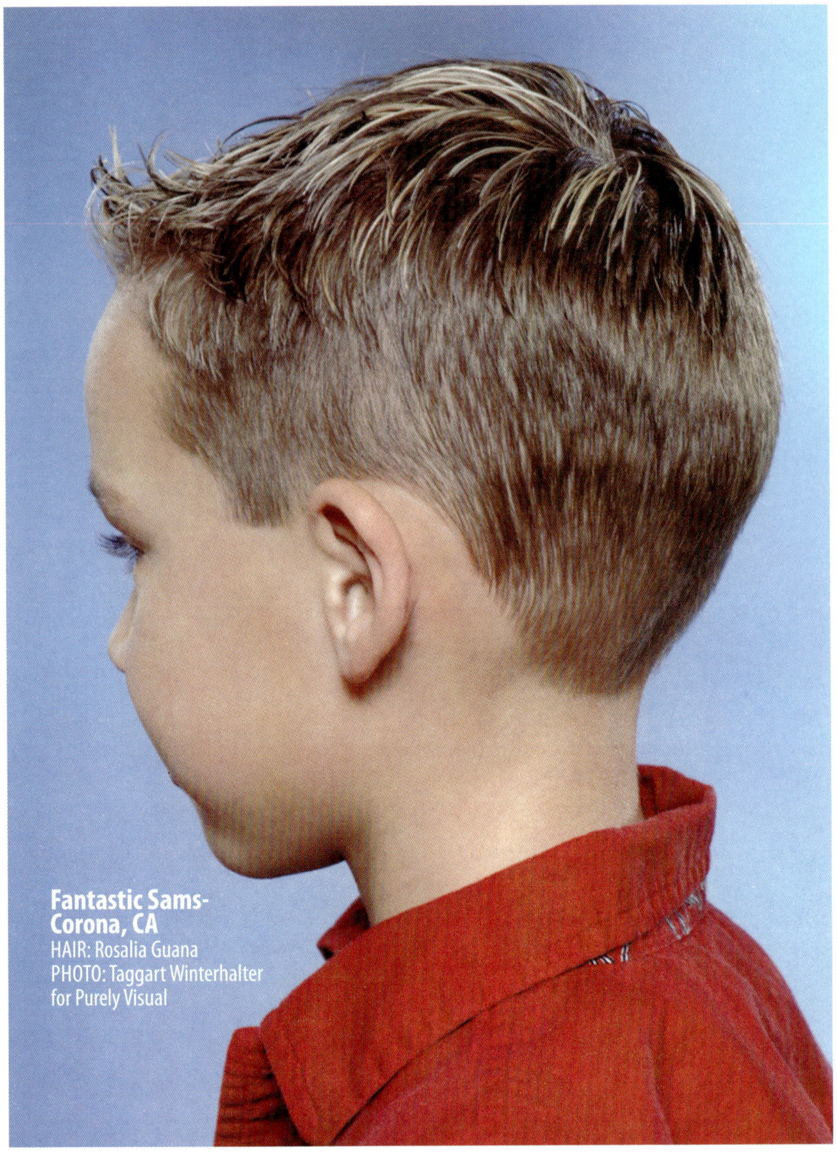

**Fantastic Sams-**
**Corona, CA**
HAIR: Rosalia Guana
PHOTO: Taggart Winterhalter
for Purely Visual

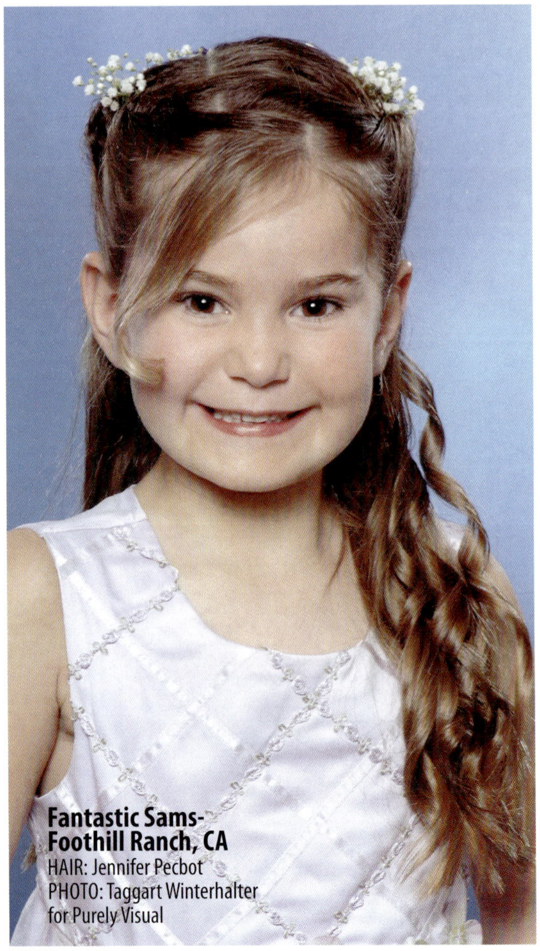

**Fantastic Sams-**
**Foothill Ranch, CA**
HAIR: Jennifer Pecbot
PHOTO: Taggart Winterhalter
for Purely Visual

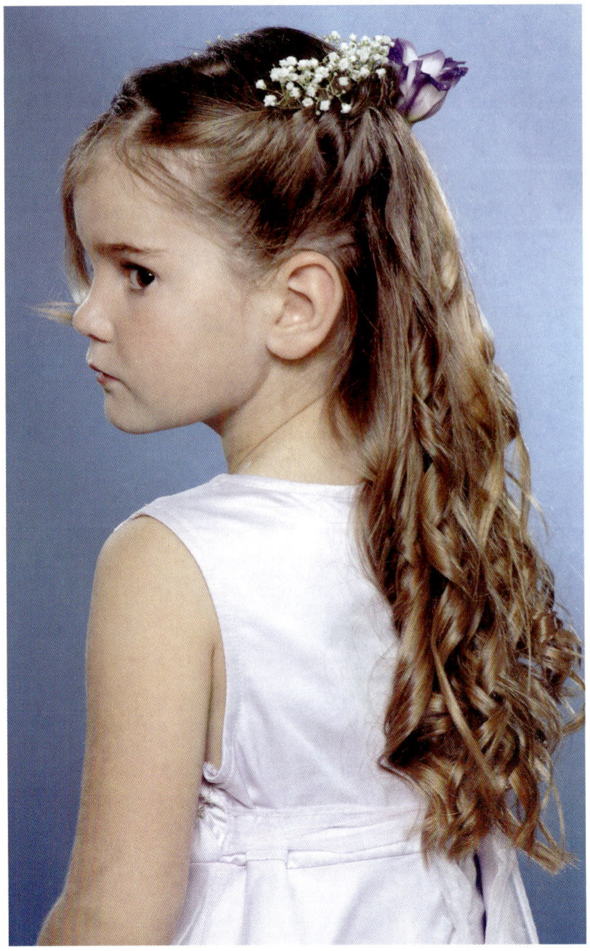

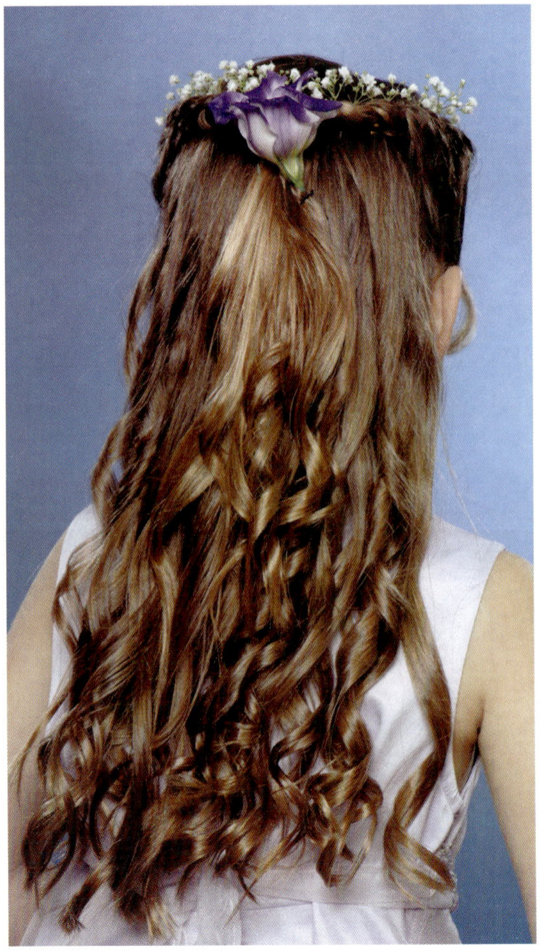

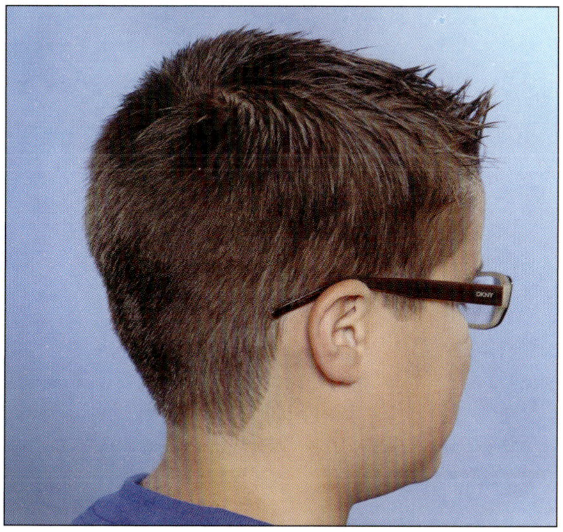

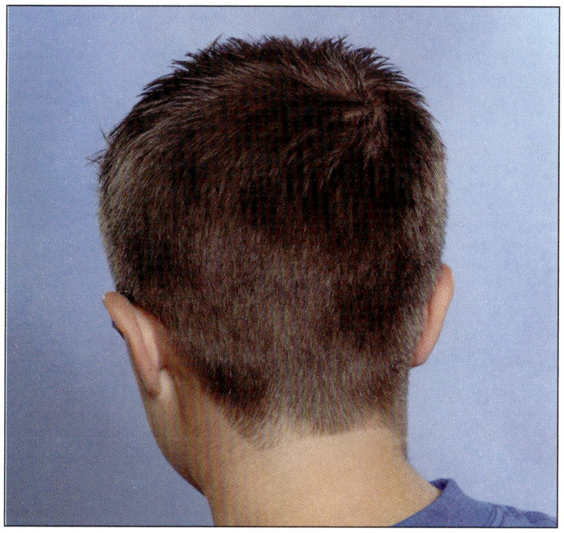

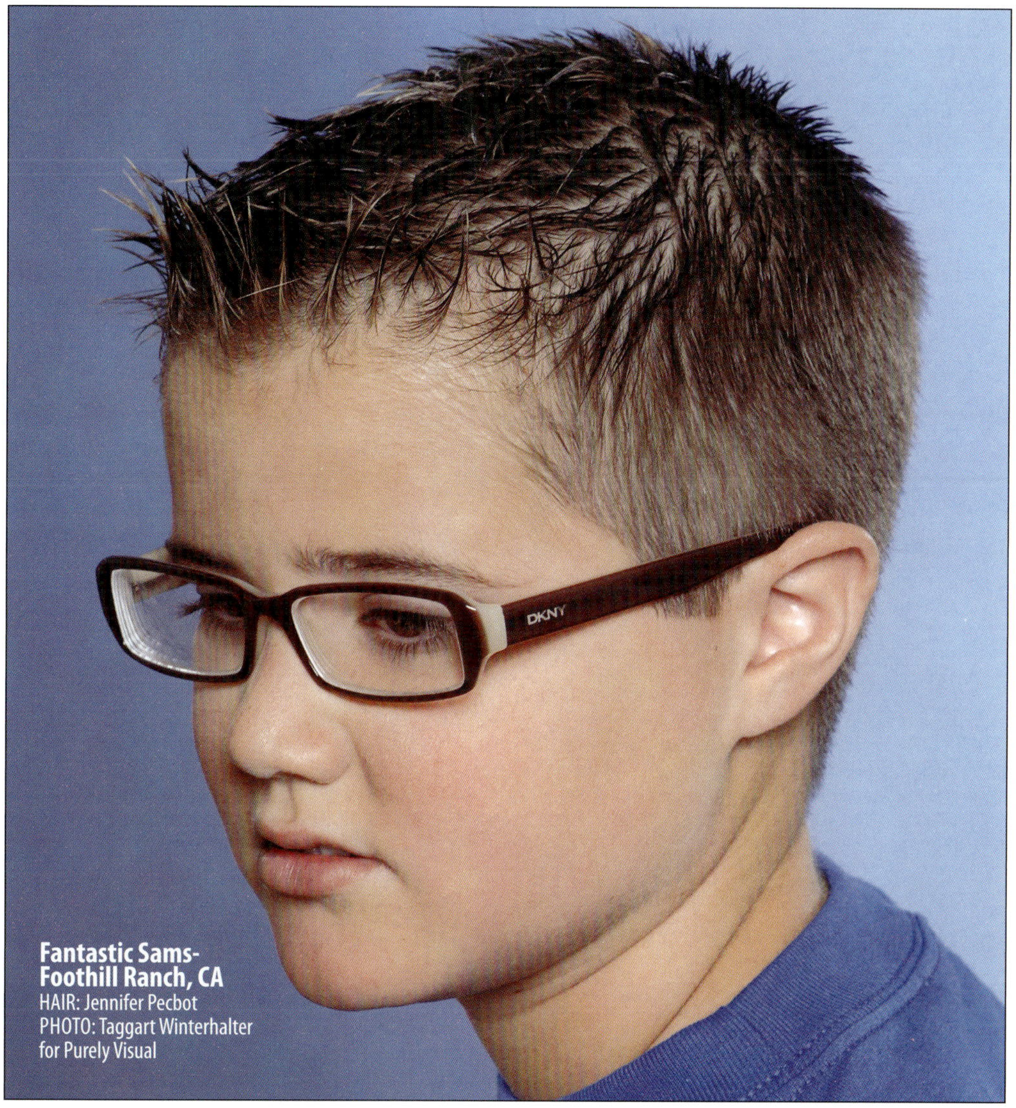


**Fantastic Sams-Foothill Ranch, CA**
HAIR: Jennifer Pecbot
PHOTO: Taggart Winterhalter for Purely Visual

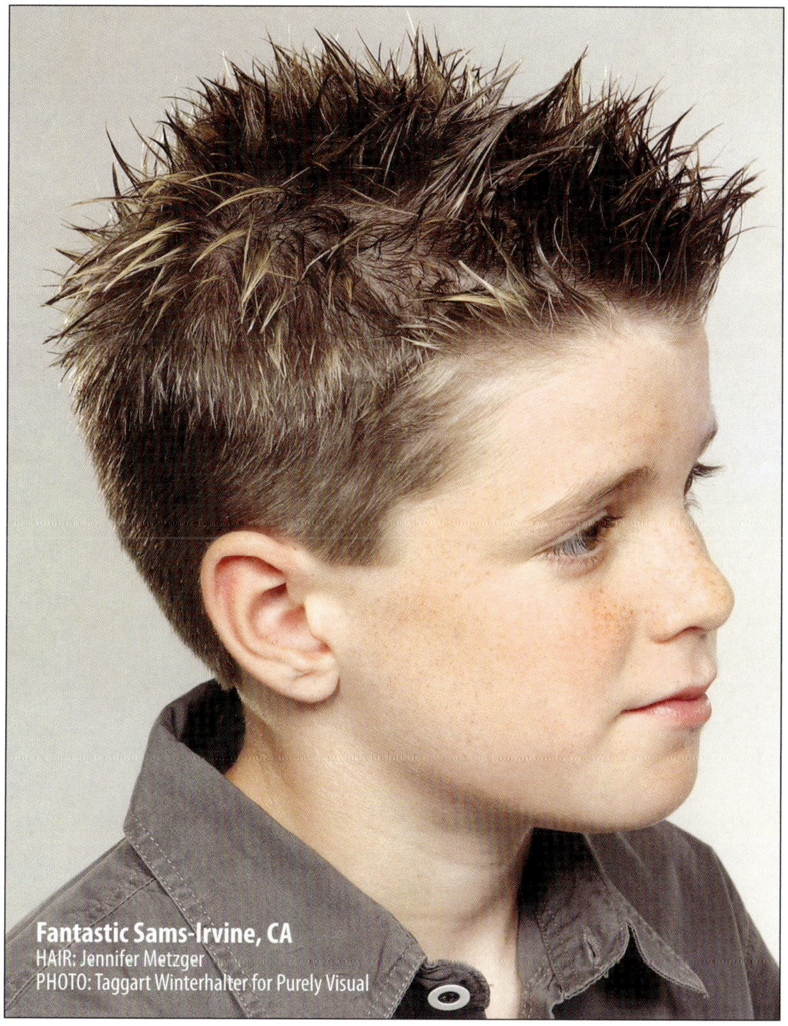

**Fantastic Sams-Irvine, CA**
HAIR: Jennifer Metzger
PHOTO: Taggart Winterhalter for Purely Visual

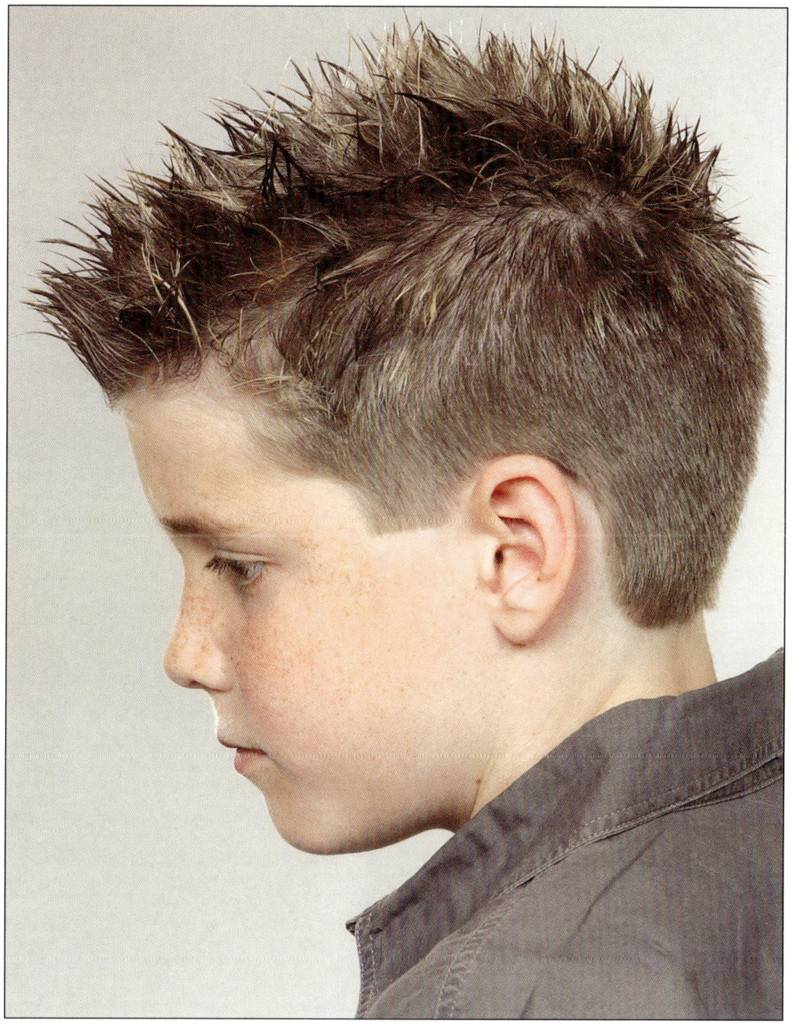

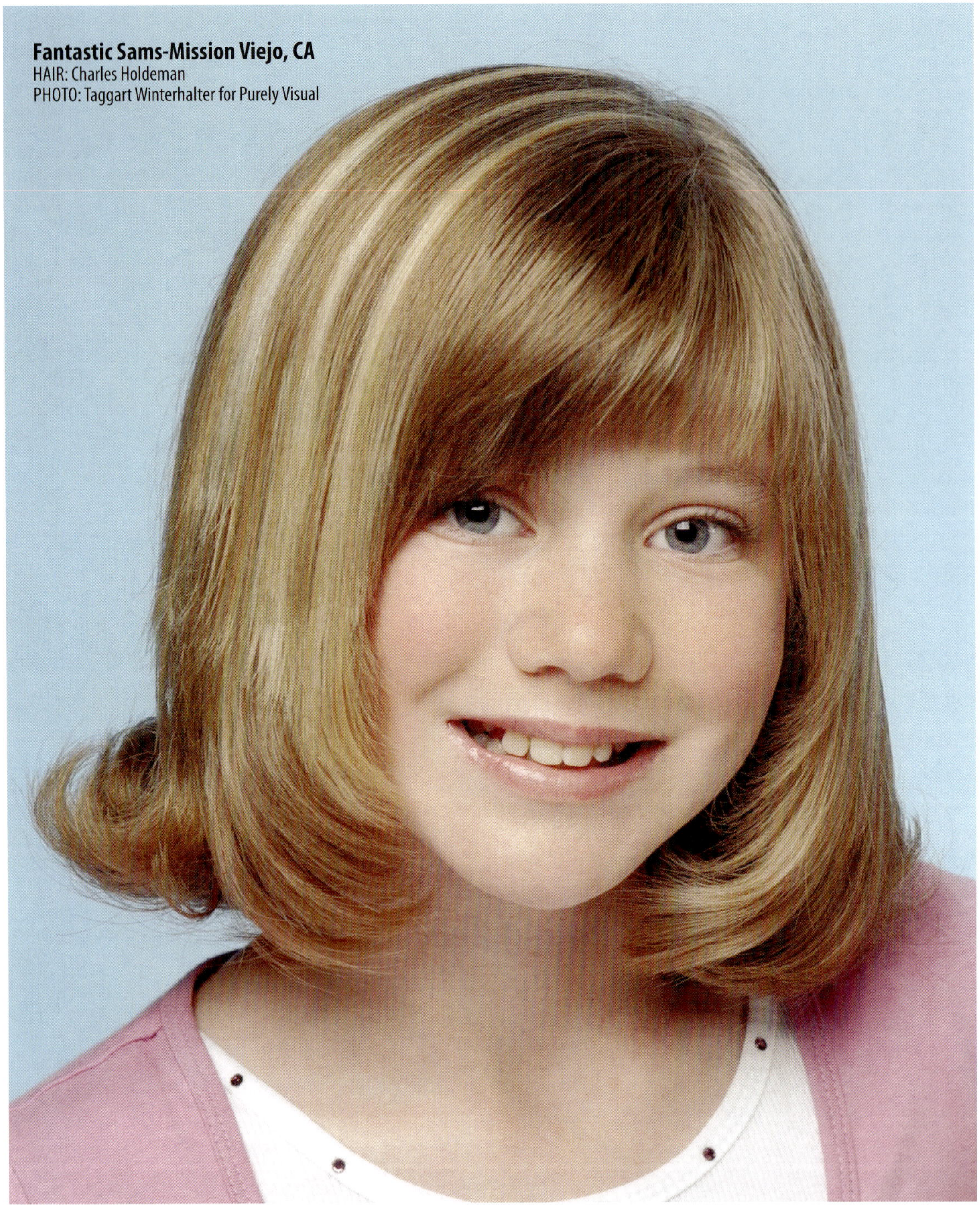

**Fantastic Sams-Mission Viejo, CA**
HAIR: Charles Holdeman
PHOTO: Taggart Winterhalter for Purely Visual

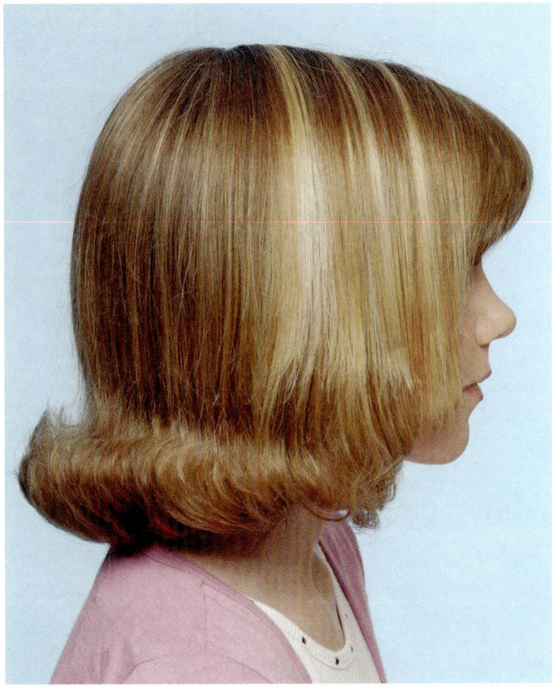

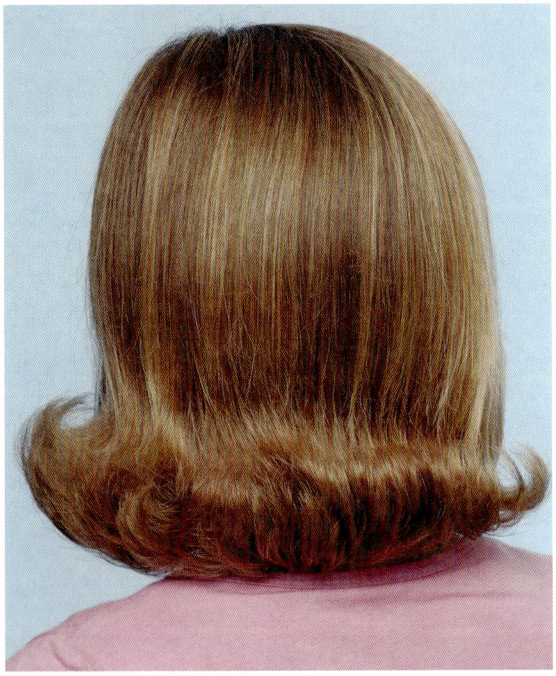

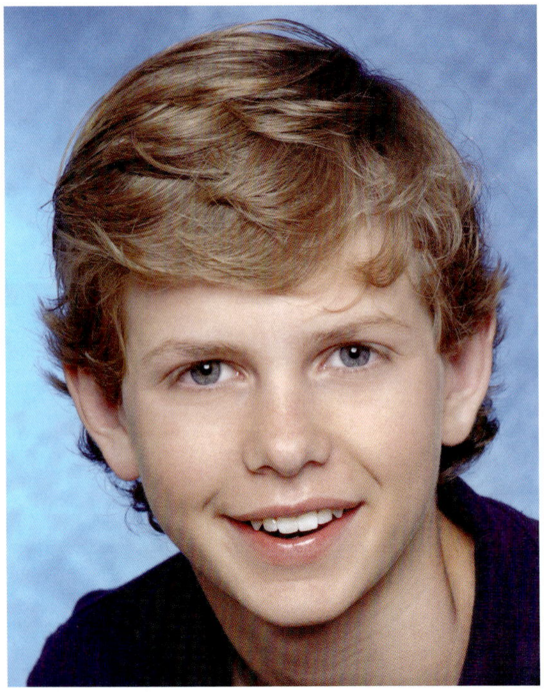

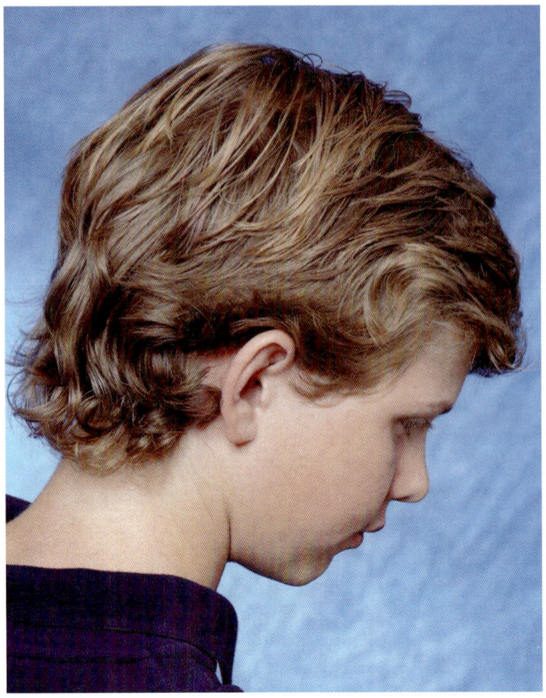

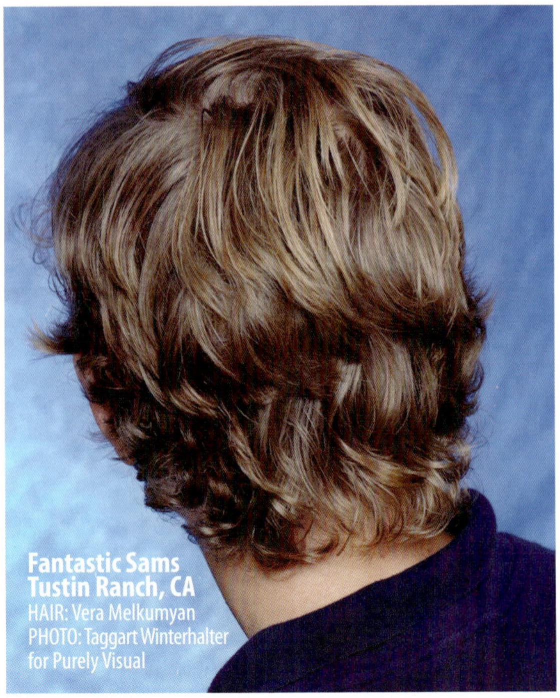

**Fantastic Sams Tustin Ranch, CA**
HAIR: Vera Melkumyan
PHOTO: Taggart Winterhalter for Purely Visual

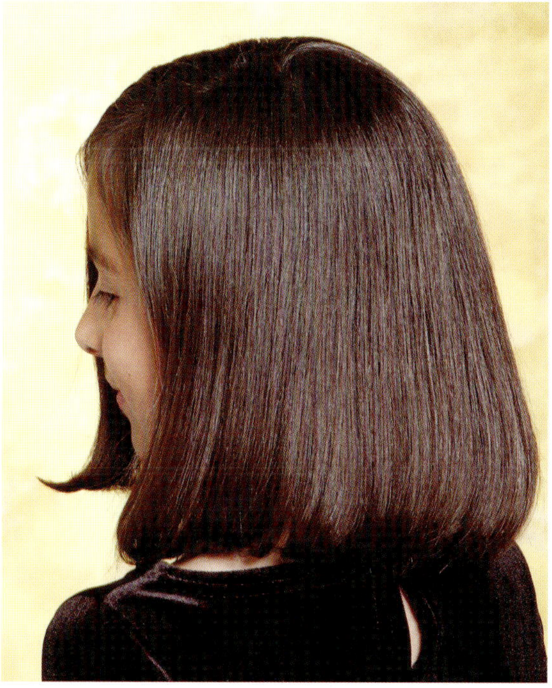

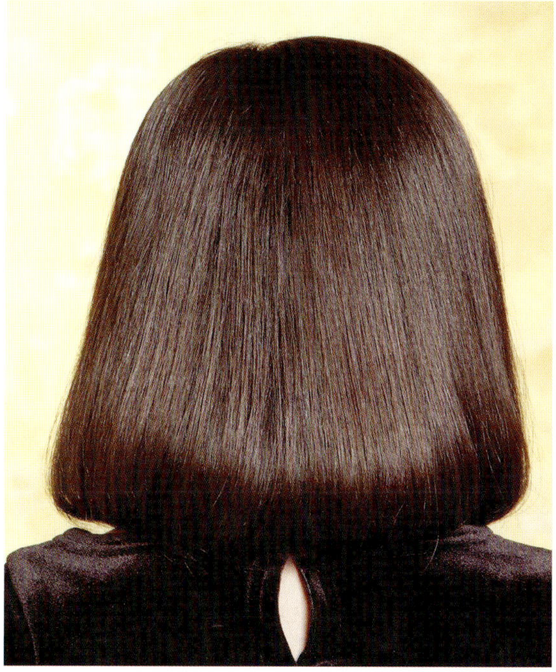

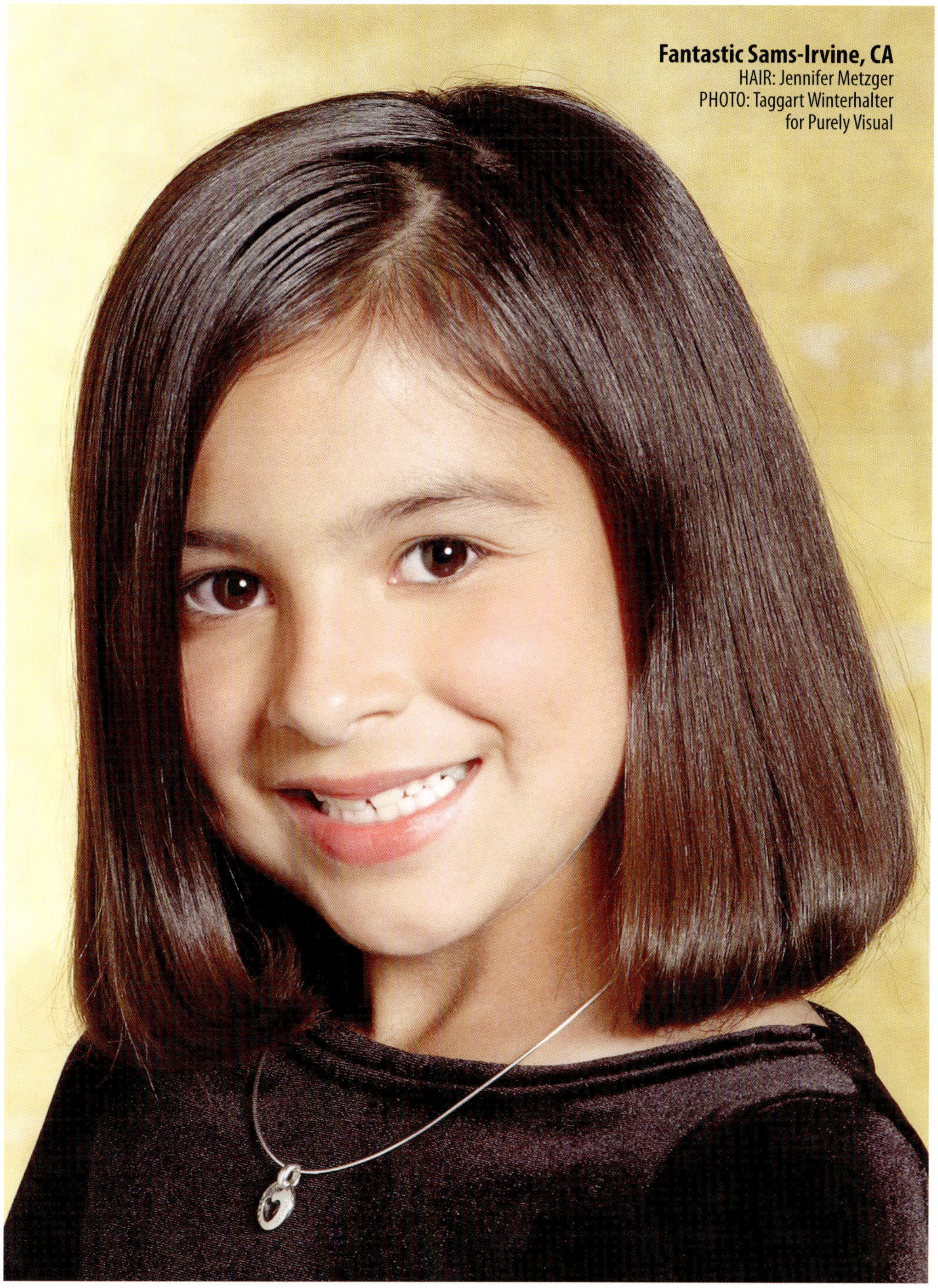

**Fantastic Sams-Irvine, CA**
HAIR: Jennifer Metzger
PHOTO: Taggart Winterhalter for Purely Visual

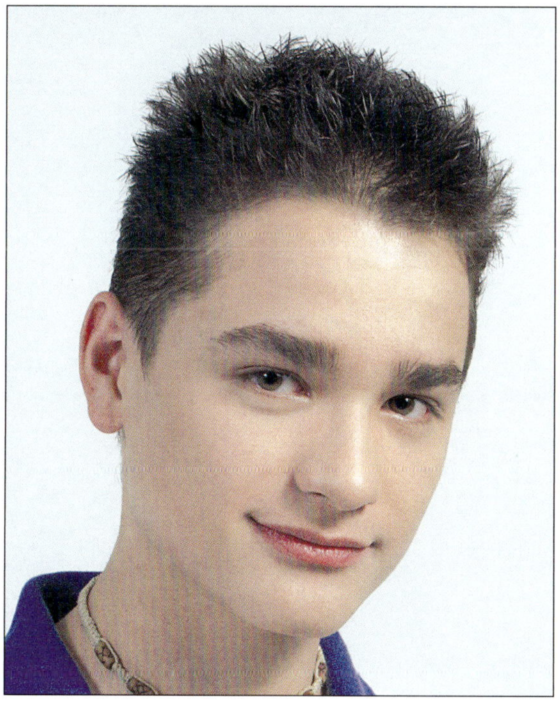

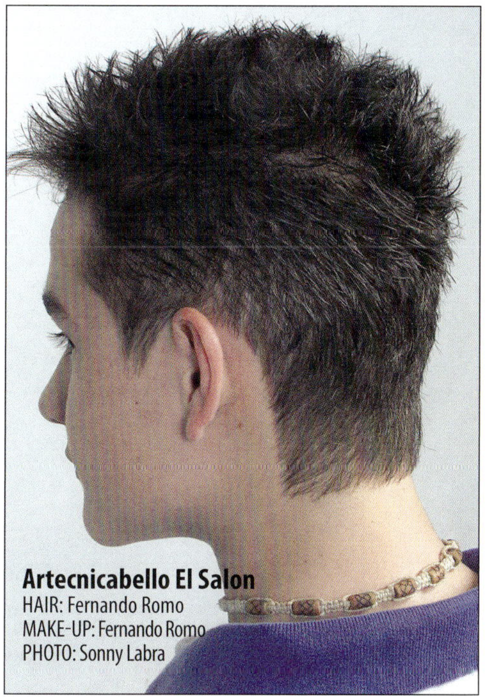

**Artecnicabello El Salon**
HAIR: Fernando Romo
MAKE-UP: Fernando Romo
PHOTO: Sonny Labra

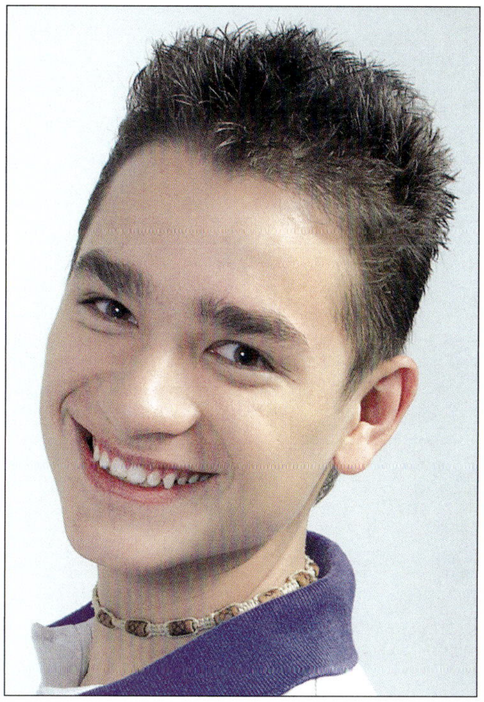

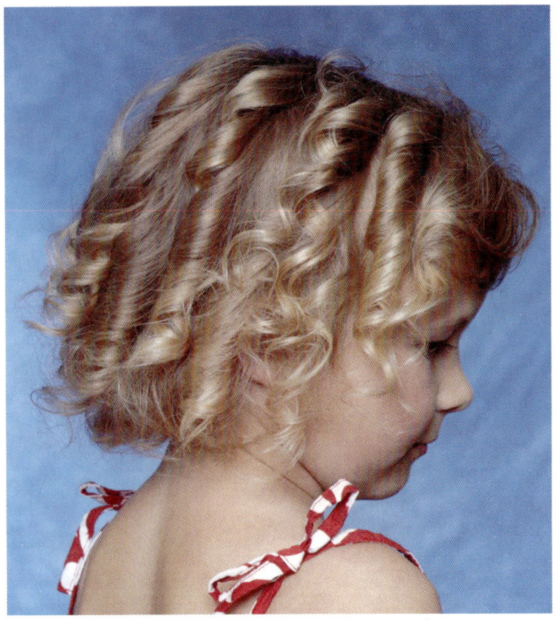

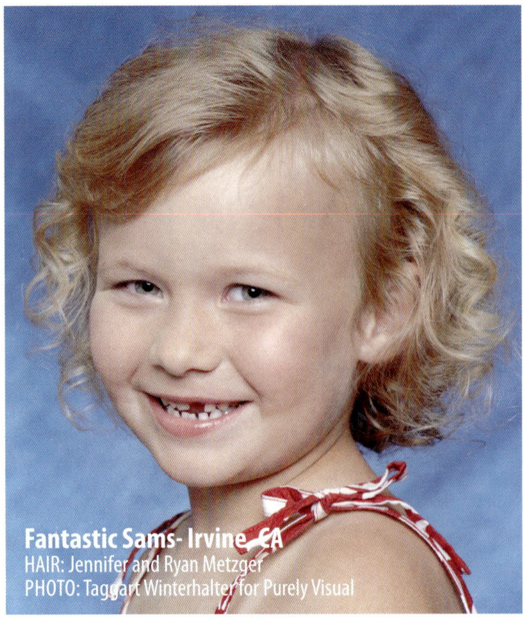

**Fantastic Sams- Irvine, CA**
HAIR: Jennifer and Ryan Metzger
PHOTO: Taggart Winterhalter for Purely Visual

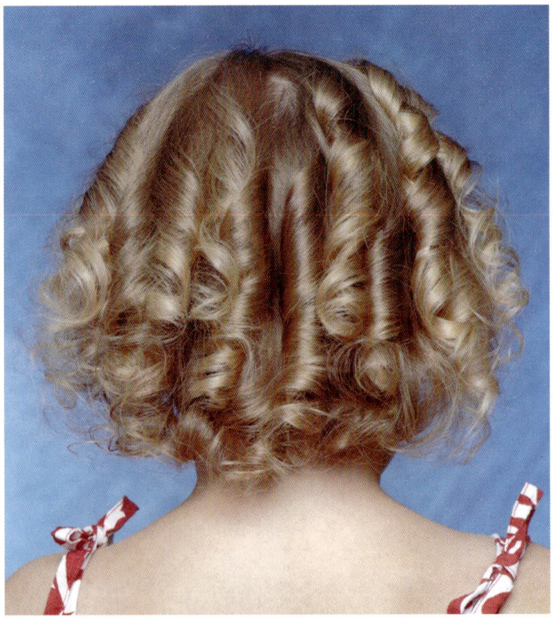

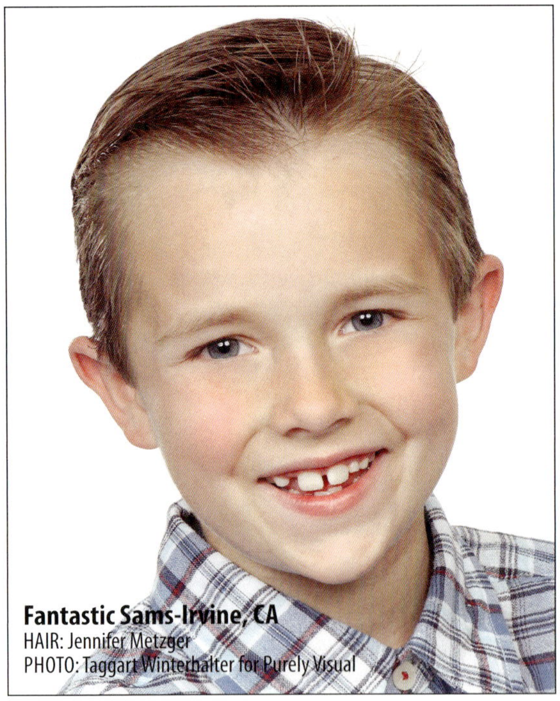

**Fantastic Sams-Irvine, CA**
HAIR: Jennifer Metzger
PHOTO: Taggart Winterhalter for Purely Visual

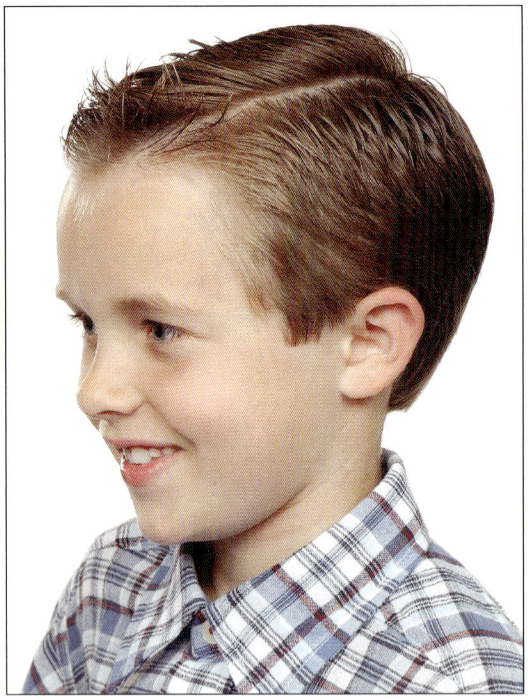

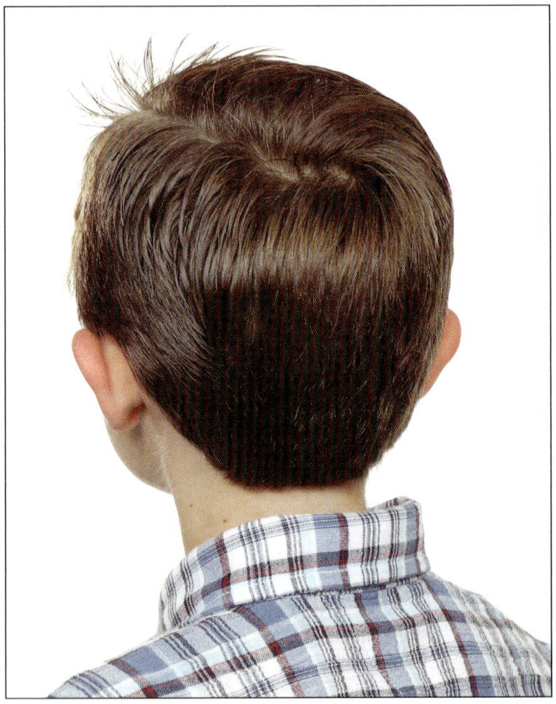

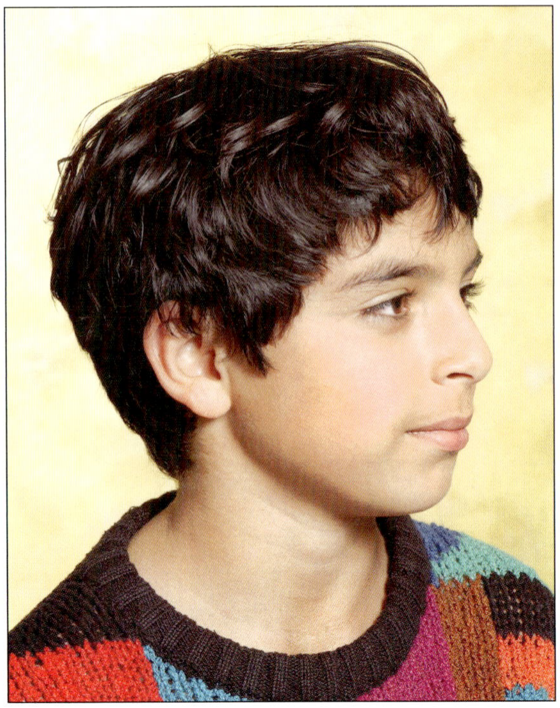

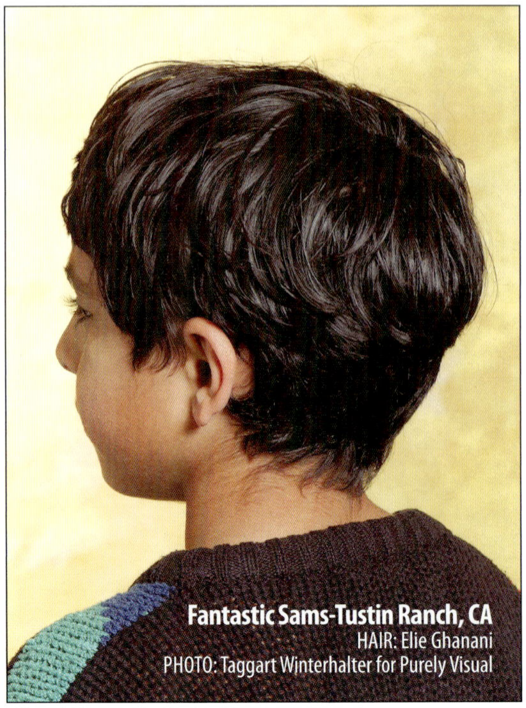

**Fantastic Sams-Tustin Ranch, CA**
HAIR: Elie Ghanani
PHOTO: Taggart Winterhalter for Purely Visual

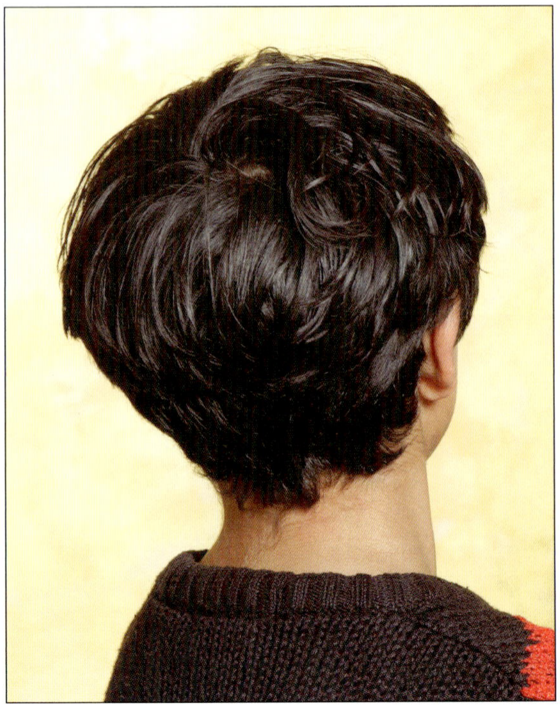

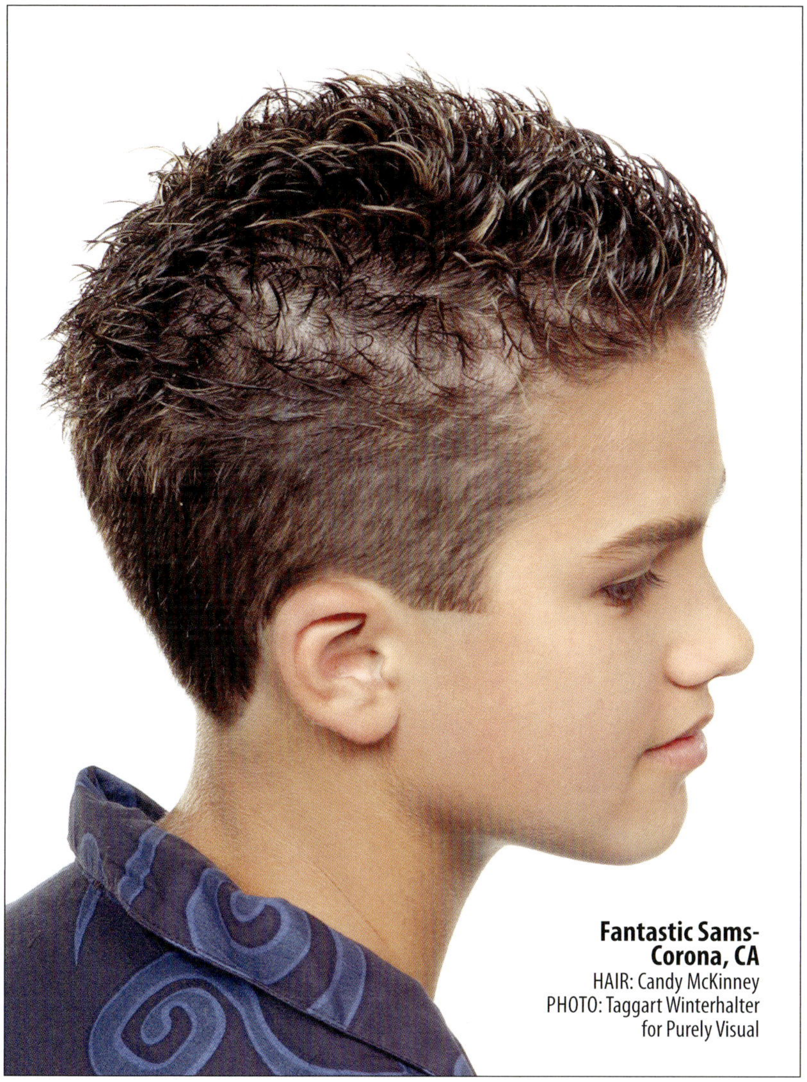

**Fantastic Sams-**
**Corona, CA**
HAIR: Candy McKinney
PHOTO: Taggart Winterhalter
for Purely Visual

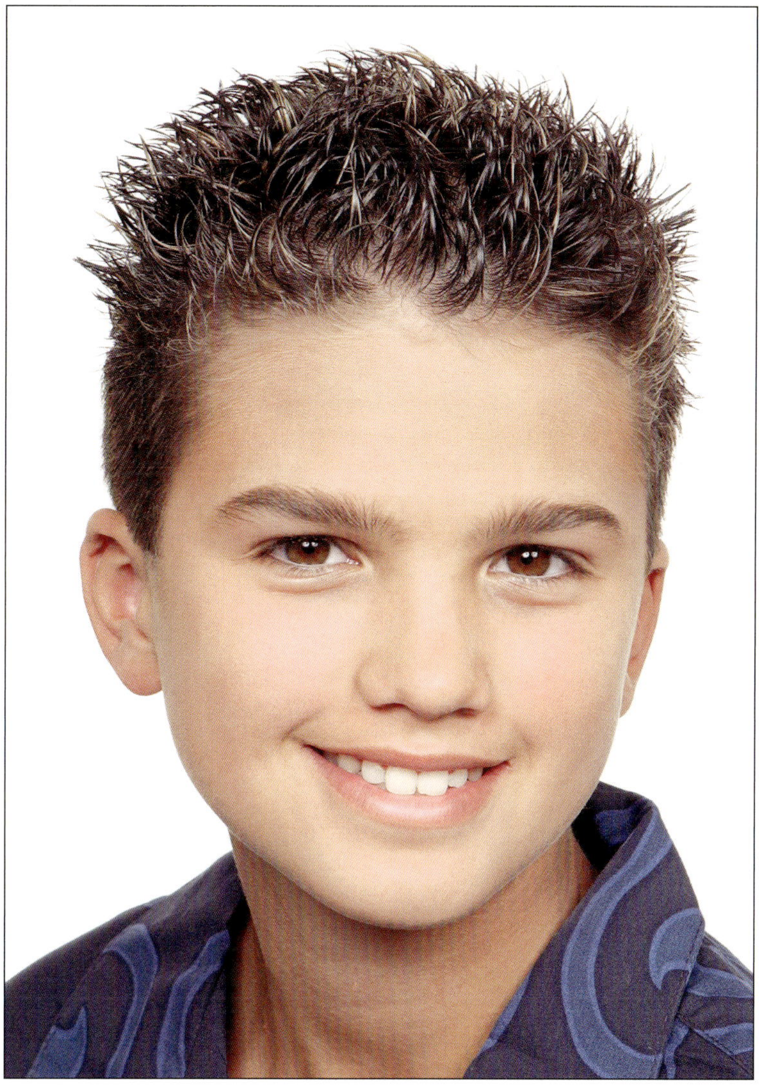

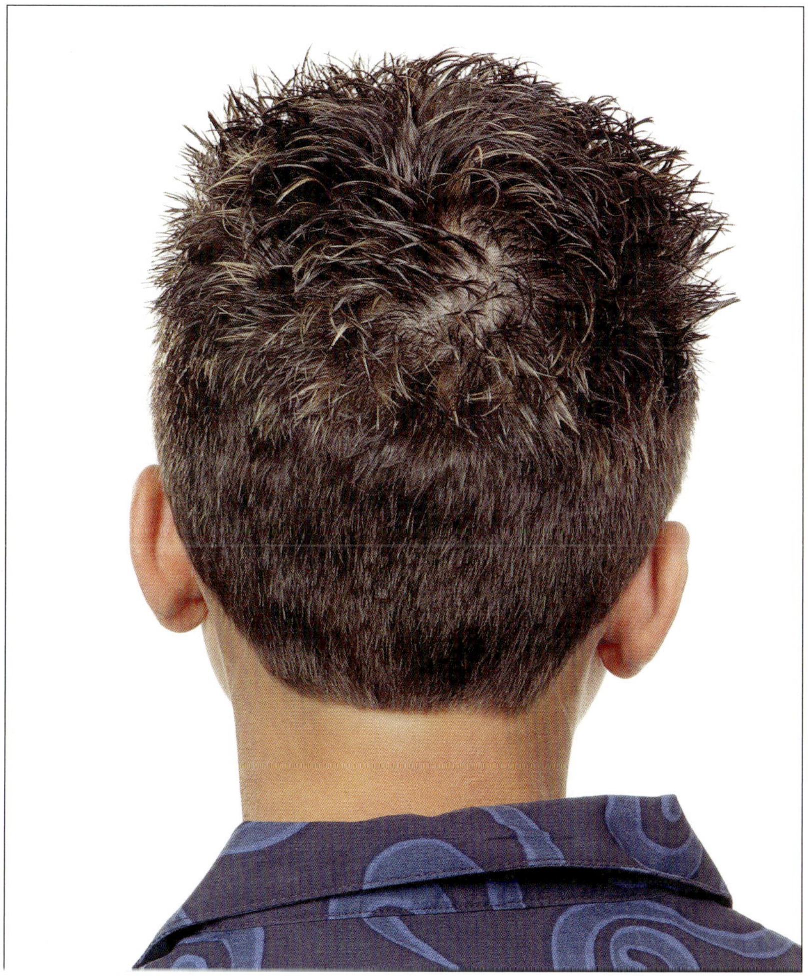

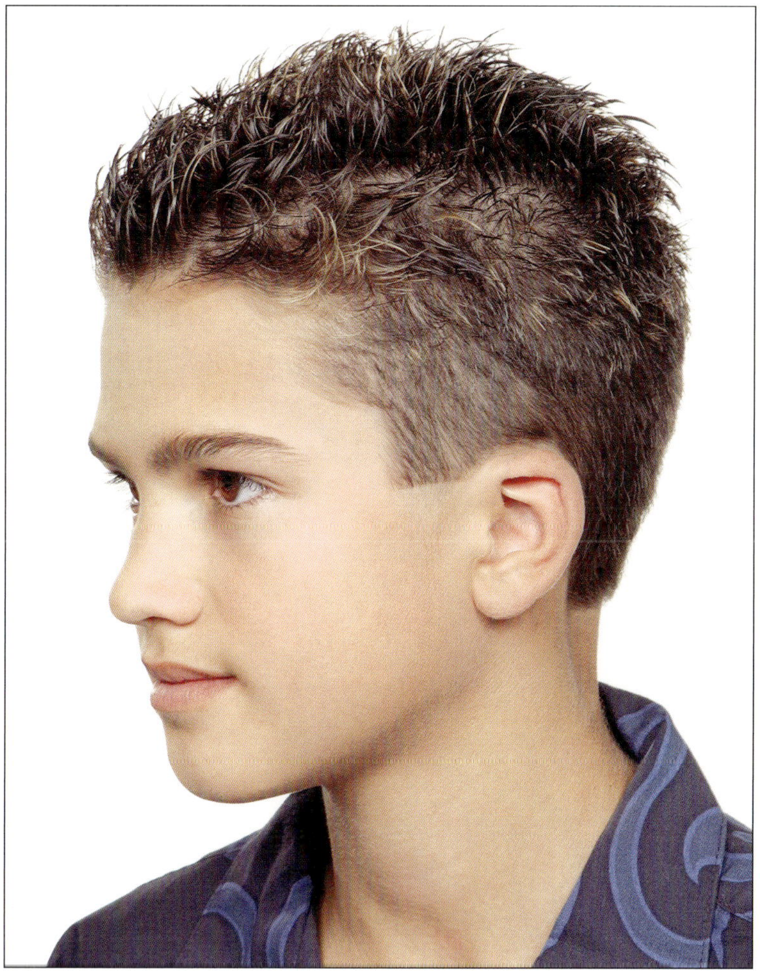

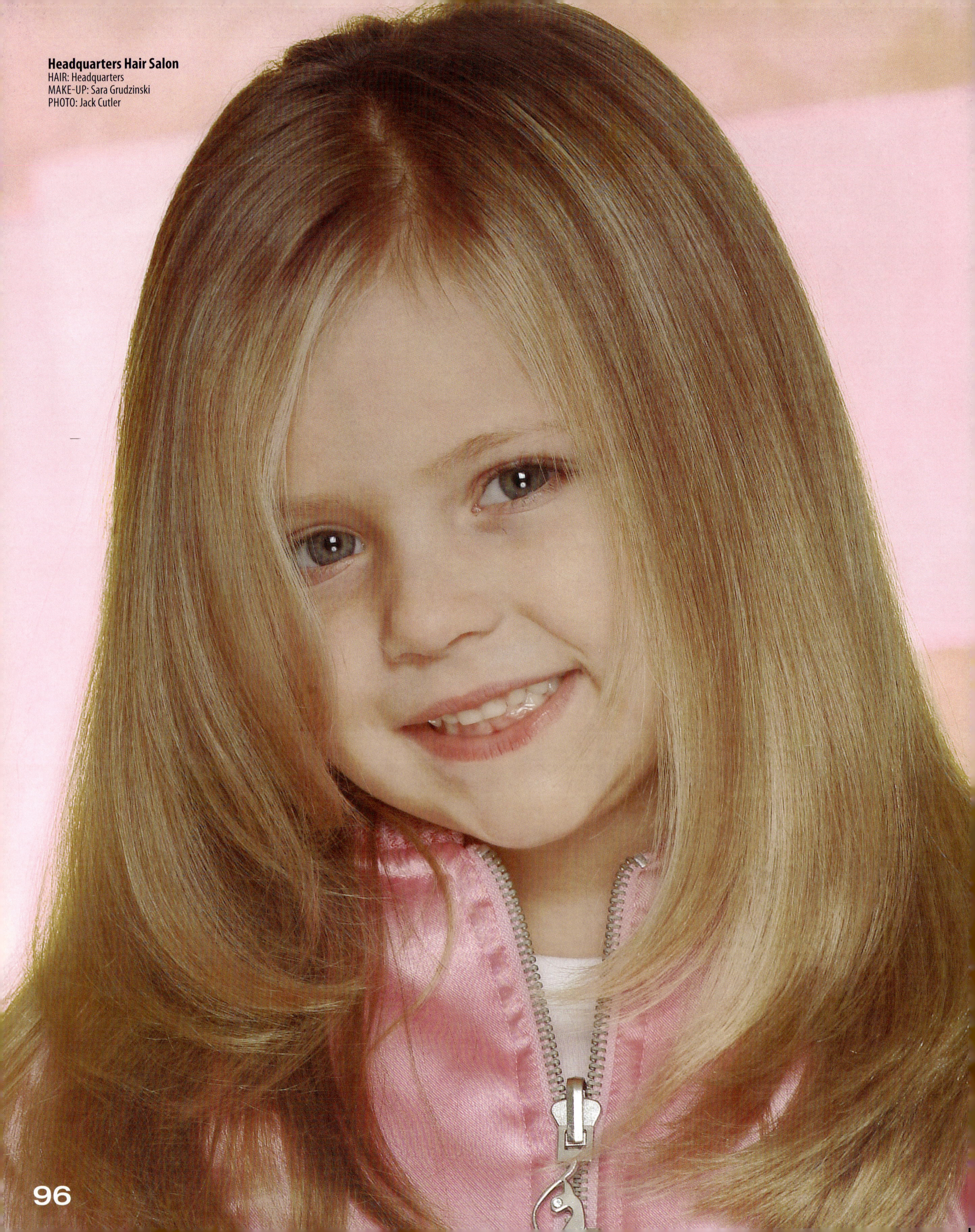

**Headquarters Hair Salon**
HAIR: Headquarters
MAKE-UP: Sara Grudzinski
PHOTO: Jack Cutler

# INSPIRE

HAIR FASHION FOR SALON CLIENTS

# INDEX VOLUME SIXTY



*Courtesy of Intercoiffure


Publisher/CEO: Deborah Carver • Managing Director: Sheryl Lenzkes • Art Director: Michae

To Contact Us: Creative Age Communications • 7628 Densmore Avenue, Van Nuys, California 914 7450

Interested in getting published . . . go to inspirebooks.com to download subr